The Biology of Antithrombins

Author

Géza Sas, M.D., D.Sc.
Professor of Medicine
First Department of Medicine
Postgraduate Medical University
Budapest, Hungary

CRC Press, Inc.
Boca Raton, Florida

Library of Congress Cataloging-in-Publication Data

Sas, Géza.
The biology of antithrombins / author, Géza Sas.
p. cm.
Includes bibliographies and index.
ISBN 0-8493-4777-7
1. Antithrombins--Physiological effect. 2. Antithrombin III-
-Physiological effect. I. Title.
[DNLM: 1. Antithrombin III--physiology. QV 193 S252b]
QC93.7.A58S27 1990
612.1′15--dc20
DNLM/DLC
for Library of Congress

89-7140
CIP

This book represents information obtained from authentic and highly regarded sources. Reprinted material is quoted with permission, and sources are indicated. A wide variety of references are listed. Every reasonable effort has been made to give reliable data and information, but the author and the publisher cannot assume responsibility for the validity of all materials or for the consequences of their use.

Direct all inquiries to CRC Press, Inc., 2000 Corporate Blvd., N.W., Boca Raton, Florida, 33431.

International Standard Book Number 0-8493-4777-7

Library of Congress Card Number 89-7140
Printed in the United States

PREFACE

At the beginning of this century, Morawitz introduced the term antithrombin for the ability of plasma or serum to neutralize thrombin.[1] A couple of years later Mellanby concluded from his experiments that a material combined chemically with thrombin (''fibrin ferment'') to form an inactive compound.[2] Furthermore, he demonstrated that fibrinogen also had an adsorptive affinity for thrombin. In 1916 McLean isolated heparin from liver and demonstrated its potent anticoagulant properties.[3] Brinkhous et al.[4] showed in 1939 that heparin was effective as an anticoagulant only in the presence of a plasma component which they termed heparin cofactor. In 1943, Astrup and Darling differentiated between the activity which inactivated thrombin progressively and the activity which functioned together with heparin immediately in the neutralization of thrombin.[5] In 1946, Gerendás analyzed the kinetics of the inactivation of thrombin and proposed a method for the determination of antithrombin activity in serum.[6,7] This assay and its further modifications rendered the first clinical investigations on antithrombin possible.

In the 1950s new antithrombin activities were described. Seegers et al.[8] proposed a number system for the various antithrombin activities, which was widely adopted for about a decade. Antithrombin I was defined as the ability of fibrin to adsorb thrombin. Antithrombin II was recommended to designate the plasma cofactor of heparin. The term antithrombin III was used to describe the substance in plasma or serum which neutralizes thrombin activity. Antithrombin IV was used to designate the material in ether-treated plasma. In 1957, Loeliger and Hers described an antithrombin activity, subsequently designated antithrombin V, in a patient with hypergammaglobulinemia.[9] Niewiarowski and Kowalski introduced the term antithrombin VI in 1958 to describe the anticoagulant activity which develops when fibrinogen is digested by plasmin.[10] In the following years this terminology became obsolete for various reasons. Some of the activities designated with Roman numerals turned out to be nonspecific or did not occur in plasma under physiological conditions. Kinetic studies supported the notion about the identity of antithrombin II and antithrombin III, i.e., plasma heparin cofactor activity and plasma antithrombin III activity.[11-13] These investigations suggested that heparin acts to accelerate the rate at which antithrombin neutralizes thrombin. In 1965, Egeberg described a family with recurrent venous thromboembolism characterized by the partial deficiency of both plasma antithrombin activity and heparin cofactor activity which also suggested the intimate relationship between these activities.[14] Abildgaard was able to isolate an alfa$_2$-globulin with both activities from human plasma 3 years later.[15] In 1973, Rosenberg and Damus, isolating large quantities of this thrombin inhibitor, provided convincing physicochemical evidence that plasma antithrombin activity and plasma heparin cofactor activity reside in the same molecular species.[16] These investigations left antithrombin III as the only plasma or serum constituent with antithrombin activity in physiological conditions. Therefore, several authors proposed to abandon the Roman numeral of antithrombin III and to designate antithrombin-heparin cofactor or simply antithrombin. However, this simplification could not be performed, because the importance of other proteins with thrombin neutralizing activity had been recognized simultaneously with the eclipse of Seegers' nomenclature. Lanchantin et al.[17] were the first to describe that alfa$_2$-macroglobulin can bind and inhibit human thrombin. According to Shapiro and Anderson, alfa$_2$-macroglobulin contributes about 25% to the overall plasma antithrombin activity.[18] Gans and Tan reported that alfa$_1$-antitrypsin inhibits thrombin slowly *in vitro*.[19] Despite its high plasma concentration it does not contribute any significant part to the overall antithrombin activity of the plasma. Saito et al.[20] described the thrombin-inhibiting activity of alfa$_2$-antiplasmin, another serine protease inhibitor, which seems to be of minor importance in inactivation of thrombin *in vivo*.

The proposed heparin-antithrombin designation for antithrombin III became surpassed by the discovery of another new heparin-dependent glycoprotein inhibiting thrombin. In

1974, Briginshaw and Shanberge hypothesized the existence of an antithrombin III-independent heparin cofactor.[21] This protein is probably identical to heparin cofactor II, isolated later by Tollefsen et al.[22]

This short historical overview has attempted to explain the development of our present terminology. The term "antithrombin" designates the proteins of normal human plasma displaying thrombin-inactivating activity. Substances which interfere with thrombin activity *in vitro,* like diisopropylfluorophosphate (DFP) or other enzyme inhibitors, are not covered by this term. Neither are antithrombins, the proteins, or degradated proteins of the plasma-like antibodies against thrombin or fibrinogen degradation products (FDP), which are produced in the course of various pathological states.

In the last 20 years we have witnessed an enormous development of knowledge on antithrombins. Hundreds of publications revealed many important features of antithrombin III, the main thrombin inhibitor of human plasma. The application of the new methods of protein chemistry rendered it possible to clarify the biochemical characteristics of antithrombin III.[15,23,24] The interaction between antithrombin III, heparin, and thrombin has been studied and disputed widely.[16,25,26] A rapid development of the methodology of the antithrombin III assays helped to establish the main features of the physiology and pathology of antithrombin III.[27-29] A great number of the clinical studies revealed the pathogenetic role of antithrombin III in the pathogenesis of thrombosis. Various forms of the congenital[30-32] and the acquired[33,34] antithrombin-III deficiencies have been described. The application of the recombinant gene techniques opened a new path in the research of the genetics of antithrombin III.[35] The production of the highly purified and safe antithrombin-III concentrates made it possible to effectively treat patients with antithrombin-III deficiency.[36,37]

The various chapters of this book discuss the biochemistry and clinical aspects of the antithrombins. However, the depth of discussion of the particular antithrombins is determined mainly by their biological importance as thrombin-inactivating proteins. This fact explains why the biochemistry, genetics, and clinical aspects of antithrombin III, the main antithrombin of human plasma, are discussed in separate chapters. The other proteins have only minor importance in the physiological inactivation of thrombin and (except for heparin cofactor II) exert their main effects in inactivation of enzymes other than thrombin. In these cases we restricted our interest to the topics related to inactivation of thrombin.

Géza Sas
Budapest, Hungary

REFERENCES

1. **Morawitz, P.,** Die Chemie der Blutgerinnung, *Ergeb. Physiol.,* 4, 307, 1905.
2. **Mellanby, J.,** The coagulation of blood, *J. Physiol.,* 38, 28, 1909.
3. **McLean, J.,** The thromboplastic action of cephalin, *Am. J. Physiol.,* 41, 250, 1916.
4. **Brinkhous, K. M., Smith, H. P., Warner, E. D., and Seegers, W. H.,** The inhibition of blood clotting: an unidentified substance which acts in conjunction with heparin to prevent the conversion of prothrombin into thrombin, *Am. J. Physiol.,* 125, 683, 1939.
5. **Astrup, T. and Darling, S.,** Antithrombin and heparin, *Acta Physiol. Scand.,* 5, 13, 1943.
6. **Gerendás, M.,** Inactivation of thrombin, *Nature,* 157, 837, 1946.
7. **Gerendás, M.,** Inactivation and stabilization of thrombin, *Hung. Acta Physiol.,* 1, 97, 1946-48.
8. **Seegers, W. H., Johnson, J. F., and Fell, C.,** An antithrombin reaction related to prothrombin inactivation, *Am. J. Physiol.,* 176, 97, 1954.
9. **Loeliger, A. and Hers, J. F. Ph.,** Chronic antithrombinaemia (antithrombin V) with haemorrhagic diathesis in a case of rheumatoid arthritis with hypergammaglobulinaemia, *Thromb. Diath. Haemorrh.,* 1, 499, 1957.

10. **Niewiarowski, S. and Kowalski, E.,** Un nouvel anticoagulant derivé du fibrinogéne, *Rev. Hématol.*, 13, 320, 1958.
11. **Waugh, D. F. and Fitzgerald, M. A.,** Quantitative aspects of antithrombin and heparin in plasma, *Am. J. Physiol.*, 184, 627, 1956.
12. **Monkhouse, F. C., France, E. S., and Seegers, W. H.,** Studies on the antithrombin and heparin cofactor activities of a fraction adsorbed from plasma by aluminium hydroxide, *Circ. Res.*, 3, 397, 1955.
13. **Gerendás, M.,** Die Thrombininaktivierung als Enzymprozess, *Thromb. Diath. Haemorrh.*, 4, 56, 1959.
14. **Egeberg, O.,** Inherited antithrombin deficiency causing thrombophilia, *Thromb. Diath. Haemorrh.*, 13, 516, 1965.
15. **Abildgaard, U.,** Highly purified antithrombin III with heparin cofactor activity prepared by disc electrophoresis, *Scand. J. Clin. Lab. Invest.*, 21, 89, 1968.
16. **Rosenberg, R. D. and Damus, P. S.,** The purification and mechanism of action of human antithrombin-heparin cofactor, *J. Biol. Chem.*, 248, 6490, 1973.
17. **Lanchantin, G. F., Plesset, M. L., Friedmann, J. A., and Hart, D. V.,** Dissociation of esterolytic and clotting activities of thrombin by Trypsin-Binding Macroglobulin, *Proc. Soc. Exp. Biol. Med.*, 121, 444, 1966.
18. **Shapiro, S. S. and Anderson, D. B.,** Thrombin inhibition in normal plasma, in *Chemistry and Biology of Thrombin,* Lundlblad, R. L., Fenton, J. W., and Mann, K. G. Eds., Ann Arbor Science Publishing, Ann Arbor, MI, 1977, 361.
19. **Gans, H. and Tan, B. H.,** α_1-Antitrypsin, an inhibitor for thrombin and plasmin, *Clin. Chim. Acta,* 17, 111, 1967.
20. **Saito, H., Goldsmith, G. H., Moroi, M., and Aoki, N.,** Inhibitory spectrum of α_2-plasmin inhibitor, *Proc. Natl. Acad. Sci. USA,* 76, 2013, 1979.
21. **Briginshaw, G. F. and Shanberge, J. N.,** Identification of two distinct heparin cofactors in human plasma. I. Separation and partial purification, *Arch. Biochem. Biophys.*, 161, 683, 1974.
22. **Tollefsen, D. M., Majerus, D. W., and Blank, M. K.,** Heparin cofactor II. Purification and properties of a heparin-dependent inhibitor of thrombin in human plasma, *J. Biol. Chem.*, 257, 2162, 1982.
23. **Miller-Andersson, M., Borg, H., and Andersson, L. O.,** Purification of antithrombin III by affinity chromatography, *Thrombos. Res.*, 5, 439, 1974.
24. **Kurachi, K., Schmer, G., Hermodson, M., Teller, D., and Davie, E. W.,** Characterization of human, bovine and horse antithrombin III, *Biochemistry,* 15, 368, 1976.
25. **Machovich, R., Blaskó, G., and Pálos, L. A.,** Action of heparin on thrombin-antithrombin reaction, *Biochem. Biophys. Acta,* 379, 193, 1975.
26. **Holmer, E., Sonderström, C., and Andressor, L. O.,** Effect of heparin in antithrombin III depleted plasma, *Thrombos. Haemostas.*, 42, 9, 1979.
27. **Sas, G., Pepper, D. S., and Cash, J. D.,** Plasma and serum antithrombin III: differentiation by crossed immunoelectrophoresis. *Thrombos. Res.*, 6, 87, 1975.
28. **Ødegard, O. R., Lie, M., and Abildgaard, U.,** Heparin cofactor activity measured with amidolytic methods, *Haemostasis,* 5, 265, 1976.
29. **Collen, D., Schetz, J., De Cock, F., Holmer, E., and Verstraete, M.,** Metabolism of antithrombin III in man: effects of venous thrombosis and of heparin administration, *Eur. J. Clin. Invest.*, 7, 27, 1977.
30. **Sas, G., Blaskó, G., Bánhegyi, D., Jákó, J., and Pálos, L. A.,** Abnormal antithrombin III (antithrombin III "Budapest") as a cause of a familial thrombophilia, *Thrombos. Diathes. Haemorrh.*, 32, 105, 1974.
31. **Sørensen, P. J., Dyerberg, J., Stoffersen, E., and Krogh Jensen, M.,** Familial functional antithrombin III deficiency, *Scand. J. Haematol.*, 24, 105, 1980.
32. **Sas, G., Petõ, I., Bánhegyi, D., Blaskó, G., and Domján, G.,** Heterogeneity of the "classical" antithrombin III deficiency, *Thrombos. Haemostas.*, 43, 133, 1980.
33. **Kauffmann, R. H., Veltkamp, J. J., van N. H. Tilburg, and van L. A. Es,** Acquired antithrombin III deficiency and thrombosis in the nephrotic syndrome, *Am. J. Med.*, 65, 607, 1978.
34. **Mannucci, L., Dioguardi, N., Del Ninno, E., and Mannucci, P. M.,** Value of normotest and antithrombin III in the assessment of liver function, *Scand. J. Gastroent.*, 8 (Suppl. 19), 103, 1973.
35. **Prochownik, E. W., Antonarakis, S., Bauer, K. A., Rosenberg, R. D., Fearon, E. R., and Orkin, S. H.,** Molecular heterogeneity of inherited antithrombin III deficiency, *New Engl. J. Med.*, 308, 1549, 1983.
36. **Thaler, E.,** Antithrombin-III-Konzentrate: Klinische Anwendung, *Haemostasis,* 3, 128, 1982.
37. **Hellgren, M., Javelin, L., Hagnevik, K., and Blombäck, M.,** Antithrombin III concentrate as adjuvant in DIC treatment. A pilot study in 9 severely ill patients, *Thrombos. Res.*, 35, 459, 1984.

THE EDITOR

Géza Sas, M.D. is Professor of Medicine in the First Department of Medicine at the Postgraduate Medical University, Budapest, Hungary.

Dr. Sas received his M.D. degree from the Medical University of Budapest in 1962. He served at the Clinical Haematological Laboratories of the National Institute for Rheumatic Diseases and the Central Military Hospital from 1962 to 1966 in Budapest. After that he was appointed an Assistant Professor of Medicine at the First Department of Medicine at the Postgraduate Medical Institute, Budapest. While there he became an Associate Professor of Medicine in 1972 and a Professor in 1980. In 1974 he worked as a Senior Research Fellow at the Blood Transfusion Center of Edinburgh, Scotland. He received his D.Sc. degree in 1978.

Dr. Sas is a member of the International Society on Thrombosis and Hemostasis, the New York Academy of Sciences, the Scientific Committee of the Danubian League Against Thrombosis and Haemorrhagic Diseases, the Hungarian Society on Internal Diseases, the Hungarian Society of Haematologists, the Hungarian Society on Clinical Laboratory Investigations, the Common Committee of the Hungarian Ministry of Health, and the Hungarian Academy of Sciences on Circulatory Diseases.

Among other awards he has received the Markusovszky Award, the title of "Distinguished Lecturer of the Higher Education," and the Golden Medal for the Service of the Fatherland.

Dr. Sas is the author of more than 100 papers and has authored two books. His current major research interests relate to the familial thrombophilias.

CONTRIBUTORS

György G. Blasko, M.D., Ph.D.
Senior Research Officer
First Department of Medicine
Postgraduate Medical University
Budapest, Hungary

Lisbet M. Javelin, M.Sc.
Clinical Trials Manager
Medical Department
KabiVitrum Haematology AB
Stockholm, Sweden

Edward V. Prochownik, Ph.D.
Associate Professor
Department of Pediatrics
University of Michigan
Ann Arbor, Michigan

István Rákóczi, M.D., Ph.D.
Associate Professor
Department of Obstetrics and Gynecology
Postgraduate Medical University
Budapest, Hungary

Géza Sas, M.D.
Professor
First Department of Medicine
Postgraduate Medical University
Budapest, Hungary

Helmut A. Vinazzer, M.D.
Professor and Director
Blood Coagulation Laboratory
Linz, Austria

TABLE OF CONTENTS

Chapter 1

THE BIOCHEMISTRY OF ANTITHROMBIN III

György Blaskó

TABLE OF CONTENTS

I. INTRODUCTION

For many years, our knowledge regarding the activation processes of blood coagulation has largely been extended due to biochemists taking over experimental work; however, the study of inhibitors of the coagulation cascade remained far behind. The term "haemostasis" is the capability of blood to maintain its fluidity and circulation within the blood vessels and it involves the existence of well-regulated compensatory system(s) acting against all the so-called procoagulatory processes. These physiological anticoagulant and/or antithrombotic mechanisms exert their activity at cellular (e.g., the production of antiaggregatory prostacyclin by endothelial cells, the proteolytic inactivation of F-Va and F-VIIIa via the endothel-bound thrombomodulin-Protein C complex, etc.) level as well as in the circulating blood plasma as the proteinase inhibitors act.*

Antithrombin III (AT-III) belongs to the last group, i.e., to proteinase inhibitors of coagulation acting in the fluid circulating phase. Antithrombin itself is an old concept originating from Morawitz, who was the first to describe the decrease in coagulant activity of clotted blood, and Weymoth, being a prophet by suggesting a complex formation of thrombin and AT-III.[1,2,3] (Regarding the nomenclature and history of the concept, see Preface.)

AT-III belongs to the protein superfamily, namely serpins, which proteins have evolved from a primitive ancestral serine protease inhibitor. As it will show in this chapter (see III.D), the common feature of plasma serpins is that they are suicidal proteins in that they form a tight 1:1 complex with their target protease, the complex being subsequently removed from the circulation and catabolized (see Table 1).

II. ISOLATION OF AT-III

A. CONVENTIONAL METHODS

A number of purification procedures were described in the early 1970s, including several adsorption/precipitation procedures and ion-exchange chromatography.[4-7]

Briginshaw and Shanberge[8] distinguished two separate heparin cofactors after PEG_{6000} precipitation and DEAE-cellulose and hydroxyapatite chromatography, but the majority of authors accepted the existence of one heparin cofactor only until the discovery and characterization of a heparin cofactor II (see Chapter 6).[4,6,8] The maximal increase in specific activity was 25- to 200-fold in these conservative procedures due to the rapid inactivation

* It is important to note that these systems are also compartmentalized, since the fibrinolytic system can act systemically as well as locally (tissue-type plasminogen activators).

TABLE 1
Plasma Serpins

Name	Concentration in plasma (μmol/l)	Molecular weight	Target enzymes, proteins
Antithrombin III (AT-III)	2	61,000	Thrombin, F-Xa, F-IXa, F-XI_a, F-XII_a, Trypsin, C_1
Heparin cofactor II	1	66,000	Mainly thrombin
Antiplasmin	1	70,000	Plasmin
Plasminogen activator-inhibitor I and II	10^{-4}	50,000	Plasminogen activator
Protein C inhibitor	10^{-2}	57,000	Activated protein C
Antitrypsin	15	51,000	Neutrophil elastase
Antichymotrypsin	7	69,000	Cathepsin G
C_1-inhibitor	2	104,000	Complement C_1s, kallikrein
Angiotensinogen	10^{-2}	50,000	They are not proteinase inhibitors
Thyroxin-binding protein	0.2	54,000	

of AT-III through the various precipitation procedures.[9,10] Using these conservative methods, the best purification procedures were described by Abildgaard, Rosenberg, and Damus (combined adsorption, gel filtration, and DEAE-Sephadex chromatography), resulting in a large-scale production of a 95% homogenous protein with a yield of 2 to 10%.[11,12,13]

B. AFFINITY CHROMATOGRAPHY

The introduction of affinity chromatography on heparin-agarose, including a PEG_{6000} precipitation, yielded a homogenous AT-III having a specific activity 4 to 500 times higher than that of plasma, and for the time being, this method is the basis of the large-scale preparation of AT-III for clinical use.[14,15,18] Wickerhauser and Williams from the American Red Cross reported that a single-step method based on heparin-sepharose affinity chromatography resulted in a highly purified AT-III concentrate with a recovery of 30%.[16] The PEG-precipitation could be replaced by the increased (0.7 *M*) salt concentration of the washing buffer and completing it with pasteurization, thus effectively reducing the risk of pyrogen development and hepatitis. Mitra et al.[17] analyzed six different coupling methods for preparing immobilized heparins to optimize the circumstances of the process and they advised a nonhazardous cyanilating agent (1-cyano-4-dim-ethyl amino pyridinium tetrafluoroborate [CDAP]) for the covalent attachment of the ligand to polysaccharide matrices having good AT-III-binding capacity.

C. PURIFICATION OF ANTITHROMBIN-III FROM ANIMAL SOURCES

Heparin-agarose chromatography was proved to be a suitable method for isolating animal antithrombins. Jordan reported the results of a series of investigations regarding the characteristics of antithrombin in vertebrate species.[19] Summarizing briefly, he found only minor differences in the molecular weights of antithrombins in mammals (chimpanzee, bovine, goat, rabbit, canine, and guinea pig), with the guinea pig showing the lowest inhibitory capacity against thrombin, and the goat against F-Xa.[15,19,21,22,24] AT-III from human, porcine, rat, and rabbit showed similar amino acid compositions with minor differences, e.g., rat antithrombin has an amino-terminal asparagine, instead of histidin as in the others.[22] The chicken-antithrombin of birds had quite different amino acids at the first four positions of the N-terminal and with a much higher inhibitory capacity against Factor Xa than that of thrombin.[23] The antithrombin-like protein of a turtle and an amphibian, namely bullfrog, showed 30% and 10% thrombin inhibitory capacities, respectively, compared to humans. A number of unsuccessful attempts have been made to isolate an antithrombin-like inhibitor from fish, i.e., from shark and carp plasma, but none could isolate a heparin-binding protein possessing a thrombin-inhibitory activity. This supports the hypothesis that the anticoagulant relationship of heparin and antithrombin was established at an early point in the evolution (more than 500 million years ago) of the coagulation system and has been highly conserved since that time.

III. THE STRUCTURE OF HUMAN AT-III

A. PHYSICOCHEMICAL PROPERTIES

The molecular weight of human AT-III has been found to differ between 54,000 and 65,000, depending on the source of the plasma and on the methods used. Gradient polyacrylamide gel electrophoresis (PAGE) in the presence of sodium duodecyl sulphate gave a value of 65,000, whereas simple PAGE resulted in a value of 60,000 and gel chromatography in the presence of 6 *M* guanidine-HCl 55,000, respectively.[26] Sedimentation equilibrium studies show a value of 58,000 ± 1000 being more reliable since the technique is more accurate.[26]

The sedimentation coefficient, $S^{O}_{20,w,}$ is 4.1 as determined in two different studies.[14,26] The intrinsic viscosity is 4.8 ml/g. Assuming the last-mentioned molecular weight, the calculated frictional ratio, $f/f_{min,}$ is 1.34, indicating that AT-III is a globular protein with an assymetric shape.[25] The partial specific volume was calculated to be 0.72 ml/g — assuming the value for β in the Scheraga-Mandelkern equation to be 2.12 x 10^6 (it is commonly accepted for globular proteins).[26] The data of the far-ultraviolet circular dichroism spectra indicated the existence of an α-helix content of only about 10%, about 40% β-structure, and 50% of random coil. Furugren et al.[27] demonstrated an ellipsoid shape of the protein with semiaxes of 1.9, 3.7, and 5.2 nm using small-angle X-ray scattering. AT-III is an acidic protein having isoelectric points ranging from 4.9 to 5.2.

Further spectroscopic investigations (using some derivatizations, i.e., S-carbamidomethylation, iodination, etc.) suggested that tyrosine and phenylalanine residues lost their rotational freedom after chemical modification. The tryptophan residues are responsible for the intrinsic fluorescence, and heparin enhances the fluorescence by 33%, indicating the binding. Villanueva and Allen determined two unfolding domains in AT-III, the first being reversible and able to renaturate, and unstable and irreversible upon renaturation, whereas the second domain was able to renaturate reversibly.[28] Using various techniques, such as fluorescene quenching, solvent perturbation, and chemical modification, they proved that some tryptophan residues are essential for the complete refolding. Furthermore, a two-step mechanism for the binding of heparin to AT-III was also suggested.

B. THE PRIMARY STRUCTURE OF AT-III

Petersen et al.[29] reported the primary sequence of human AT-III in 1979. Summarizing their results briefly, the protein contains 425 amino acids (plus 4 to 5 yet undetermined between 210- and 211-residue stretches). The carboxy-terminal end is responsible for the binding to thrombin and other enzymes, whereas heparin and/or other mucopolysaccharides bind to the amino-terminal region. Three disulfide bridges are located between Cys 8 to Cys-128, Cys-21 to Cys-95, and Cys-239 to Cys-422, resulting in the formation of a structure which is roughly outlined on Figure 1. The mild reduction of AT-III with dithiothreitol resulted in a cleavage of presumably Cys-21 to Cys-95 bridge only, as it has been reported by Longas et al.,[30] however, these changes were accompanied by the loss of affinity of AT-III to heparin. It was one of the first suggestions regarding the existence of different heparin- and thrombin-binding sites in this inhibitor.

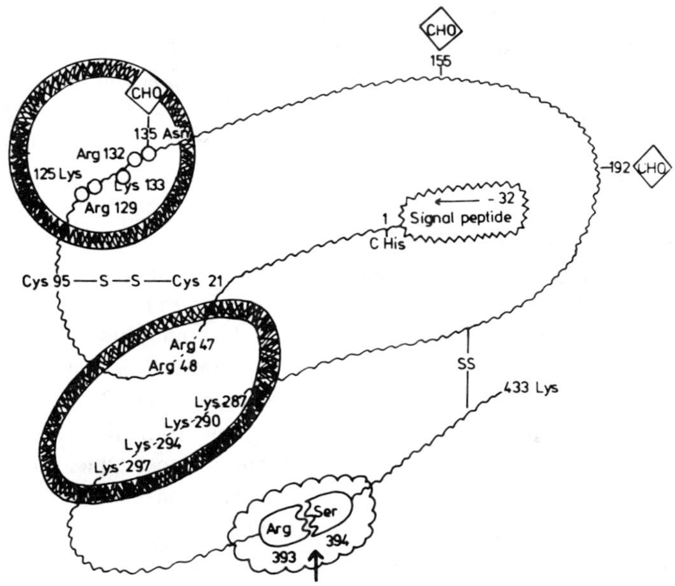

FIGURE 1. The rough structure of antithrombin-III. The oval circle shows the most important primary heparin-binding site, the round circle represents the secondary heparin-binding site. The arrow indicates the site of thrombin-proteolysis, surrounded by the enzyme-binding area of antithrombin-III. CHO = carbohydrate moieties.

1. The Active Site of AT-III

Since AT-III inhibits all the serine proteinases primarily in the coagulation cascade (as it will be discussed in detail in this chapter) by forming extremely stable equimolar complexes with the enzymes, it has been suggested that the mechanism of this inhibition is very similar in the case of various enzymes. It has also been observed that the formation of this complex is accompanied by the rapid appearance of a free, proteolytically slightly modified form of the inhibitor.[32] Heparin accelerated the formation of this modified AT-III. Amino acid analysis showed that only a single peptide bond was cleaved between Arg-385 and Ser-386 in the splitted AT-III. The two resulting fragments (molecular weight of about 50,000 and 5000) are held together by a disulfide bridge at Cys-239 to Cys-422. Björk et al.[31] demonstrated that in the case of the reactions with factors Xa, IXa, and thrombin, the cleavage site remains the same, but the specificity of the reaction differs. This strongly suggests that the observed Arg-Ser cleavage site is the active site of AT-III. These experiments gave an indication of the state of the active-site peptide bond of AT-III because the cleavage excludes the existence of a tetrahedral intermediate, it suggests the formation of an acyl-intermediate. In the acyl-intermediate state, the liberated carboxy-terminal arginyl residue of the large fragment of the cleaved AT-III remains attached to the active site Ser of the enzyme(s) by an acyl bond, while no covalent bonds contribute to the stability of the complex in the fully hydrolyzed state.[33] In a forthcoming step, several experiments prove the formation of a covalent, irreversible bond at this site between the active center of Ser in thrombin and Arg-385 of AT-III.[13,34-36] α_1-antitrypsin was split by trypsin at a Met-Ser bond 37 residue from the C-terminal, giving evidence that this is the active site for trypsin inhibition. The analysis of the C-terminal end of the inhibitor showed a 30% identity with human AT-III, but a much stronger homology was observed in the neighborhood of the active site.[37] Chandra et al.[38] identified a number of human α_1-antichymotrypsin cDNA clones using a baboon cDNA insert as a hybridization probe until finally the amino acid sequence of human α_1-antichymotrypsin was deduced. It showed a 42% homology with α_1-antitrypsin and 33% with AT-III. Griffith et al.[39] demonstrated a structural similarity in the reactive site peptide between AT-III and heparin cofactor II (see Chapter 6). However, a disulfide bond linking the carboxy-terminal (reactive site) region of AT-III to the remainder of the molecule, which is important for the heparin-induced conformational change in the protein and high-affinity binding of heparin, does not appear to exist in heparin cofactor II.

2. The Heparin-Binding Site of AT-III

The essential role of tryptophan residues in heparin binding is known.[40] After the modification of one tryptophan per molecule of AT-III with dimethyl (2-hydroxy-5-nitrobenzyl) sulfonium bromide,[41] the derivatized inhibitor does not exhibit the heparin-accelerated inactivation of thrombin, however, it does not loose its specific activity against thrombin alone. It did not bind to the heparin-agarose column, too. The exact place of this tryptophan is not yet determined. This heparin-binding region of the protein contains one or more lysine residues as well as this critical tryptophan residue. Other basic amino acids like arginine also take place in heparin binding, however, an extensive modification is necessary in the numbers of amino acids to block heparin binding. The importance of arginines in heparin binding is well-proved in the cases of AT-III variants having a loss or decrease in heparin affinity. AT-III "Toyama" (47 Arg → Cys,) AT-III "Rouen 1" (47 Arg → His), and AT-III "Rouen 2" (47 Arg → Ser) demonstrate it well. A fourth variant with reduced heparin affinity is AT-III "Basel" (41 Pro → Leu), which can be predicted to cause a perturbation in the region of residue 47. If the positions of the basic amino acids mentioned above are mapped on a computer projection of AT-III, seven important basic amino acid residues, including Arg-47, Lys-125, Arg-129, Arg-132, and Lys-133, are seen to form a closely related sphere of positive charge. This sphere of the surface of AT-III seems likely to be the major binding site of heparin. Olson et al.[43,44] measured the kinetics of heparin binding to AT-III using stopped-flow fluorescence measurement, etc. and agreed with Villanueva and Allen in suggesting a two-step procedure for binding (it will be discussed here as the "inhibitor-fitting theory").[28]

3. The Carbohydrate Components of AT-III

As it can be seen on Figure 1, four glucosamine-based oligosaccharide units are coupled to Asn-96, Asn-135, Asn-155, and Asn-192, respectively.[29,45] All the oligosaccharides contain N-acetylneuraminic acid, N-Acetyl-glucosamine, mannose, galactose in a molar ratio of approximately 1:1:1:0.6; however, Danishefsky at al.[46] reported a glycolipid associated with AT-III, defined as glucocerebroside, but Dale and Westwood[47] excluded the possibility of the coupling of this major plasma glycolipid to AT-III. Mizuochi et al.[45] determined the carbohydrate sequences almost completely in AT-III and they stated that the sugar chain of the inhibitor has a typical complex-type structure as found in human transferrin, human J chain, C_{1q}, and α_1-protease inhibitor, but there are some minor differences since AT-III does not contain fucose, but IgG and C_{1q} do. (The AT-III-producing cells do not have fucosyltransferase.) Nonenzymatic glycosylation may occur under pathological conditions, i.e., in the case of diabetes mellitus. The presence of glucose and appropriate circumstances result in the formation of a glycosilated AT-III, which has a decreased thrombin-inhibiting activity even in the presence of heparin. The nonenzymatic glycation of AT-III *in vivo* accounts for the hypercoagulable state observed in diabetics.[48] Sugar preservatives, which are used in AT-III preparates, can also cause a loss of the heparin cofactor activity, but they stabilize AT-III against thermal denaturation.[49] Mitra et al.[50] determined exactly that the calculated activation energies during the thermal denaturation of AT-III, which denaturates the hepatitis B virus, were estimated to be at least four times lower than that associated with the unfolding of the tertiary structure of the protein — this decreases the risk of transmission of the virus reliably. At 65°C for 16.5 h, only a 16.4% aggregate formation was seen in the presence of sucrose. (On the contrary to this, we described earlier that purified AT-III completely lost its activity at the same temperature within 3 min.[51] Heparin did not prevent AT-III against heat inactivation, but it did so in the case of α-thrombin.)[51,52] Bushby et al.[53] showed a slight stabilizing effect of heparin, phosphate, sulphate, and EDTA, but the heparin concentration applied was extremely high, such as 10mg/ml, and T_d increased by 7°C. Therefore, pasteurization could result in minor alterations in the interactions with heparin and/or thrombin.

C. HETEROGENITY OF PURIFIED HUMAN AT-III

Borsodi and Narasimhan were the first who reported the microheterogeneity of purified human AT-III with the use of isoelectric focusing in 1978.[54] It has been confirmed since then by a number of reports.[55,57] The profile of the isoelectric focusing pattern of purified AT-III changed immediately after lyophilization (it changed entirely after storage at 4°C for 2 years).[55] About 8 to 10 bands are observable by isoelectric focusing and immuno-fixation — alterations in microheterogeneity were seen in patients undergoing surgery and those with nephrotic syndrome and liver diseases.

D. HOMOLOGY WITH α_1-ANTITRYPSIN

After the appearance of the first publication regarding the amino acid sequence of a domain of α_1-antitrypsin consisting of 109 amino acids,[58] a sequence homology was found between this and the sequence of 265 to 379 of AT-III (see Section III.A). Between the 108 residue stretches of AT-III (positions 268 to 375) and positions 4 to 106 of the 109 residues of the α_1-antitrypsin fragment,[29] 36 identities were observable. This means that these two proteins may have a common ancestor. It is interesting to note that the amino acid sequence homology between trypsin and chymotrypsin, the representative target proteases inhibited by α_1-antitrypsin and α_1-antichymotrypsin, respectively, is also 42%.[38] Thus, the serpin antiprotease superfamily of proteins consists of AT-III, heparin cofactor II, α_1-antitrypsin, α_1-antichymotrypsin, and ovalbumin.[39] But ovalbumin diverged approximately 500 million years ago,[59] whereas α_1-antitrypsin diverged approximately 300 million years ago, and the divergence of α_1-antichymotrypsin was much more recent. With the exception of AT-III, all the antiproteinases mentioned earlier are increased in the plasma level under acute conditions, i.e., inflammation, surgery, or infections. It would be interesting to determine the gene signals for acute-phase response and to find out when during the evolutionary process the AT-III gene lost its capability to respond.

IV. BIOSYNTHESIS OF AT-III

Previous studies of AT-III biosynthesis gave some contradictory data regarding the exact place of the synthesis. Losito et al.[60] failed to demonstrate a net synthesis, Koj et al.[61] and Owens and Miller[62] could detect AT-III in liver perfusates, and puromycin, an inhibitor of protein synthesis, was capable of inhibiting the appearance of AT-III in the organ perfusate. The immunofluorescence studies gave controversial results. Chan and Chan did not find AT-III in the hepatocytes.[63] Watada et al.[64] and Léon et al.[65] reported that AT-III was detectable in hepatocytes by an immunoperoxidase technique. Using the method of the incorporation of radiolabeled amino acids into AT-III, ^{75}S-methionin incorporation was observed in hepatocytes as well as into the endothelial cells-derived AT-III. [63,65] ^{14}C-glycin incorporation could be demonstrated especially in liver-, spleen-, and kidney-derived AT-III fractions,[66,67] and the use of inhibitor(s) showed that the chief site of AT-III synthesis was in the liver. It is a supporting evidence that the plasma AT-III level is remarkably decreased in liver disorders.[66] A suggestion was proposed that AT-III released from hepatocytes probably binds to endogenous heparin or glycosaminoglycanes immediately, protecting the vessel wall against thrombosis.[63] The decrease in the level of AT-III during heparin treatment is also explainable, i.e., the inhibitor-heparin or the inhibitor-heparin-enzyme complex gets trapped into the reticuloendothelial cells of the tissues.

Fair and Bahnak clarified the cellular origin of AT-III utilizing a human hepatoma cell-line, namely Hep G2, which was capable of synthesizing a variety of plasma proteins including coagulation factors, fibrinolytic and complement proteins, etc.[68] The secreted AT-III was biologically active, and the activity could be inhibited by monospecific antibodies. Interestingly, Warfarin has a transient inhibitory effect on the secretion of AT-III, however, its intracellular and extracellular concentrations are not affected by this drug. Amrani and coworkers showed that AT-III in chicken and perhaps in mammals is a developmentally regulated glycoprotein.[82] The concentration of AT-III in plasma rises from approximately 26 μ/ml to the normal level, from the 16th day until hatching. The degree of sialilation also changes because the "early" AT-III does contain a subminimal sialic acid, in contrast to the adult form (3.5 residue per moles). Gross and Stuart have made similar observations in humans between the 7th and 9th month of gestation.[83] The sialization-glycosylation process might protect glycoproteins against intracellular proteolytic degradation.[84]

V. DISTRIBUTION AND FATE OF AT-III

The normal plasma concentration of AT-III in human beings is 2 to 3 μ*M* (150 to 200 mg/l).[69,70] Collen et al.[71] determined the half-life of radiolabeled AT-III in healthy subjects: it was found to be 2.83 ± 0.26 d. They demonstrated first a significantly shortened value for patients suffering from venous thrombosis and treated with heparin. Reeve et al.[72] described a three-compartment steady-state model for AT-III, thrombin, and F-Xa with a mathematically proved very rapid breakdown of the antithrombin portion of the labeled protease AT-III complex. Marciniak and Gockerman published shorter elimination times for AT-III using a nonisotopic method — 8.4 to 13.6 hours.[73] No differences were found between untreated and previously heparinized patients for several days, but the rate of elimination increased threefold when AT-III and heparin were given simultaneously. The injected AT-III could be demonstrated immunologically, but it was not active biologically. They proved the regulating role of heparin in AT-III catabolism.

The distribution volume of AT-III between the intravascular and extravascular compartments is similar to that of albumin, having an intravascular fraction of 0.45.[71] The concentration of AT-III in the cerebrospinal fluid is 80 to 400 n*M*.Urine does not contain active AT-III. The excreted amount of the protein is 50 to 50 μg/d.[74] There are controversial reports regarding the existence of AT-III within the platelets.[74,75] The intracellular concentration was found to be about 1 p*M*. AT-III is also distributed in the lymph. The distribution of this protein in the intracellular compartment is specific or receptor-mediated because the competition experiments show identical clearance curves even at a 10,000-fold molar excess of unlabeled AT-III. The clearance did not show alteration when the reactive site of the inhibitor was blocked.[76] The identical clearance of the lysine-blocked human AT-III suggests that *in vivo* it does not bind to tissue glycosaminoglycanes via the heparin-binding domain as a factor in distribution.

If AT-III has already formed a complex with thrombin, the clearance of this complex is shown to be more rapid than AT-III alone. It was demonstrated in rabbits, mice, and in humans, but there are remarkable species differences.[77,90] The rapid clearence of the complexes was not affected by reticuloendothelial system blockade, i.e., mannan or asialoorosomucoide. This also argues for the receptor-mediated clearance of the complexes, similar to that of the clearance of α_2-macroglobulin-trypsin complex.[78] Several data suggest the formation of a neoantigenic determinant(s) when AT-III binds to thrombin and/or proteases, and these new, neoantigenic complex(es) are recognized and result in an uptake by the hepatocytes. Changes in the clearence data when turnover properties of the heparin-AT-III complex (chemically stabilized by covalent bonds) were studied show that possibly heparin should dissociate from the complex.[79] No differences were found in the distribution and catabolism of AT-III between patients with congenital AT-III deficiency and normals, but the half-life of the AT-III in the deficient patients was longer[80] (see details in Chapter 2). Recently, Knot et al.[81] published that neither the plasma disappearance half-times nor fractional catabolic rate constants differed significantly between members of AT-III-deficient families and normal subjects. However, the mean absolute catabolic rate in the patients' group was lower. The application of these results to the three-compartment model may suggest that the deficient protein binds less to the endothelial cell surface. Marciniak and Romond administered commercial AT-III concentrate and dysfunctional AT-III, incapable of binding enzymes or heparin, to normal and AT-III deficient subjects and they found a significantly faster disappearance of the excess functional AT-III as compared to that of the AT-III antigen.[86] They supported the previous hypothesis of Carlson and his co-workers that a heparin-like endothelial receptor may control the transport and even the turnover of AT-III.[85,87,88] AT-III shows an increased reactivity with serine proteinases in the presence of endothelial cells: the exact characteristics of such an endothelial receptor are not clear and until now no clinical conditions have been elucidated with such an abnormal receptor. Savion and Farzame recently emphasized the important role of human skin fibroblasts in the removal of AT-III-protease complexes from extravascular spaces in the body.[147] A specific binding of the complexes to hepatocytes has been confirmed, accompanied by their subsequent internalization and degradation.[148,149] However, the potential regulatory role of this receptor in the prevention of thrombosis has strongly been emphasized.[89]

VI. THE MECHANISM OF ACTION OF AT-III

Since thrombin is a product of an amplifying enzyme cascade, its production and disappearance should be precisely regulated. It is a well-known fact that thrombosis occurs if the clearance mechanism of thrombin is defected. There are two separate pathways for the removal of thrombin from circulation:[85]

1. The direct binding of thrombin to the endothelial cell receptor, followed by internalization and degradation.
2. Rapid formation of thrombin (or active clotting enzyme) to the inhibitor complex, which is recognized, removed, and degraded.

At this part of the chapter, we discuss in detail the mechanism of the latter pathway, describing the binding mechanisms of AT-III to thrombin first, followed by the presentation of data regarding the binding of F-Xa and other enzymes to AT-III, and finally the involvement of heparin in these interactions.

A. THE INTERACTION AND BINDING OF THROMBIN TO AT-III

Early investigations showed that thrombin and AT-III form a 1:1 stoichiometric complex in a purified system, and this complex is relatively stable against reducing and denaturing agents.[13,34,36] Abildgaard was the first[91] to describe the second-order reaction kinetics of the inactivation of thrombin by AT-III in 1969. The covalent nature of this binding was supported by Longas and Finlay, indicating that during the formation of this complex, the inhibitor is cleaved at an arginine-X bond and this arginine forms a carboxylic ester with thrombin.[36] The excised polypeptide of AT-III remains bound via disulphide bridges. The circular dichroism and optical rotatory dispersion studies[92] demonstrate that when thrombin binds to

AT-III, the complex undergoes considerable conformational changes. In the absence of heparin, the velocity of the complex formation is relatively slow. The solvent perturbation results indicated an exposure of approximately seven tyrosine residues. These residues are relatively distant from certain tryptophans which undergo an exposure in the presence of heparin. It was conceivable that the susceptibility of the complex to further degradation is due to an unfolding process which exposes more thrombin-sensitive bonds to the surface of the complex. When the carbohydrate moieties of AT-III were labeled and fluorescent polarization was measured at a higher temperature, the complex did not show any change in polarization at 70°C, indicating a conformational change in the glycosylated part of the inhibitor.[93]

1. Factors Regulating Thrombin-AT-III Binding

An early suggestion from Esmon was to search for blood components which may regulate the reaction of enzymes to AT-III.[94] Such a protein was prothrombin Fragment 2, which inhibited the complex formation of thrombin and AT-III. This interaction would favor the localization of the clot, protecting thrombin against inactivation at the place of the formation of the enzyme.

Two polypeptides of 74 and 55 kDa present on the surface of platelets are known to specifically enhance the activity of thrombin towards different synthetic substrates. These platelet proteins protect thrombin against AT-III either in the absence or in the presence of heparin. In contrast, the inhibition of trypsin by AT-III was not affected by these proteins. Therefore, one may say that platelet proteins may regulate the inhibition of thrombin by AT-III.[95]

The sugar residues of thrombin and AT-III are not required for the formation of the complex and their existence (or change) does not regulate the complex formation.[96]

The molecular form of thrombin and the species origin of this enzyme may also influence the complex formation. α-Thrombin (E.C. 3.4.21.5) having a 36-residue A-chain and a 259-residue B-chain polypeptide linked by an S-S bridge, may undergo a limited proteolysis (autolytic or tryptic) to β-thrombin, resulting in the formation of γ-thrombin with an accompanying loss of clotting activity.[97,98] The apparent second-order rate constants differ in human α-, bovine α-, bovine β-, and human γ-thrombins depending on ionic strengths.[99] The γ-thrombin-AT-III complex did not inhibit clotting catalyzed by α-thrombin and fibrinogen, and did not affect the reaction of γ-thrombins with AT-III.[99] These indicate the importance of any proteolyzed form of thrombin which, in circulation, may reduce the content and efficacy of AT-III.[98] The regulatory role of ionic strengths in the complex formation *in vitro* was published earlier, but the importance of their standardization in functional tests has not been emphasized in the past decade.[99-101] Using the chromogenic substrates, the catalytic role of heparin and the inhibitory effect of AT-III could be suspended in extreme high ionic strength, indicating the availability of these substrates for the active center under these circumstances.[101]

Lipid peroxides inhibit the activity of AT-III. Heparin-Sepharose binding studies and heparin cofactor assays suggested that the heparin-binding site of AT-III is the target of lipid peroxides.[102] Being increasingly recognized in atherosclerotic processes, lipid peroxides may contribute locally to AT-III functions.

As far as other components of the hemostatic system are concerned, regarding their effect on the thrombin-AT-III reaction, Jesty demonstrated that purified prothrombin and phospholipid have no effect. Ca ions inhibit it slightly at 5 mmol/l, whereas in the presence of calcium, fibrinogen reduced the rate of inhibition.[103,104] Unstimulated platelets increased the rate of inhibition by 40%; ADP-stimulated platelets increased it by 55%. The explanation of this finding was discussed earlier.[95]

Interestingly, the complex of thrombin-AT-III binds to vitronectin, which is present in tissues, at cell surfaces, and in the plasma, being in strong interaction with glycosaminoglycanes, promoting the attachment and spreading of normal and neoplastic cells.[105] The constituents of the complex alone do not bind to it, and the binding occurs at the cryptic site in the inhibitor after the formation of the complex. However, the significance of this phenomenon is speculatory; the interaction of vitronectin in creating a mitogenic signal on the cell surface, its strong binding site for heparin, suggests that it has yet an unknown role in clotting and atherosclerosis.

Although the effect of aspirin on haemostasis is mainly concerned to its ability to inhibit platelet functions, recently it has been demonstrated that acetylsalycylic acid inhibits AT-III irreversibly via a specific acetylation of two lysines in AT-III.[113] This modification of AT-III may result in a negative effect on the activity of this drug as an antithrombotic agent.

We can find some data regarding the influence of calcium ions on the inactivation of thrombin by AT-III in literature: Ca^{++} ions enhance the rate of inactivation in the absence of heparin, too.[114,115] This effect of Ca^{++} could be suspended with Na^{+} ions. The physiological role of these findings has not yet been elucidated. Electronegative ions have a much greater role in the purification of AT-III.[116]

Surface-bound thrombin has a quite different effect from AT-III: immobilized thrombin splits AT-III, resulting in the formation of an inactive 50 kDa molecule without biological or heparin-binding activity.[117] Therefore, thrombin bound to endothelial cells might have a different effect on soluble AT-III.

2. Kinetics of the Formation and Dissociation of Thrombin-AT-III Complexes

A previous study of F-Xa confirmed that the inactivation of this enzyme follows second-order kinetics.[106] So in the plasma, where AT-III is in large excess over the levels of activated factors that may be normally generated, we may expect pseudo-first-order conditions to exist. Jesty demonstrated that the initial rate of inhibition would be independent of enzyme concentration and in contrast to the low (5×10^{-10} *M*) dissociation constant, free F-Xa was measurable by bioassay.[106] He suggested that the formation of the complex is perhaps not irreversible.

Taking into consideration that the total amount of thrombin generated during glass-activation is approximately 160 pmol/ml and the concentration of AT-III in plasma is known to be about 2 to 4.5 μM, Jesty gave direct evidence for the existence of reversibility of the thrombin-antithrombin complex. The plots of the pseudo-first-order rate constants were linear to 20 μM AT-III concentration.[107] He suggested the existence of a very rapid first step and a lower second one. He emphasized the dubious authenticity of the kinetic data using the S-2238 substrate, because it is expected to compete with AT-III for thrombin. In plasma, the obvious substrates are fibrinogen, F-XIII, F-V, F-VIII, and possibly prothrombin, all reducing the rate of inhibition. The extent of this competition depends on the binding constants for each substrate and these are not yet known. The reversibility of the complex formation could maintain a low, but definite level of free thrombin in plasma (i.e., if 20% of prothrombin became activated, a minimum equilibrium level of 1 milliunit per ml of thrombin may be present, which is sufficient to split F-VIII or other natural substrates, despite the low K_d) and may regulate the level of other factors, too. A bovine system parallels the human one at excess amounts of AT-III. The second-order rate constants are 1.43×10^4 *M*/s and 5.7×10^3 *M*/s, respectively.

Using a very potent inactivator for thrombin, Ile-Pro-Arg-CH_2Cl, Griffith and Lundblad also proved the reversibility of the complex, demonstrating that active AT-III can be released from the complex.[108] Measurable thrombin can be released too, depending on the pH. A peptide bond hydrolizes in AT-III during this dissociation. Their results also suggest that the rate of thrombin release via acylation-deacylation is limited by the rate of the formation of an acylated enzyme-inhibitor complex, whereas the inhibition of thrombin by AT-III appears to be affected by the formation of a nonacylated enzyme-inhibitor complex.

Stability of the thrombin-AT-III complex has been measured by numerous authors, demonstrating a direct evidence that a covalent bond is formed between AT-III and thrombin.[108-110] It is also possible that this bond does not involve the active-site serine. If the complex is denatured with 0.1% sodium dodecyl sulfate, 1 *M* hydroxylamine will dissociate it.[109] Hydroxylamine is known to split Arg-Gly bonds in proteins,[110] however, the exact site and nature of this bond is not known. The mechanism of action of α_2-macroglobulin entraps the enzyme and it undergoes a conformational change. It is possible that "trapping" of thrombin by AT-III occurs in such a way that the substrate is no longer accessible (or only under extreme conditions) to the active center of thrombin.

Thrombin is capable of modifying AT-III proteolytically during the formation of the complex, even in the presence of heparin.[112] This modification is rather different from proteinase inhibitors observed in plants or animal tissues because modified AT-III is formed at neutral pH and at a near-equimolar amount of enzyme and inhibitor react. This modification of AT-III is of significance in the heparin-accelerated reactions discussed here.

When all the known thrombin-inhibitors are present, e.g., as it is the case in plasma, α_2-macroglobulin is responsible for approximately 20%, AT-III for 70%, α_1-proteinase inhibitor 8 to 10%, and heparin cofactor II, for one third of that of AT-III of the total enzyme inhibiting capacity of the plasma.[98,111]

B. THE INTERACTION OF F-Xa WITH AT-III

Seegers and Marciniak were the first, in 1962, to find that AT-III inhibits F-Xa.[118] Yin et al.[119-121] have proved that the inhibitor of F-Xa is identical with AT-III. By calculations on weight basis, they suggested that purified rabbit AT-III should neutralize much more Factor Xa than thrombin, however, Biggs et al.[122] demonstrated that human F-Xa is neutralized much more slowly than the bovine one. The divergence of opinions resulted in the creation of a debate in literature. It has been shown that if F-Xa was associated with phospholipids, platelets, or complexes with other factors, it became protected against inactivation by AT-III.[123,124,132] Furthermore, after the release of thrombin from the prothrombin activation complex, F-Xa remains attached to the phospholipid surface, being capable of converting more prothrombin to thrombin.[131] On the other hand, Ødegard and Lie, and Yin and Wessler pointed out that an iv injection of 5 units of F-Xa was more explosive in generating endogenous thrombin *in vivo* than giving 100 units of purified thrombin, i.e., they suggested very early that the inhibitory system may be primed by early events in the coagulation cascade.[125,126] These suggestions will be considered in detail when the heparin-accelerated inactivation of coagulation enzymes will be discussed in this chapter.

1. The Kinetics of Inhibition of Factor Xa by AT-III

The inhibition of human F-Xa by AT-III follows second-order kinetics. In the case of plasma, this translates to the pseudo first-order decay of enzyme activity at any given level of AT-III because the inhibitor is present in large excess: the apparent first-order rate constant is proportional to the concentration of AT-III. Jesty found it to be 3.9 x 10^{-3} *M*/s at 37°C.[127] However, the first-order plots of log F-Xa concentration against time do not remain linear, but become concave, indicating the presence of free F-Xa (similar to that of thrombin). Early suggestions were made and proved later that F-Xa is capable of splitting AT-III during the complex formation; however, the complex is quite stable. The apparent association constant of F-Xa to AT-III is 2 x 10^{-9} *M*. Under physiological circumstances and in the absence of heparin, the relative roles of other plasma proteinase inhibitors become conspicuous, i.e., a partition of F-Xa between AT-III and the α_1-proteinase inhibitor occurs. Jesty and his co-workers studied the kinetics of the inhibition of F-Xa in the presence of all the inhibitors present in plasma as well as the F-Xa-AT-III complex.[128,129] As far as the physiological significance is concerned, oestrogen-treated rabbits have a reduced Xa inhibitory activity, accompanied by an increased thrombogenicity and hypercoagulability.[130]

Summarizing the mechanism of the complex formation of the two coagulation enzymes most intensively investigated, i.e., F-Xa and thrombin, the most comprehensive scheme can be proposed based on the data of Wong et al.,[133] Jesty,[107] and Griffith and Lundblad:[108]

$$E + AT\text{-}III \rightleftharpoons E \cdot AT\text{-}III_1 \rightleftharpoons E \cdot AT\text{-}III_c \rightarrow E + AT\text{-}III_m$$

where E stands for Factor Xa or thrombin, AT-III for antithrombin-III, E· $AT\text{-}III_1$ for a labile enzyme-inhibitor complex, E· $AT\text{-}III_c$ for a covalent enzyme-inhibitor complex, and $AT\text{-}III_m$ for proteolytically modified antithrombin-III.[134] The kinetics of the inactivation of other enzymes participating in the action of AT-III, as discussed here have not been clarified so exhaustively.

C. AT-III AND OTHER ENZYMES

Damus et al.[135] showed that AT-III (human) was inhibited not only by thrombin and F-Xa, but it was able to neutralize Factors XIIa, XIa, and IXa.

AT-III forms inactive complexes with the following enzymes:

trypsin[136,137,133]
chymotrypsin[138]
thrombin[13]
Factor IXa[139] (F-IXa)
Factor Xa (see Section VI.B.1) (F-Xa)
Factor XIa[135] (F-XIa)
Factor Va[140] (F-Va)
Factor XIIa[135,146] (F-XIIa)
Factor VIIa[127] (F-VIIa)
Kallikrein[140]
Complement C_1[140]
Plasmin[141-144]
Granulocyte elastase[145]

The mechanism of the complex formation of AT-III with trypsin is very similar, if not identical, with thrombin and F-Xa. They form an equimolar complex which is inactive, and the noncomplexed compartment of AT-III becomes proteolytically modified. The reaction of the complex formation is 20 times faster than the inactivation of thrombin:[137] the second-order rate constant is 1.5 x 10^5 *M*/s at 25°C. Dissociation of the complex followed first-order kinetics with a $T^{1/2}$ of 80 h. Interestingly, the dissociation of the complex resulted in the formation of a two-chain modified inhibitor, cleaved at the same Arg-Ser bond as in modified AT-III released from complexes with thrombin, F-Xa, and F-IX.[36,139] The role of AT-III in the inactivation of chymotrypsin is not important *in vivo* since this inhibitor is very weak for this enzyme; nevertheless, heparin doubles the rate of its inactivation.[138] The activators of plasminogen are not influenced by AT-III, but plasmin is progressively inhibited by AT-III, whereas heparin increases the rate of inactivation.[134,144] AT-III does not inhibit the activation of glu-plasminogen to glu-plasmin or the conversion of glu-plasmin to lys-plasmin.[144] Collen et al.[142] and Semeraro et al.[141] demonstrated that the AT-III-heparin complex seems to play a very limited role in the inactivation of plasmin under physiological conditions and at therapeutic levels of heparin. Recently, it has also been demonstrated that contrary to previous suggestions, AT-III contributes only by 2 to 3% to the inhibition of F-XII, hence, the major inhibitor of this coagulation enzyme is the CI inhibitor, even in the presence of heparin.[135,146,171]

Granulocyte elastase is not inhibited by AT-III, but depending on the concentration of the enzyme, it destroys the thrombin-inhibiting activity of AT-III.[145] Granulocytic proteinase inhibitors (eglin, Bowman-Birk inhibitor) were effective in preventing the AT-III inactivation due to elastase. Maybe the thrombin-directed reactive site could be cleaved by this enzyme.

S-protein, the inhibitor of the membrane attack complex of complement, forms a trimolecular complex with thrombin and AT-III, and at a low concentration of heparin, it protects thrombin against inactivation.[171] Furthermore, in addition to its role as a heparin-neutralizing factor, it can incorporate into the nascent thrombin-antithrombin complex or can bind to the preformed thrombin-antithrombin complex during the inactivation reaction.[222]

D. THE INTERACTION OF HEPARIN WITH AT-III

Heparin was discovered and isolated from liver 70 years ago.[150,151] However, its exact chemical structure and all the structure-activity relationships have not yet been elucidated despite the huge amount of data collected.

Heparins are a family of linear anionic polysaccharides, specifically glycosaminoglucuronan sulphate esters, having highly variable chain-lengths and molecular weights. The major constituent of heparin is 2,6-disulfoglycosamine, which alternates with uronic acid residues having a larger amount of sulfated iduronate and a lesser part unsulfated glucuronate. The residues are joined by 1-4 glycosidic bonds. The distribution of acid groups and sulfate groups is highly variable on the carbohydrate skeleton; furthermore, additional sugar residues, e.g., acetylglucosamine, 2,3-disulfoglucosamine, and some amino acids, are covalently incorporated in the heparin coil, resulting in a wide variability of binding, size, charge, and biological functions.[152] Jaques demonstrated from the data in literature that heparinoids affect or modify the functions of more than 50 enzymes; they bind to various types of cells, proteins, etc.[152]

1. The AT-III Binding Sequence of Heparin

Lindahl et al.[153] demonstrated that an octasacharide small fragment is responsible for the AT-III binding: it has the highest affinity for AT-III. This unit contains two N-sulfate groups and both are necessary for AT-III binding. The loss of either one (with or without subsequent N-acetylation) results in a distinct and appreciable decrease of AT-III binding affinity. The free carboxyl groups in uronic acid residues are also essential.[155] Recently, a pentasaccharide unit has been chemically synthesized which corresponds to the antithrombin-III binding fragment of heparin.[156] The application of this AT-III binding fragment in affinity isolation of the inhibitor is very suitable for large-scale production of AT-III.[157] Danielsson and Björk investigated the binding of heparin fractions to AT-III and demonstrated a low- and a high-affinity fraction of heparins to AT-III.[158] Fluorescence titration showed that each binding site of heparin showed a stoichiometry 1:1 and there were no big differences in binding constants. They varied between 6 and 26 x 10^{-6} *M*. The variations in binding changed with molecular weight, whereas the differences in the number of heparin molecules bound to AT-III and in the affinity of binding could not be the main reason for molecular weight dependence of the anticoagulant actions of high-affinity heparins since the high-affinity molecules with essentially identical binding properties to AT-III have also changed in their activity depending upon molecular weight. The authors suggested that maybe at least one high-affinity heparin molecule should bind to the outer site of the inhibitor, either ready for binding thrombin or forming an additional binding site for AT-III. Piepkorn et al.[159] also found that a single molecule of high-molecular weight, high-affinity heparin attaches to two sites when it binds to AT-III, whereas low-molecular weight, low-affinity heparin binds to the two sites separately. Since the AT-III molecule by low-angle X-ray diffraction studies is less than 6 nm in maximal diameter, the two separate heparins should or may exhibit an energy transfer.

Hoylaerts et al.[175] coupled covalently two high-affinity heparin fragments to AT-III with an apparent 1:1 stoichiometry and found that they inhibited F-Xa with second-order rate kinetics, very similar to the one obtained by covalent complexes with native heparin. The covalent coupling of heparin resulted in the stabilization of heparin in circulation since the approximately 2.4 h of native half-life time increased 3.5-fold, approaching that of free AT-III and resulting in a 30 fold longer life time of F-Xa inhibitory activity in plasma, as compared to that of free intact heparin.

The binding of high-affinity heparin to AT-III has been studied by several spectroscopic techniques. Heparin binding results in a 40% increase of the protein fluorescence.[160] However, the question, whether the binding does cause a conformational change in AT-III or not, has been solved by Olson et al.,[43,44] who demonstrated that the positions of the buried tryptophan residues change during the heparin-AT-III interaction. The fluorescence of exposed tryptophans is unaffected by heparin binding; the shifting of their emission spectra to blue indicates that heparin does perturb their environment. Their stopped-flow kinetic studies demonstrated that heparin binding is a two-step procedure where the initial binding step results in a rapid equilibrium with a K_D of 4.3 x 10^{-5} M and it causes a conformational change in the AT-III molecule. This conformational change is accompanied (it is its function) by a significant — greater than 300 fold — increase in the affinity of heparin to AT-III, a K_D of 7.2 x 10^{-8} M. The equilibrium constants are very sensitive to ionic strength. The importance of charge interactions between the highly negative heparin and a presumed lysine-rich binding site on AT-III has also been demonstrated.[44,154] The authors emphasize that the formation of the second, tight binding of heparin to AT-III occurs only at the interaction of heparin with the inhibitor alone, hence the first, relatively weak complex, which subsequently undergoes a highly favorable conformational change, is essential for the anticoagulant action of heparin. Probably, it favors the approximation of AT-III and a coagulation enzyme on the surface of heparin. After the involvement of the clotting factor in the formation of a ternary complex, the binding interaction becomes weaker after the protease-AT-III complex is formed, resulting in the possibility of the release of heparin from the complex. Therefore, the conformational change of AT-III plays an important role in modulating heparin-binding affinity during the catalytic cycle of heparin (as it will be discussed later in this chapter).

Heparin preparates from different animal sources, i.e., hog intestinal, bovine lung, pig intestinal mucosa, or whale-intestinal heparins show only minor differences in AT-III binding sites; however, whale-heparin differs in this respect from the others. Presumably, it contains a hitherto underscribed saccharide sequence at the site other than the well-characterized AT-III-binding site.[161]

2. Enzyme-Binding Sequence of Heparin

As the detailed description of all the molecular interactions of heparin are beside the mark owing to its central role in regulating coagulation, we should like to touch upon its binding to enzymes having a key role in the coagulation cascade. It was a very early observation that heparin binds to thrombin as well as to F-Xa.[162,164] Later, the binding constants were found also be very tight: 1.5 $\times$ 10^{-9} M for thrombin. Heparin also forms complexes with trypsin, plasmin, F-XIIa, and F-XIa.[165] The exact region of the polysaccharide, at which it binds to these enzymes, is not known; but, recently Casu et al.[166] described an oligosaccharide fragment of heparin with a high anti-Xa activity containing the minimal AT-III-binding sequence. The ^{13}C-NMR data suggested the presence of an unusual 2-deoxy-2sulfamino-α-D-glucopyranoside-6-0-sulphate and other acetamido-sugars which are present at those sequences of the heparin coil where AT-III does not bind. Being sulfated, these regions are able to bind enzymes. These enzyme-binding sites of heparin are nonspecific[134] and may result in a conformational change in the enzymes as well as in heparin (it was the so-called "enzyme fitting" hypothesis for the mechanism of the action of heparin, proposed first in 1975).[162]

3. Heparin and Enzyme-Binding Sites of AT-III

Theoretical predictions of the secondary structure of AT-III suggest that Lys-290, Lys-294, and Lys-297, located in a helical region of the inhibitor, may bind to the active saccharide sequence of heparin.[167] Tryptophan residues were also found to be involved in the AT-III-heparin interaction.[168] Furthermore, the modification of Try-49 in AT-III resulted in the loss of heparin binding.[169] The naturally occuring molecular disorder of AT-III, i.e., the substitution of Arg-47 by cysteine, also resulted in an inability of heparin binding.[42] With respect to the reaction of AT-III and thrombin, the enzyme cleaves the inhibitor between Arg-393 and Ser-394.

After a CNBr-degradation, Rosenfeld and Danishefsky isolated a fragment of AT-III, characterized as a disulphide-bridged, three-chain structure.[170] This fragment showed a competition with heparin as well as with thrombin: the part with residues 104 to 251 of this fragment was responsible for the competition.

AT-III forms a complex with S-protein (an inhibitor of the complement system), but the site of binding is not known.[171] Interestingly, in this case, thrombin remains to be protected against inactivation in this ternary complex, even in the presence of heparin. S-protein, scavenging heparin, may play a regulatory role in thrombin inactivation. It is accepted that very low concentrations of thrombin in circulation have an anticoagulant action due to the thrombin binding to the endothelial cell surface receptor thrombomodulin and Protein C, thus S-protein advances to reach thrombin, being protected against AT-III to the endothelial cell surface.

VII. AT-III AND PLATELETS

Kim at al.[173] found that the neutralization of thrombin by AT-III is highly accelerated in the presence of platelets. They demonstrated that platelets are able to bind AT-III at specific binding sites with a rapid equilibrium. The K_D for binding was estimated to be 3.2 $\times$ $10^{-7}M$, and the binding capacity was 3800 AT-III molecules per platelet. Previously in this chapter, we mentioned that the main place for biosynthesis of AT-III is the hepatocytes, much less than endothelial cells. Recently, it was shown that platelets are able to synthesize AT-III and they contain about 70 ng per 10^9 cells. After stimulation with arachidonic acid, AT-III antigen is released from platelets accompanied by immunoreactive fibrinogen.[174] It is contained in the storage granules of platelets. The physiological significance of platelet-derived AT-III is not yet clarified, since the AT-III present in platelet corresponds to aproximately 0.01% of the total AT-III in normal blood. It may, however, not be excluded that since platelets are concentrated in fibrin clots, the release of AT-III from the platelets can contribute to the action of AT-III.

VIII. INACTIVATION OF COAGULATION FACTORS BY AT-III IN THE PRESENCE OF HEPARIN—THE PHYSIOLOGICAL SIGNIFICANCE OF AT-III

A. THROMBIN

It was a very old observation that if trace amounts of heparin were present in the mixture of thrombin and AT-III, the rate of the inactivation reaction significantly increased. Exact measurements have proved that this rate enhancement was about 50,000 fold.[176] The sequence of component interaction was an unresolved question for many years. In this three-component system, there are three possible binding sequences:

1. heparin + AT-III [H·AT]* + thrombin → [heparin-AT-III-thrombin]
2. heparin + thrombin [H·T]** + AT-III → [heparin-AT-III-thrombin]
3. AT-III + thrombin → [T − AT-III] + heparin → [heparin-AT-III-thrombin]

The first two possibilities have been confronted in literature since 1975, i.e., the "inhibitor fitting" hypothesis, assuming that heparin primarily binds to AT-III and activates it.[177] The "enzyme fitting" theory suggested a primary role of the enzyme-heparin interaction leading to a subsequent conformational change in the enzyme, rendering it more susceptible for the inhibitor.[164] Another complication was an apparent variation of the inactivation rate constants, depending on the concentration of the constituents.

Summarizing all available data regarding the accelerating effect of heparin in the inhibition of the coagulation enzymes by AT-III, the "inhibitor fitting" theory is one that has been accepted worldwide. However, recent publications tried to emphasize the equal importance of the enzyme as well as the inhibitor in this reaction. The "inhibitor fitting" theory gives primary importance to the interaction of heparin with AT-III (see binding sequence 1). This tight interaction results in a conformational change in the inhibitor. This possibility has been suggested and investigated by many authors.[13,44,92,186-188]This interaction appears to be sufficient for accelerating the rate of inactivation of other coagulation enzymes such as F-Xa. The exact description of the kinetics of inactivation has also been reported. Pletcher and Nelsestuen have reported a transition from first- to zero-order kinetics (overall) with increasing protein to heparin concentration ratios and they published zero-order kinetics with respect to thrombin at all thrombin-to-heparin ratios studied.[178] According to this, the rate-limiting step for the heparin-catalyzed AT-III-thrombin reaction is independent of thrombin. K_m was 10×10^{-8} M for the formation of kinetically active heparin-AT-III complex in a saturation kinetics model and an overall rate constant of 13.3×10^{7} M^{-1} s^{-1} for the heparin-AT-III interaction.[178] However, Nesheim emphasized that in both models of heparin action, secondary nonproductive interactions of thrombin with heparin were invoked to account for decreased reaction rates at high concentrations of heparin, i.e., the decrease of the biphasic reaction rate curve in the function of heparin concentrations did not follow the pseudo first-order kinetics, described earlier.[179] Using fluorescence and dansylarginine-N-(3ethyl-1,5 pentanediyl) amid displacement (a specific, active-site-directed thrombin inhibitor) experiments, he described that if concentrations of thrombin and the inhibitor were fixed as a function of increasing heparin concentration, the initial rates of reaction increased up to a maximum and then decreased. Both the maximum rate and the concentration of heparin had to obtain a maximum increase with increasing concentration of the proteins. The reaction appeared second order overall, first order with respect to each protein when heparin was in excess, and zero order overall when the proteins were in excess. This indicated that the proteins may have been saturated. The rate equation suggested that interactions of both proteins with heparin were involved in the expression of catalytic activity through a template mechanism. The template mechanism was first proposed by Pomerantz and Owen and Griffith.[183-185] Earlier, Olsen and Shore presented evidence for a two-step mechanism involving the initial formation of a Michaelis complex, followed by covalent bond formation between the two proteins.[180] Heparin has little effect (according to them) in the rate constant of the reaction, however, the apparent dissociation constant for the complex formation is markedly decreased from 500 μM in the absence of heparin to 4 μM in its presence. This apparent increase in affinity may be the result of the coconcentration of reactants by virtue of their mutual interaction with heparin.[180]

The template model considers heparin more as an enzyme in a bireactant system.[182] In this model, thrombin and AT-III are substrates which react more rapidly bound simultaneouly

* H·AT: Heparin-antithrombin complex.

** H·T: Thrombin-heparin complex (or serine protease-heparin complex).

to the same heparin molecule. More recently, Danielsson et al.[181] proved that the formation of ternary complexes between thrombin and AT-III, as well as F-Xa and AT-III and heparin, have a primary role in enzyme inactivation, but the length of the heparin chain is of importance, too. The minimum heparin sequence capable of binding both thrombin and F-Xa comprises of at least 18 saccharide units. Interestingly, the F-Xa-AT-III interaction does not require long heparin chains for acceleration of the reaction. The ability of heparins of increasing size to form a ternary complex with AT-III and thrombin goes strictly parallel to the ability of the fractions to accelerate the inactivation reaction.[181] In a pure system, the size dependence of the accelerating ability is similar to that of anticoagulant activity. All oligosaccharides tested, from dodecasaccharide upward, showed an appreciable ability to accelerate the inactivation of the enzymes by AT-III. In the case of F-Xa, as it has previously been mentioned, there is no contradiction to this theory, since the increase may partly reflect the increasing occurence of two AT-III-binding sites in heparin chains, longer than 30 monosaccharide units. The bindings constants for the interaction between AT-III and high-affinity heparins were found to be largely independent of the size of the heparin. It has also been shown that the AT-III-heparin interacti on is restricted to a specific pentasaccharide-binding region.[166] It appears likely that about 12 additional monosaccharide units are required to participate in the acceleration reaction, due to the binding of the thrombin to heparin by less specific interactions. However, the modification of the basic amino acid residues in thrombin has demonstrated the importance of these amino acids in the heparin-thrombin interaction, too.[189] In the thrombin-AT-III reaction, a heparin chain, sufficiently long to bind both the inhibitor and the enzyme, may remain bound in the ternary complex, past the intermedier stage of the reaction, at which two possibilities may occur: a stable complex is formed between the two proteins or AT-III may serve as a substrate for thrombin proteolysis, resulting in the formation of cleaved AT-III. Heparin may accelerate both possibilities. The regulation of these two pathways may be due to the conformal change induced in AT-III. In the F-Xa reaction, presumably neither the inhibitor-enzyme complex formation nor the increase in the production of cleaved AT-III play important roles. Both effects can be ascribed only to the conformational change in AT-III induced by the bound heparin.[181] Analysis of the molecular weights of the complexes mentioned earlier as a function of time has shown that at the initial phase of the reactions there is an opportunity for the formation of a 2:1 complex between AT-III and heparin, but only one molecule in this complex undergoes a conformational change. The complex formation shows species differences, too: bovine AT-III and thrombin form a 1:1 complex, but in the presence of stoichiometric amounts of heparin, high molecular-weight aggregates (molecular weight of 230,000, i.e., a dimer, heparin-thrombin-AT-III complex) are formed. Similar observations were made with human proteins.[182] The length of the heparin chains are also very important in heparin-catalyzed reactions. Using 12 and 16 monosaccharide units (M_r: 3200 and 4300) and high-affinity heparin (M: 15,000), Hoylaerts et. al.[176] found that the AT-III-heparin complexes inhibited thrombin in the manner of the active-site-directed, irreversible inhibitors, and the values determined for K_i were molecular-weight dependent. They concluded that all the activity of high-affinity, high-molecular weight heparin depends upon binding both thrombin and AT-III to heparin, and the exceptionally high activity of heparin results partly from the capacity of thrombin, bound nonspecifically to heparin, to diffuse in the dimension of the heparin chain towards the bound AT-III. They determined all the kinetic constants for the heparin-catalyzed inhibition of thrombin by AT-III and stated that the association of the enzyme and inhibitor on the heparin chain was strongly dependent upon the full chain length, whereas the dissociation rate constant of thrombin form the AT-III binding site on heparin was independent of the heparin's chain length.[176] Since the molecular weight of heparin varied form 10,000 to 30,000, the average number of AT-III binding sites per heparin molecule varied from 1.0 to 2.1 and 2.4 to 6.8, furthermore, the molar-specific activity increased

5.7 -fold. The rate of the reaction was proportional to the number of AT-III molecules bound to heparin. All bound thrombin and AT-III molecules were accessible to each other.[190] Nesheim et al.[190] raised an issue that there was a formal similarity between heparin as a template for the interaction of AT-III and thrombin, and negatively charged phospholipids (or cellular surface) in the prothrombinase-catalyzed activation of prothrombin. In both reactions, the concentration of the template(s) had an optimum, above which the rate of reaction decreased.

''Template model'' is an excellent, well-proved compromise between the ''inhibitor-, and enzyme-fitting'' theories, with the latter also gaining some experimental support:

1. The binding of thrombin to heparin is extremely tight (K_d for thrombin is 1.5×10^{-9} *M*.
2. Employing kinetic analysis, Griffith demonstrated that by using fixed amounts of thrombin and heparin, the increase in AT-III concentration results in a displacement of heparin from thrombin, accompanied by a decrease in the inhibition rate.[191] Similar suggestions were made by others.[192-194]
3. The results of amino acid modification experiments: a random modification of 4 to 6 arginine residues of thrombin with 1,2-cyclohexanedione resulted in a selective loss of the rate enhancement effect of heparin, but did not alter the rate of inactivation in the presence of AT-III alone.[189]

Similar phenomenon was demonstrated in the case of F-Xa; however, 12 arginines had to be modified.[195] As it was expected, modification of other basic amino acids, i.e., lysines in thrombin with trinitrobenzenesulphonic acid caused a loss of 40% in the specific activity, but the ability of AT-III to inactivate it remained unchanged. The catalytic activity of heparin was grossly reduced, suggesting the importance of intact lysines in the thrombin-heparin interaction.[196] The modification of basic amino acids in proteins may be accompanied by a decreased thermal stability.[197] However, the binding of heparin to α-thrombin via the arginyl and lysyl residues resulted in a protection against thermal denaturation.[52] On contrary to these, prominent authors demonstrated similar effects in the case of the modification of basic amino acids in AT-III, serving as good arguments for the inhibitor-fitting theory.[198-201] The trinitrophenylation of lysines in AT-III and the modification of arginines with phenylglyoxal (7 Arg per AT-III) resulted in the predominant loss of the heparin cofactor activity.[201] The modification of tryptophans with N-bromosuccimide or dimethyl (2-hydroxy-5-nitrobenzyl) sulfonium bromide in AT-III markedly decreased the binding and interaction between high-affinity heparin to AT-III as it was shown by spectroscopic studies.[190,198,200,201] The S-carbamidomethylation of disulphide bridges in AT-III altered the tertiary structure of the molecule, effectively modifying the inhibitory activity, heparin binding, etc.[199] Danishefsky et al.[202] modified heparin chemically, producing various derivatives and they have found that all types of modification decreased (i.e., carboxymodification) or resulted in a loss of catalytic activity (N-desulfatation). N-sulfates are critical in the interaction of heparin with AT-III.

Based on various considerations, the enzyme-fitting theory was supported by several teams and created a fruitful debate in literature in the 1970s.[203-206] The modifying effects of various ions (K^+, Na^+, Ca^{++}) and ionic strength on the heparin effect has been widely studied, and publications aided both theories.[100,104,205,206,218-220] Here is the opportunity to mention that calcium ions decrease the binding of heparin to both the proteins, and in contrast to this, the physiological concentrations of K and Na are optimal for heparin action. When the ionic strength is low, the usual 1:1 molar ratio of thrombin to AT-III may be altered 9.8:1,[206] and under these circumstances, AT-III becomes a suitable substrate for thrombin-proteolysis.

B. OTHER COAGULATION FACTORS

Heparin has a rate-enhancing effect on those inactivation reactions where AT-III is involved. It was a very early finding that the inactivation of factors Xa and XIa is accelerated by heparin.[135] However, Scott et al.[211] demonstrated that in the case of F-XIa, it is probably not true vs. under physiological and clinically used heparin concentrations. Holmer et al.[208] found a molecular weight dependence in heparin regarding this aspect. Low molecular-weight heparins were found to potentiate the inactivation of F-Xa and F-XIIa only; at the same time, they did not exert any effect on the inactivation of Factors IXa and XIa. Pixley et al.[146] showed that therapeutically used, an approximate 0.7 U/ml concentration of plasma heparin, the accelerating effect of heparin on the inactivation of Hageman factor, was only fourfold: this implies only a 6% contribution to the inhibitory effect of plasma. At extremely high heparin concentrations, the rate of inactivation has markedly increased. The heparin-F-Xa interaction was also suggested to be less important since the high anti-Xa activity of the AT-III-bound tetrasaccharide unit of heparin did not show a significant binding to thrombin.[128,129,217] Pentosan polysulphate probably acts primarily through F-Xa (early support of the template model of heparin action).[210] However, others could not differentiate between the priority of reactions by using high-affinity heparins to both thrombin and Factor Xa.

The fibrinolytic serin protease-plasmin may also interact with heparin, but the kinetic analysis of the reaction (pseudo first-order) showed that the rate-enhancement effect of heparin is about 20-fold, and heparin must bind to plasmin to accelerate the inactivation.[212]

C. HEPARIN AS A BIOCATALYST

Pomerantz and Owen were the first to suggest and express their opinion regarding the catalytic role of heparin.[184] Earlier, Owen and Kowalski and Finlay mentioned that heparin, exerting its effect in nonstoichiometric amounts, may be a catalyst.[213,216] Heparin fulfills some criteria of a catalyst: (1) in binding nature, affinity, and K_d values to proteins; (2) reaction-rate enhancement through increasing activation entropy; and (3) in specificity, Michaelis-Menten kinetics, and recyclization.[134,192,212,214,215] It is a unique representative of a nonprotein biocatalyst.

In summary, heparin forms a weak ionic complex with AT-III ($K_d = 10^{-4}$ *M*), which induces a highly favored conformational change in AT-III that enhances the binding affinity by about 300- to 400-fold.[44] A noncovalent ternary complex between [AT-III and heparin] and thrombin is then formed with an affinity that is about three orders of magnitude higher than was found in a similar complex between thrombin and AT-III in the absence of heparin.[43] The ternary complex undergoes an irreversible covalent reaction between the enzyme and the inhibitor with a rate constant of 5/sec, which triggers a loss of the heparin-induced conformational change in AT-III, either as a concerted process or else as a very rapid event. The resulting complex of thrombin and AT-III binds heparin with a weak affinity, compatible with rapid heparin dissociation.[180] Since AT-III binds heparin with a 100-fold greater affinity than the product thrombin-AT-III complex, rebinding of heparin to AT-III will initiate a new catalytic cycle. This differential binding affinity between AT-III and the thrombin-AT-III complex means that the thrombin-AT-III complex concentration must reach at least 100 times dissociation constant of the complex of heparin and conformationally change AT-III before the reaction velocity would be decreased by 50% due to the nonproductive binding of heparin to the product thrombin-AT-III complex. Thus, the catalytic efficiency of heparin is linked to changes in the heparin-binding affinity, which are mediated by conformational changes in AT-III.[180]

IX. AT-III AND HEPARIN IN THE ACTIVATION OF THE COAGULATION CASCADE

Lindhout et al.[132] determined the rate constants of the inactivation of F-Xa and thrombin by AT-III and heparin during the process of prothrombin activation. If the reaction mixture was saturated by F-Va or phospholipid, the second-order rate constant of Xa was 1.1 to 1.2 x $10^{-6}M$/min in the presence of AT-III, too. If both F-Va and phospholipid were present, the F-Xa inhibition by AT-III was reduced about ten fold. When F-Xa acts in the prothrombinase complex on prothrombin in the presence of heparin, it was shown that it is profoundly protected from inhibition by AT-III in the absence, as well as in the presence, of heparin. Surprisingly, heparin hardly enhanced the AT-III-dependent rate of the inhibition of thrombin activity formed during the initial phase of prothrombin activation. In his brilliant review, Hemker also emphasized that heparin primarily acts on the inactivation of thrombin and on free F-IXa, if it gets a change, but not on F-Xa in the prothrombinase complex, nor on F-IXa in the tenase complex.[225] As far as the order of reactions is concerned, the random ordered bireactant (template) reaction mechanism was favored by him. The synthetic pentasaccharide of Choay did not act on thrombin, but it did inhibit prothrombinase in the presence of AT-III. The potential therapeutical role of this product is very promising, but is not the topic of this paper.

Ofosu et al.[207,223] demonstrated an AT-III-independent anticoagulant effect of heparin on the activation of F-Xa and prothrombin, but these effects seemed negligible in the case of normal plasma.

Mohan Rao and Rapaport described a plasma component — not identical with AT-III — which inhibits F-VIIa-tissue factor activity and F-Xa.[224] This extrinsic pathway inhibitor may play a regulatory role in the formation of F-Xa, hence it may be able to bind to the F-VIIa-tissue-factor complex irreversibly. According to them, it may play a key role in the regulation of the extrinsic pathway of activation.

Marciniak[226,227] reported an enhancing effect of heparin on AT-III proteolysis, induced by thrombin. This phenomenon was dependent upon the molecular weight of heparin fractions and may have resulted in a decrease of the functional amount of AT-III, even due to the high-affinity heparin which was highly active in the induction of thrombin-proteolysis.

X. THE INTERACTION OF AT-III (AND HEPARIN) WITH NATURAL (ENDOTHELIUM) AND ARTIFICIAL SURFACES

A. AT-III AND ENDOTHELIUM

The nonthrombogenic property of the blood vessel lumen surface has been attributed to the pericellular localization of certain proteoglycans of the endothelial cell membrane. The endothelial cells possess proteoglycans chemically similar to that of heparin (oids) degradable by heparinase and other glycosaminoglycan-specific enzymes.[228,229] The thrombin-AT-III complexes are attracted by these materials, however, no direct binding of AT-III to the endothelium has been reported. So far only speculations suggested an interaction between them via the pericellular heparin-like proteoglycans. Hatton et al.[228,230] have studied the binding and interaction of thrombin and AT-III to different immobilized glycosaminoglycanes and showed that thrombin binds firmly to these, but AT-III binds only to heparin (oids). Interestingly, numerous studies showed that blood vessels contain dermatan sulfate and heparan sulfate, but not heparin, and cultured endothelial cells retain this property, too.

Thrombin has a great affinity to endothelial cells. This cell-bound thrombin could rapidly be inactivated by AT-III.[231] By using labeled AT-III, relatively small amounts of AT-III were found to bind to the endothelium as compared to thrombin. Desendothelialized vessels have been found to bind AT-III to a much higher extent, and this bound-AT-III could also be replaced by heparin(oids).[230] Probably, there is a difference between the large vessels and the microvasculature in this respect: (1) possibly, the endothelial cells of the microvasculature possess pericellular proteoglycans acting as binding sites for attracting AT-III and thrombin, to catalyze thrombin inactivation; (2) in contrast to this, endothelium of the aorta and large vessels attracts only thrombin through the proteoglycane-binding sites, and the inactivation of the endothelium-bound thrombin is carried out by plasma antitrombin.[230] These mechanisms may have evolved so as to reflect the various different blood flow conditions: microvasculature gives 95% of the total vascular surface, but contains only 5% of the entire blood volume, circulating very slowly (0.07 cm/sec). Arteries have a surface of less than 1% of the vascular surface area but transport about 20% of the blood volume at a speed of 40 to 50 cm/sec. A rapid rise in the circulating AT-III level after heparin administration could be explained by the suggestion that heparin displaces glycosaminoglycane-bound AT-III. The endothelial cell surface-bound thrombin has a special importance in Protein C activation; therefore, the regulatory role of AT-III in this reaction has a primary role. If AT-III is in excess in the plasma, the activation of Protein C by thrombin is not influenced because in the thrombomodulin complex, thrombin is protected against the action of AT-III and heparin. Delvos et al.[232] suggest that in microvasculature, the cleavage of Factors VIIIa and Va by activated Protein C is a more effective approach in preventing a procoagulant state when compared to the role of AT-III.

B. AT-III AND ANTICOAGULANT BIOMATERIALS

Efforts to improve the nonthrombogenecity of vascular drafts and biomaterials were made very early. Miura et. al.,[233] Goosen et. al.,[234] and Hatton et. al.[235] reported results regarding the inactivation of thrombin after the exposure of heparinized biomaterials. AT-III and heparin were coimmobilized to various polymers: Sepharose 4B, polyvinyl alcohol, polyhydroxyethyl-ethacrylate, silicone-coated nylon, etc. These coimmobilized preparations actively neutralized both F-Xa and thrombin. Hatton et. al.[235] demonstrated the formation of a complex between covalent-bound heparin, thrombin, and AT-III. Using labeled thrombin, the displacement of thrombin from the complex was measured and surprisingly, α_2-macroglobulin-thrombin complexes appeared after elution: they suggested an unknown mechanism by which thrombin got released from the complex from the heparinized surface and reacted with α_2-macroglobulin. Plasma may contain component(s) which displace the thrombin-AT-III complex from immobilized heparin.

The plasma proteins may have different binding sites to artificial surfaces, including the hydrophilic haemodialysis membrane, Cuprophane, and hydrophobic PVC tubings.[236] Crassous et. al.[237,238] prepared a polystyrene derivative with antocoagulant activity only in the presence of AT-III. The active surface was extremely large.[237] Soluble polymethacrylic acid was also found to be heparin-like.[239] Japanese authors came up with a good antithrombogenic material group—heparinized polyetherurethanes (via their quaterner ammonium groups)—by using a novel technique. It releases heparin for a very long period of time, continuously.[240] This technique seems to be very promising for producing thromboresistant materials for cardiac prostheses or total artificial hearts.

ACKNOWLEDGMENT

The author is grateful to Dr. Susanna B. Turi for her advice and helpful criticism. The excellent preparation of this manuscript by Mrs. Ibolya Turi is also thankfully appreciated.

REFERENCES

1. **Morawitz, P.,** Die Chemie der Blutgerinnung, *Ergebnis Physiol.*, 4, 307, 1905.
2. **Schmidt, A.,** Zur Blutlehre, Leipzig, F. C. W. Vogel, 1892.
3. **Weymouth, F. W.,** The relation of metathrombin to thrombin, *Am. J. Physiol.*, 32, 266, 1913.
4. **Hensen, A. and Loeliger, E. A.,** Antithrombin III. Its metabolism and its function in blood coagulation, *Thromb. Diath. Haemorrh. Suppl.*, 19, 1, 1963.
5. **Loeb, J.,** Le cofacteur plasmatique de l'heparine et ses rapports avec l'antithrombine, *Arch. Sci. Physiol.*, 10, 129, 1956.
6. **Markwardt, F. and Walsmann, P.,** Untersuchungen über den Mechanismus der Antithrombinwirkung des Heparins, *Hoppe-Seyler's Z. Physiol. Chem.*, 317, 64, 1959.
7. **Heimburger, N.,** On the proteinase inhibitors of the human plasma with special reference to antithrombin, *1st Int. Symp. on Tissue Factors in the Homeostasis of Coagulation — Fibrinolysis System,* Florence, Abstr. No. 174, Springer-Verlag, Berlin, 1967.
8. **Briginshaw, G. F. and Shanberge, J. N.,** Identification of two distinct heparin cofactors in human plasma. Seperation and partial purification, *Arch. Biochem. Biophys.* 161, 683, 1974.
9. **Machovich, R., Blaskó, Gy., Himer, A., and Szikla, K.,** Effect of sodium and potassium ions on the human antithrombin-heparin cofactor, *Thromb. Res.*, 7, 305, 1975.
10. **Abildgaard, U.,** A review of antithrombin-III, in The physiological Inhibitors of Coagulation and Fibrinolysis, Collen, D., Wiman, B., Verstraete, M., Eds., Elsevier, Amsterdam, 1979, 19.
11. **Abildgaard, U.,** Purification of two progressive antithrombins of human plasma, *Scand. J. Clin. Lab. Invest.*, 19, 190, 1967.
12. **Fagerhol, M. K. and Abildgaard, U.,** Immunological studies on human antithrombin III. Influence of age, sex and use of oral contraceptives on serum concentration, *Scand. J. Haematol.* 7, 10, 1970.
13. **Rosenberg, R. D. and Damus, P. S.,** The purification and mechanism of action of human antithrombin-heparin cofactor, *J. Biol. Chem.*, 248, 6490, 1973.
14. **Miller-Andersson, M., Borg, H., and Andersson L. O.,** Purification of antithrombin III by affinity chromatography, *Thromb. Res.*, 5, 439, 1974.
15. **Thaler, E. and Schmer, G.,** A simple two-step isolation procedure for human and bovine antithrombin II/III (heparin cofactor): a comparison of two methods, *Br. J. Haematol.*, 31, 233, 1975.
16. **Wickerhauser, M. and Williams, C.,** A single-step method for the isolation of antithrombin-III, *Vox Sang.*, 47, 397, 1984.
17. **Mitra, G., Hall, E., and Mitra, I.,** Application of immobilized heparins for isolation of human antithrombin-III, *Biotechnol. Bioeng.*, 28, 217, 1986.
18. **Trobisch, H., Wüst, Th., and Rustige, H.,** Möglichkeiten der Isolierung und Charakterisierung des menschlichen Antithrombin III, *Behring Inst. Res. Comm.*, 79, 177, 1986.
19. **Jordan, R. E.,** Antithrombin in vertebrate species: conservation of the heparin-dependent anticoagulant mechanism, *Arch. Biochem. Biochem. Biophys.*, 227, 587, 1983.
20. **Pellegrini, A., Zweifel H.-R., and von Fellenberg, R.,** Identification of the second α_2-antiprotease of equine serum as antithrombin III, *Int. J. Biochem.*, 15, 917, 1983.
21. **Carlson, T. H. and Atencio, A. C.,** Isolation and partial characterization of two distinct types of antithrombin III from rabbit, *Thromb. Res.*, 27, 23, 1982.
22. **Koide, T.** Isolation and characterization of antithrombin III from human, porcine and rabbit plasma and rat serum, *J. Biochem.*, 86, 1841, 1979.
23. **Koide, T., Ohta, Y., Odani, S., and Ono, T.,** Chicken antithrombin. Isolation, characterization and comparison with mammalian antithrombins and chicken ovalbumin, *J. Biochem.*, 91, 1223, 1982.
24. **Damus, P. S. and Wallace, G. A.,** Purification of canine antithrombin-III-heparin cofactor using affinity chromatography, *Biochem. Biophys. Res. Comm.*, 61, 1147, 1974.
25. **Andersson, L.-O.,** Pysicochemical properties of antithrombin III, in The Physiological Inhibitors of Coagulation and Fibrinolysis, Collen, D., Wiman, B., Verstraete, M., Eds., Elsevier, Amsterdam, 1979, 39.
26. **Nordenman, B., Nyström, C., and Björk, I.,** The size and shape of human and bovine antithrombin III, *Eur. J. Biochem.*, 78, 195, 1977.
27. **Furugren, B., Andersson, L. -O., and Einarsson, L.,** Small-angle X-ray scattering studies on human antithrombin III and its complex with heparin, *Arch. Biochem, Biophys.*, 178, 419, 1977.
28. **Villanueva, G. B. and Allen, N.,** Refolding properties of antithrombin III. Mechanism of binding to heparin, *J. Biol. Chem.*, 258, 14048, 1983.
29. **Petersen, T. E., Dudek-Wojciechowska, G., Sottrup-Jensen, L., and Magnusson, S.,** Primary structure of antithrombin III (heparin cofactor). Partial homology between α_1-antitrypsin and antithrombin III, in The Physiological Inhibitors of Coagulation and Fibrinolysis, Collen, D., Wiman, B., Verstraete, M., Eds., Elsevier, Amsterdam, 1979, 43.

30. **Longas, M. O., Ferguson, W. S., and Finlay, T. H.,** A disulfide bond in antithrombin is required for heparin-accelerated thrombin inactivation, *J. Biol. Chem.*, 255, 3436, 1980.
31. **Björk, I., Jackson, C. M., Jörnvall, H., Lavine, K. K., Nordling, K., and Salsgiver, W. J.,** The active site of antithrombin. Release of the same proteolytically cleaved form of the inhibitor from complexes with Factor IXa, Factor Xa and thrombin, *J. Biol. Chem.*, 257, 2406, 1982.
32. **Björk, I., Danielsson, A., Fenton, J. W., II and Jörnvall, H.,** The site in human antithrombin for functional proteolytic cleavage by thrombin, *FEBS Lett.*, 126, 257, 1981.
33. **Wallgren, P., Nordling, K., and Björk, I.,** Immunological evidence for a proteolytic cleavage at the active site of antithrombin in the mechanism of inhibition of coagulation serine proteases, *Eur. J. Biochem.*, 116, 493, 1981.
34. **Owen, W. G.,** Evidence for the formation of an ester between thrombin and heparin cofactor, *Biochim. Biophys. Acta*, 405, 380, 1975
35. **Barrowcliffe, T. W., and Thomas, D. P.,** Antithrombin III and heparin, in Haemostasis and Thrombosis, Bloom, A. L. and Thomas, D. P., Eds., Churchill Livingstone, New York, 1981, 712.
36. **Longas, M. O. and Finlay, T. H.,** The covalent nature of the human antithrombin III-thrombin bond, *Biochem. J.*, 189, 481, 1980.
37. **Carrell, R. W., Boswell, R. D., Brennan, S. O., and Owen, M. C.,** Active site of α_1-antitrypsin: homologus site in antithrombin III, *Biochem. Biophys. Res. Comm.*, 93, 399, 1980.
38. **Chandra, T., Stackhouse, R., Kidd, V. J., Robson, K. J. H., and Woo, S. K. C.,** Sequence homology between human α_1-antichymotrypsin, α_1-antitrypsin annd antithrombin III, *Biochemistry*, 22, 5055, 1983.
39. **Griffith, M. J., Noyes, C. M., and Church, F. D.,** Reactive site peptide structural similarities between heparin cofactor II and antithrombin III, *J. Biol Chem.*, 260, 2218, 1985.
40. **Einarsson, R.,** The increase in human antithrombin III tryptophan fluorescence produced by heparin, *Biochim. Biophys. Acta*, 534, 156, 1978.
41. **Blackburn, M. N. and Sibley, C. C.,** The heparin binding site of antithrombin III. Evidence for a critical tryptophan residue, *J. Biol. Chem.*, 255, 824, 1980.
42. **Koide, T., Odani, S., Takahoshi, K., Ono, T., and Sakuragawa, N.,** Antithrombin III_{Toyama}: replacement of arginine-47 by cysteine in hereditary abnormal antithrombin that lacks heparin-binding ability, *Proc. Natl. Acad. Sci. U.S.A.* 81, 289, 1984.
43. **Olson, S. T. and Shore, J. D.,** Binding of high affinity heparin to antithrombin-III. Characterization of the protein fluorescence enhancement, *J. Biol. Chem.*, 256, 11065, 1981.
44. **Olson, S. T., Srinivasan, K. R., Björk, I., and Shore, J. D.,** Binding of high affinity heparin to antithrombin III. Stopped flow kinetic studies of the binding reaction., *J. Biol. Chem.*, 256, 11073, 1981.
45. **Mizuochi, T., Fuji, J., Kurachi, K., and Kobata, A.,** Structural studies of the carbohydrate moiety of human antithrombin III, *Arch. Biochem. Biophys.*, 203, 458, 1980.
46. **Danishefsky, I., Zweben, A., and Slominay, B. L.,** Human antithrombin III. Carbohydrate components and associated glycolipid, *J. Biol. Chem.*, 253, 32, 1978.
47. **Dale, G. L. and Westwood, B.,** Antithrombin III does not have bound glucocerebroside, *Biochim. Biophys. Acta*, 669, 260, 1981.
48. **Ducrocq, R., Bachour, H., Belkhodja, R., Berriche, S., and Elion, J.,** Evidence for non-enzymatic glycation of antithrombin III in diabetic patients, *Clin. Chem.*, 31, 338, 1985.
49. **Busby, T. F. and Ingham, K. C.,** Thermal stabilization of antithrombin III by sugars and sugar derivatives and the effect of non-enzymatic glycosilation, *Biochim. Biophys. Acta*, 799, 80, 1984.
50. **Mitra, G., Schneider, P. M., and Lundblad, J. L.,** Kinetics of thermal denaturation of antithrombin III, *Biotechnol. Bioeng.*, 24, 97, 1982.
51. **Pálos, Á. L., Blaskó, G., and Machovich, R.,** Some properties of human progressive antithrombin, *Acta Physiol. Acad. Sci. Hung.*, 49, 95, 1977.
52. **Machovich, R., Blaskó, G., and Arányi, P.,** The interaction of thrombin and heparin. Heat inactivation kinetics, *Thromb. Res.*, 7, 253, 1975.
53. **Bushby, T. F., Atha, D. H., and Ingham, K. C.,** Thermal denaturation of antithrombin III. Stabilization by heparin and lyotropic anions, *J. Biol. Chem.*, 256, 12140, 1981.
54. **Borsodi, A. and Narasimhan, T. R.,** Microheterogeneity of human antithrombin III, *Br. J. Haematol.*, 39, 121, 1978.
55. **Murano, G., Miller-Andersson, M., and Williams, L.,** Heterogeneity of purified human antithrombin-III, *Thromb. Res.*, 24, 489, 1981.
56. **Milner, A. E., Burnett, D., Rutter, J., and Bradwell, A. R.,** Detection of antithrombin III microheterogeneity, *Thromb. Res.*, 37, 127, 1985.
57. **Daly, M. and Hallinan, F.,** Analysis of antithrombin III microheterogeneity by isoelectric focusing in polyacrylamide gels and immunoblotting, *Thromb. Res.*, 40, 207, 1985.
58. **Owen, M. C., Lorier, M., and Carrell, R. W.,** α_1-antitrypsin: structural relationship of the substitutions of the S and Z variants, *FEBS Lett.*, 88, 234, 1978.

59. **Hunt, L. T. and Dayhoff, M. O.,** A surprising new protein superfamily containing ovalbumin, antithrombin III and alpha-l-proteinase inhibitor, *Biochem. Biophys. Res. Comm.*, 95, 864, 1980.
60. **Losito, R., Barlow, G., and Lemieux, E.,** ^{3}H-heparin and antithrombin III in the isolated liver perfusion, *Thromb. Res.*, 10, 83, 1977.
61. **Koj, A., Regoeczi, E., Toews, C. J., Leveille, R., and Gauldie, J.,** Synthesis of antithrombin III and α_1-antitrypsin by the perfused rat liver, *Biochim. Biophys. Acta*, 539, 496, 1978.
62. **Owens, M. R. and Miller, L. L.,** Net biosynthesis of antithrombin-III by the isolated rat liver perfused for 12-24 hours compared with rat fibrinogen and α_2 (acut phase) globulin. Antithrombin III is not an acut phase protein, *Biochim. Biophys. Acta*, 627, 30, 1980.
63. **Chan, T. K. and Chan, V.,** Antithrombin III, the major modulator of intravascular coagulation is synthesized by human endothelial cells, *Thromb. Haemost.*, 46, 504, 1981.
64. **Watada, M., Nagakawa, M., Kitani, T., Okajima, Y., Maeda, Y., Urano, S., and Ijichi, H.,** Identification of the AT III synthesizing hepatocytes by immunofluorescent technique, *Thromb. Haemost.*, 46, 284, 1981.
65. **Léon, M., Aiach, M., Coezy, E., Guennec, J.-Y., and Fiessinger, J.-N.,** Antithrombin III synthesis in rat liver parenchymal cells, *Thromb. Res.*, 30, 369, 1983.
66. **Nakagawa, M., Kitani, T., Watada, M., Okuda, S., Urano, S., Okajima, Y., Rin, K., Osamura, K., Maeda, Y., and Ijichi, H.,** Biosynthesis and metabolism of rat antithrombin III, *Acta Haematol. Jpn.*, 44, 1479, 1981.
67. **Lee, A. K. Y., Chan, V., and Chan, T. K.,** The identification and localization of antithrombin III in human tissues, *Thromb. Res.*, 14, 209, 1979.
68. **Fair, D. S. and Bahnak, B. R.,** Human hepatoma cells secrete single chain Factor X, prothrombin, and antithrombin III, *Blood*, 64, 194, 1984.
69. **Róka, L. and Bleyl, H.,** Die Rolle von Antithrombin bei gestörter Haemostase, *Folia Haematol.*, 104, 707, 1977.
70. **Marciniak, E. and Gora-Maslak, G.,** High molecular weight forms of antithrombin III complexes in blood, *Thromb. Haemost.*, 49, 32, 1983.
71. **Collen, D., Schezt, J., De Cock, F., Holmer, E., and Verstraete, M.,** Metabolism of antithrombin III (heparin cofactor), in Man: Effects of Venous Thrombosis and of Heparin Administration, *Eur. J. Clin. Invest.*, 7, 27, 1977.
72. **Reeve, B. E., Leonard, B., and Carlson, T.,** Kinetic studies of antithrombin III, *Ann. N.Y. Acad. Sci.*, 370, 680, 1981.
73. **Marciniak, E. and Gockerman, J. P.,** Kinetics and elimination of antithrombin III concentrate in heparinized patients, *Br. J. Haematol.*, 48, 617, 1981.
74. **Bleyl, H.,** Radioimmunologische Antithrombin-Bestimmung im Liquor cerebrospinalis, Urin, Dialysate und Thrombocyten, in Mikrozirculation und Prostaglandinstoffwechsel, Blumel, G. and Haas, S., Eds., F. K. Schattauer Verl., New York, 1981, 433.
75. **Gursoy, A. and Ulutin, O. N.,** Platelet antithrombin III, *Ann. Univ. Sarav. Med. Suppl.*, 3, 75, 1983.
76. **Shifman, M. A. and Pizzo, S. V.,** The *in vivo* metabolism of antithrombin III and antithrombin III complexes, *J. Biol. Chem.*, 257, 3243, 1982.
77. **Lam, L. S. L., Regoeczi, E., and Hatton, M. W. C.,** *In vivo* behaviour of some antithrombin III — protease complexes, *Br. J. Exp. Pathol.*, 60, 151, 1979
78. **Abildgaard, U., Lie, M., and Ødegard, O. R.,** Antithrombin (heparin cofactor) assay with "new" chromogenic substrates (S-2238 and Chromozym TH), *Thromb. Res.*, 11, 549, 1977.
79. **Ceustermans, R., Hoylaerts, M., Del Mol, M., and Collen, D.,** Preparation, characterization and turnover properties of heparin-antithrombin III complexes stabilized by covalent bonds, *J. Biol. Chem.*, 257, 3401, 1982.
80. **Tengborn, L., Frohm, B., Nilsson, L. E., and Nilsson I. M.,** On antithrombin III concentrate: its catabolism in congenital antithrombin III deficiency and in health, *Scand. J. Clin. Lab. Invest.*, 41, 469, 1981.
81. **Knot, E. A. R., De Jong, E., ten Cate, J. W., Iburg, A. H. C., Henny, Ch., P., Bruin, T., and Stibbe, J.,** Purified radiolabelled antithrombin III metabolism in three families with hereditary AT III deficiency. Application of a three-compartment model, *Blood*, 67, 93, 1986.
82. **Amrani, D. L., Mosesson, M. W., and Koide, T.,** Evidence that chicken antithrombin III is a developmentally regulated glycoprotein synthesized by hepatocytes, *Biochim. Biophys. Acta*, 847, 324, 1985.
83. **Gross, S. J. and Stuart, M. J.,** Haemostasis in the premature infant, *Clin. Perinatol.*, 4, 259, 1977.
84. **Olden, K., Parent, J. B., and White, S. L.,** Carbohydrate moieties of glycoproteine. A re-evaluation of their function, *Biochim. Biophys. Acta*, 650, 209, 1982.
85. **Carlson, T. H.,** Clearance of thrombin *in vivo:* significance of alternative pathways, *Mol. Cell. Biochem.*, 7, 97, 1986.
86. **Marciniak, E. and Romod, E. H.,** Catabolism and distribution of functionally heterogenous human antithrombin III, *J. Lab. Clin. Med.*, 109, 89, 1987.

87. **Carlson, T. H., Atencio, A. C., and Simon, T. L.,** Comparison of the behavior *in vivo* of two forms of antithrombin III, *Biochem. J.*, 225, 557, 1985.
88. **Carlson, T. H., Simon, T. L., and Atencio, A. C.,** *In vivo* behavior of human radiolabeled antithrombin III: distribution among three physiologic pools, *Blood,* 66, 13, 1985.
89. **Rosenberg, R. D.,** Role of heparin-like molecules in thrombosis and atherosclerosis, *Fed. Proc.*, 44, 404, 1985.
90. **Sié, P., Lansen, J., Lacheretz, F., Verschuere, B., and Boneu, B.,** Comparative turn-over of heparin cofactor II and antithrombin III in baboons, *Thromb. Haemost.*, 56, 302, 1986.
91. **Abildgaard, U.,** Binding of thrombin to antithrombin III, *Scand. J. Clin. Lab. Invest.*, 24, 23, 1969.
92. **Villanueva, G. and Danishefsky, I.,** Conformational changes accompanying the binding of antithrombin III to thrombin, *Biochemistry,* 18, 810, 1979.
93. **Atha, D. H., Brew, S. A., and Ingham, K. C.,** Interaction and thermal stability of fluorescent labeled derivatives of thrombin and antithrombin III, *Biochim. Biophys. Acta,* 785, 1, 1984.
94. **Esmon, C. T.,** Factors regulating the inhibition of thrombin by antithrombin III, in The Chemistry and Biology of Thrombin, Lundblad, R. L., Fenton, J. W., and Mann, K. G., Eds., Ann Arbor Science, Ann Arbor, MI, 1977, 403.
95. **Chelladurai, M. and Ganguly, P.,** Thrombin-reactive polypeptides may regulate inhibition of thrombin by antithrombin, *Biochim. Biophys. Acta,* 870, 204, 1986.
96. **Rosenfeld, R. and Danishefsky, I.,** Effects of enzymatic deglycosylation on the biological activities of human thrombin and antithrombin, *Arch. Biochem. Biophys.*, 229, 359, 1984.
97. **Chang, T., Feinman, R. D., Landis, B. H., and Fenton, J. W., II,** Antithrombin reactions with β and γ-thrombins, *Biochemistry,* 18, 113, 1979.
98. **Machovich, R., Borsodi, A., Blaskó, G., and Orakzai, S.,** Inactivation of α- and β-thrombin by antithrombin III, α_2-macroglobulin and α_1-proteinase inhibitor, *Biochem. J.*, 167, 393, 1977.
99. **Latallo, Z. S. and Jackson, C. M.,** Reaction of thrombin with human antithrombin III. II. Dependence of rate of inhibition on molecular form and origin of thrombin, *Thromb. Res.*, 43, 523, 1986.
100. **Latallo, Z. S. and Hall, J. A.,** Reaction of thrombins with human antithrombin III. I. Enzyme activity losses unrelated to the inhibitory reaction and their prevention, *Thromb. Res.*, 43, 507, 1986.
101. **Blaskó, Gy.,** On the inactivation of Factor Xa, Symposium on Chromogenic substrates, AB Kabi, Budapest, *Lab. Diagn. Med.*, 6, 126, 1979.
102. **Gray, E. and Barrowcliffe, T. W.,** Inhibition of antithrombin III by lipid peroxides, *Thromb. Res.*, 37, 241, 1985.
103. **Jesty, J.,** The kinetics of inhibition of thrombin by antithrombin in the presence of components of the hemostatic system, *Blood,* 66, 1189, 1985.
104. **Blaskó, Gy.,** Natural antithrombotics (antithrombin-III, heparin, prostacyclin). Ph.D. thesis, Hungarian Academy of Sciences, Budapest, 1980, 50.
105. **Ill, C. R. and Ruoslahti, E.,** Association of thrombin-antithrombin III complex with vitronectin in serum, *J. Biol. Chem.*, 260, 15610, 1985.
106. **Jesty, J.,** Dissociation of complexes and their derivatives formed during inhibition of bovine thrombin and activated Factor X by antithrombin III, *J. Biol. Chem.*, 254, 1044, 1979.
107. **Jesty, J.,** The kinetics of formation and dissociation of bovine thrombin-antithrombin-III complex, *J. Biol. Chem.*, 254, 10044, 1979.
108. **Griffith, M. J. and Lundblad, R. L.,** Dissociation of antithrombin III-thrombin complex. Formation of active and inactive antithrombin-III, *Biochemistry,* 20, 105, 1981.
109. **Owen, W. G., Penick, G. D., Yoder, E., and Poole, B. L.,** Evidence for an ester bond between thrombin and heparin cofactor, *Thromb. Haemost.*, 35, 87, 1976.
110. **Bornstein, P. and Balian, G.,** Cleavage at Asn-Gly bonds with hydroxylamine, *Methods Enzymol.*, 47, 132, 1977.
111. **Jesty, J.,** The kinetics of inhibition of α-thrombin in human plasma, *J. Biol. Chem.*, 261, 10313, 1986.
112. **Björk, I. and Fish, W. W.,** Production *in vitro* and properties of a modified form of bovine antithrombin, cleaved at the active site by thrombin, *J. Biol. Chem.*, 257, 9487, 1982.
113. **Villanueva, G. B. and Allen, N.,** Acetylation of antithrombin III by aspirin, *Semin. Thromb. Haemost.*, 12, 213, 1986.
114. **Machovich, R.,** Effect of calcium phosphate on thrombin and on its sensitivity to heparin and antithrombin-III, *Thromb. Res.*, 9, 123, 1976.
115. **Lundblad, R. L., Roberts, J. C., Johnston, K. D., Featherstone, G. F., and Griffith, M. J.,** Acceleration by calcium of the inactivation of thrombin by plasma proteinase inhibitors, *Thromb. Res.*, 22, 135, 1981.
116. **Oshima, G. and Nagasawa, K.,** Effects of different ions on the interactions of heparin with bovine antithrombin III and thrombin, *Thromb. Res.*, 42, 375, 1986.
117. **Marciniak, E. and Gora-Masiak, G.,** The interaction of immobilized thrombin with human antithrombin III, *Thromb. Haemost.*, 51, 27, 1984.

118. **Seegers, W. H. and Marciniak, E.,** Inhibition of autoprothrombin C activity with plasma, *Nature,* 193, 1188, 1962.
119. **Yin, E. T., Wessler, S., and Stoll, P. J.,** Identity of plasma activated Factor X inhibitor with antithrombin III and heparin cofactor, *J. Biol. Chem.,* 246, 3712, 1971.
120. **Yin, E. T., Wessler, S., and Stoll, P. J.,** Biological properties of the naturally occuring plasma inhibitor to activated Factor X, *J. Biol. Chem.,* 246, 3703, 1971
121. **Yin, E. T., Wessler, S., and Stoll, P. J.,** Rabbit plasma inhibitor of the activated species of blood coagulation Factor X, *J. Biol. Chem.,* 246, 3694, 1971.
122. **Biggs, R., Denson, K. W. E., Akman, N., Barrett, R., and Hadden, M.,** Antithrombin III, antifactor Xa and heparin, *Br. J. Haematol.,* 19, 283, 1970.
123. **Yin, E. T.,** Effect of heparin on the neutralization of Factor Xa and thrombin by plasma alpha-2globulin inhibitor, *Thromb. Diath. Haemorrh.,* 33, 43, 1974.
124. **Jackson, C. M.,** The biochemistry of prothrombin activation, in Heparin: Chemistry and Clinical Usage, Kakkar, V. V. and Thomas, D. P., Eds., Academic Press, London, 1976, 61.
125. **Ødegard, O. R. and Lie, M.,** Simultaneous inactivation of thrombin and Factor Xa by AT-III: influence of heparin, *Thromb. Res.,* 12, 697, 1978.
126. **Yin, E. T. and Wessler, S.,** Heparin accelerated inhibition of activated Factor X by its natural plasma inhibitor, *Biochim. Biophys. Acta,* 201, 387, 1970.
127. **Jesty, J.,** The inhibition of bovine coagulation factors X and VII by antithrombin III, *Arch. Biochem. Biophys.,* 185, 165, 1978.
128. **Jesty, J., Morrison, S. A., and Harpel, P. C.,** Measurement of human activated Factor X-antithrombin complex by enzyme-linked differential-antibody immunosorbent assay, *Anal. Biochem.,* 139, 158, 1984.
129. **Jesty, J.,** Measurement of the kinetics of inhibition of activated coagulation Factor X in human plasma: the effect of plasma and inhibitor concentration, *Anal. Biochem.,* 152, 402, 1986.
130. **Gitel, S. N., Stephenson, R. C., and Wessler, S.,** The activated Factor X — antithrombin III reaction rate: a measure of the increased thrombotic tendency induced by estrogen-containing oral contraceptives in rabbits, *Haemostasis,* 7, 10, 1978.
131. **Bajwa, S. S.,** Mechanism of action of an antithrombotic agent antithrombin III-Factor Xa complex, *Proc. West. Pharmacol. Soc.,* 25, 1, 1982.
132. **Lindhout, T., Baruch, D., Schoen, P., Franssen, J., and Hemker, H. C.,** Thrombin generation and inactivation in the presence of antithrombin III and heparin, *Biochemistry,* 25, 5962, 1986.
133. **Wong, R. F., Chang, T., and Feinman, R. D.,** Reaction of antithrombin with proteases: nature of the reaction with trypsin, *Biochemistry,* 21, 6, 1982.
134. **Machovich, R.,** Inactivation of thrombin by plasma proteinase inhibitors, in The Thrombin, Vol. 2, Machovich, R., Ed., CRC Press, Boca Raton, FL, 1984, 1.
135. **Damus, P. S., Hicks, M., and Rosenbert, R. D.,** Anticoagulant action of heparin, *Nature,* 246, 355, 1973.
136. **Jacobsson and Lindahl, U.,** Biosynthesis of heparin. Concerted action of late polymer-modification reactions, *J. Biol. Chem.,* 255, 5094, 1980.
137. **Danielsson, A. and Björk, I.,** Mechanism of inactivation of trypsin by antithrombin, *Biochem. J.,* 207, 21, 1982.
138. **Oshima, G.,** Inactivation of bovine chymotrypsin by bovine antithrombin III, *Thromb. Res.,* 44, 315, 1986.
139. **Rosenberg, J. S., McKenna, P. W., and Rosenberg, R. D.,** Inhibition of human Factor IXa by human antithrombin, *J. Biol. Chem.,* 250, 8883, 1975.
140. **Fareed, J.,** New methods in coagulation testing, in Perspectives in Haemostasis, Fareed, J., Messmore, H. L., Fenton, J. W., II, and Brinkhous, K. M., Eds., Pergamon Press, New York, 1981, 310.
141. **Semeraro, N., Colucci, M., Telesforo, P., and Collen, D.,** The inhibition of plasmin by antithrombin-heparin complex I. In human plasma *in vitro, Br. J. Haematol.,* 39, 91, 1978.
142. **Collen, D., Semeraro, N., Telesforo, P., and Verstraete, M.,** Inhibition of plasmin by antithrombin-heparin complex III. During thrombolytic therapy in man, *Br. J. Haematol., 39,* 101, 1978.
143. **Crawford, G. P. M. and Ogston, D.,** The action of antithrombin III on plasmin and activators of plasminogen, *Biochim. Biophys. Acta,* 391, 189, 1975.
144. **Summaria, L., Boreisha, I. G., Arzadon, L., and Robbins, K. C.,** Activation of human Glu-plasminogen to Glu-plasmin by urokinase in presence of plasmin inhibitors, *J. Biol. Chem.,* 252, 3945, 1977.
145. **Jochum, M., Lander, S., Heimburger, N., and Fritz, H.,** Effect of human granulocytic elastase on isolated human antithrombin III, *Hoppe-Seyler's Z. Physiol. Chem.,* 362, 103, 1981.
146. **Pixley, R. A., Schapira, M., and Colman, R. W.,** Effect of heparin on the inactivation rate of human activated Factor XII by antithrombin III, *Blood,* 66, 198, 1985.
147. **Savion, N. and Farzame, N.,** Comparative study of antithrombin III protease complex metabolism by fibroblasts and vascular endothelial cells, *Thromb. Res.,* 41, 459, 1986.
148. **Bauer, P. I., Mandl, J., Machovich, R., Antoni, F., Garzó, T., and Horváth, I.,** Specific binding of thrombin-antithrombin III complex to hepatocytes, *Thromb. Res.,* 28, 595, 1982.

149. **Fuchs, H. E., Shifman, M. A., Michalopoulos, G., and Pizzo, S. V.,** Hepatocyte receptors for antithrombin III proteinase complexes, *J. Cell Biochem.*, 24, 197, 1984.
150. **McLean, J.,** The thromboplastic activity of cephalin, *Am. J. Physiol.*, 41, 250, 1916.
151. **Howell, W. H. and Holt, E. A.,** Two new factors in blood coagulation: heparin and pro-antithrombin, *Am. J. Physiol.*, 47, 328, 1918.
152. **Jaques, L. B.,** Perspectives on heparin research, in Perspectives in Haemostasis, Fareed, J., Messmore, H. L., Fenton J. W., II, and Brinkhous, K. M., Eds., Pergamon Press, New York, 1981, 168.
153. **Lindahl, U., Bäckström, G., Höök, M., Fransson, L.-A., and Linker, A.,** Structure of the antithrombin-binding site of heparin, *Proc. Natl. Acad. Sci. U.S.A.*, 76, 3198, 1979.
154. **Riesenfeld, J., Thunberg, L., Höök, M., and Lindhal, U.,** The antithrombin-binding sequence of heparin. Location of essential N-sulfate groups, *J. Biol. Chem.*, 256, 2389, 1981.
155. **Agarwal, A. and Danishefsky, I.,** Requirement of free carboxyl groups for the anticoagulant activity of heparin, *Thromb. Res.*, 42, 673, 1986.
156. **van Boeckel, C. A. A., Beetz, T., Vos, J. N., de Jong, A. J. M., van Aelst, S. F., van den Bosch, R. H., Martens, J. M. R., and van der Vlugt, F. A.,** Synthesis of a pentasaccharide corresponding to the antithrombin III binding fragment of heparin, *J. Carbohydrate Chem.*, 4, 293, 1985.
157. **Tomono, T., Igarashi, S., and Sawada, E.,** Synthesis of an affinity chromatography gel for AT-III — Effect of purification of AT-III-binding sequence of heparin, *Thromb. Res.*, 35, 467, 1984.
158. **Danielsson, A. and Björk, I.,** Binding to antithrombin of heparin fraction with different molecular weights, *Biochem. J.*, 193, 427, 1981.
159. **Piepkorn, M. W., Lagunoff, D., and Schmer, G.,** Binding of heparin to antithrombin III: the use of dansyl and rhodamine labels, *Arch. Biochem. Biophys.*, 205, 315, 1980.
160. **Einarsson, R.,** The increase in human antithrombin III tryptophan fluorescence produced by heparin, *Biochim. Biophys. Acta*, 534, 165, 1978.
161. **Nagasawa, K. and Uchiyama, H.,** Anticoagulant properties of heparin preparations from different animal sources with equivalent high affinity for antithrombin III, *J. Biochem.*, 95, 619, 1984.
162. **Mahovich, R., Blaskó, Gy., and Pálos, L. Á.,** Action of heparin on thrombin-antithrombin reaction, *Biochim. Biophys. Acta*, 379, 193, 1975.
163. **Barrowcliffe, T. W., Johnson, E. A., and Thomas, D.,** Antithrombin and heparin, *Br. Med. Bull.*, 34, 143, 1978.
164. **Machovich, R.,** Mechanism of action of heparin through thrombin on blood coagulation, *Biochim. Biophys. Acta*, 412, 13, 1975.
165. **Smith, G. F. and Sundboom, J. L.,** Heparin and protease inhibition. I. Heparin complexes with thrombin, plasmin and trypsin, *Thromb. Res.*, 22, 103, 1981.
166. **Casu, B., Oreste, P., Torri, G., Zoppetti, G., Choay, J., Lormeau, J. C., and Petitou, M.,** The structure of heparin oligosaccharide fragments with high anti-factor-Xa activity containing the minimal antithrombin III-binding sequence, *Biochem. J.*, 197, 599, 1981.
167. **Villanueva, G. B.,** Predictions of the secondary structure of antithrombin III and the location of the heparin-binding site, *J. Biol. Chem.*, 259, 2531, 1984.
168. **Karp, G. I., Marcum, J. A., and Rosenberg, R. D.,** The role of tryptophan residnes in heparin-antithrombin interactions, *Arch. Biochem. Biophys.*, 233, 712, 1984.
169. **Blackburn, M. N., Smith, R. L., Carson, J., and Sibley, C. C.,** The heparin-binding site of antithrombin III. Identification of a critical tryptophan in the amino acid sequence, *J. Biol. Chem.*, 259, 939, 1984.
170. **Rosenfeld, L. and Danishefsky, I.,** A fragment of antithrombin that binds both heparin and thrombin, *Biochem. J.*, 237, 639, 1986.
171. **Schapira, M.,** Major inhibitor of the contact phase coagulation factors, *Semin. Thromb. Haemost.*, 13, 69, 1987.
172. **Podack, E. R., Dahlbäck, B., and Griffin, J. H.,** Interaction of S-protein of complement with thrombin and antithrombin III during coagulation. Protection of thrombin by S-protein from antithrombin III inactivation, *J. Biol. Chem.*, 261, 7387, 1986.
173. **Kim, B. K., Steiner, M., and Baldini, M. G.,** Antithrombin III binds to human platelets, *Biochem. Biophys. Res. Comm.*, 97, 1227, 1980.
174. **Alhenc-Gelas, M. L., Aiach, M., Gorenflot, A., and Andreux, J. P.,** Antithrombin III antigen in human platelets, *Thromb. Haemost.*, 54, 599, 1985.
175. **Hoylaerts, M., Holmer, E., De Mol, M., and Collen, D.,** Covalent complexes between low molecular weight heparin fragments and antithrombin III — inhibition kinetics and turnover parameters, *Thromb. Haemost.*, 49, 109, 1983.
176. **Hoylaerts, M., Owen, W. G., and Collen, D.,** Involvement of heparin chain length in the heparin-catalyzed inhibition of thrombin by antithrombin III, *J. Biol. Chem.*, 259, 5670, 1984.
177. **Jordan, R. E., Costa, G. M., Gardmer, W. T., and Rosenberg, R. D.,** The kinetics of haemostatic enzyme-antithrombin interactions in the presence of low molecular weight heparin, *J. Biol. Chem.*, 255, 10081, 1980.

178. **Pletcher, C. H. and Nelsestuen, G. L.,** The rate determining step of the heparin-catalyzed antithrombin/thrombin reaction is independent of thrombin, *J. Biol. Chem.*, 257, 5342, 1982.
179. **Nesheim, M. E.,** A simple rate law that describes the kinetics of the heparin-catalyzed reaction between antithrombin III and thrombin, *J. Biol. Chem.*, 258, 14717, 1983.
180. **Olson, S. T. and Shore, J. D.,** Transient kinetics of heparin-catalyzed protease inactivation by antithrombin III. The reaction step limiting heparin turnover in thrombin neutralization, *J. Biol. Chem.*, 261, 13151, 1986.
181. **Danielsson, A., Raub, E., Lindahl, U., and Björk, I.,** Role of ternary complexes, in which heparin binds both antithrombin and proteinase, in the acceleration of the reactions between antithrombin and thrombin or Factor Xa, *J. Biol. Chem.*, 261, 15467, 1986.
182. **Pletcher, C. H., Cunningham, M. T., and Nelsestuen, G. L.,** Molecular weight analysis of antithrombin-III-heparin and antithrombin III-thrombin-heparin complexes, *J. Biol. Chem.*, 261, 4143, 1986.
183. **Griffith, M. J.,** The heparin-enhanced antithrombin III/thrombin reaction is saturable with respect to both thrombin and antithrombin III, *J. Biol. Chem.*, 257, 13899, 1982.
184. **Pomerantz, M. W. and Owen, W. G.,** A catalytic role of heparin. Evidence for a ternary complex of heparin cofactor, thrombin and heparin, *Biochim. Biophys. Acta,* 535, 66, 1978.
185. **Griffith, M. J.,** Kinetics of the heparin-enhanced antithrombin III/thrombin reaction. Evidence for a template model for the mechanism of action of heparin, *J. Biol. Chem.*, 257, 7360, 1982.
186. **Björk, I. and Nordenman, B.,** Acceleration of the reaction between thrombin and antithrombin III by non-stoichiometric amounts of heparin, *Eur. J. Biochem.*, 68, 507, 1976.
187. **Holmer, E., Söderström, G., and Andersson, L.-O.,** Studies on the mechanism of the rate-enhancing effect of heparin on the thrombin-antithrombin III reaction, *Eur. J. Biochem.*, 93, 1, 1979.
188. **Villanueva, G. B. and Danishefsky, I.,** Evidence for a heparin-induced conformational change on antithrombin III, *Biochemistry,* 18, 810, 1979.
189. **Machovich, R., Staub, M., and Patthy, L.,** Decreased heparin-sensitivity of cyclohexanedione-modified thrombin, *Eur. J. Biochem.*, 83, 473, 1978.
190. **Nesheim, M., Blackburn, M. N., Lawler, C. M., and Mann, K. G.,** Dependence of antithrombin III and thrombin binding stoichiometries and catalytic activity on the molecular weight of affinity-purified heparin, *J. Biol. Chem.*, 261, 3214, 1986.
191. **Griffith, M. J.,** Kinetic analysis of the heparin-enhanced antithrombin III/thrombin reaction. Reaction rate enhancement by heparin-thrombin association, *J. Biol. Chem.*, 254, 12044, 1979.
192. **Smith, G. F. and Sundboom, J. L.,** Heparin and protease inhibition. II. The role of heparin in the AT-III inactivation of thrombin plasmin and trypsin, *Thromb. Res.*, 22, 115, 1981.
193. **Stürzebecher, J. and Markwardt, F.,** Role of heparin in the inactivation of thrombin, Factor Xa and plasmin by antithrombin III, *Thromb. Res.*, 11, 835, 1977.
194. **Griffith, M. J., Kingdon, H. S., and Lundblad, R. L.,** Inhibition of the heparin-antithrombin III/thrombin reaction by active-site blocked-thrombin, *Biochem. Biophys. Res. Comm.*, 87, 686, 1979.
195. **Blaskó, Gy. and Machovich, R.,** Decreased heparin sensitivity of cyclohexadione-modified Factor Xa, *Thromb. Haemost.*, 42, 556, 1979.
196. **Machovich, R., Regoeczi, E., and Hatton, M. W. C.,** Altered inactivation of trinitrophenylated thrombin by antithrombin III in the presence of heparin, *Thromb. Res.*, 17, 383, 1980.
197. **Qaw, F. S. and Brewer, J. M.,** Arginyl residues and thermal stability in proteins, *Mol. Cell Biochem.*, 71, 121, 1986.
198. **Blackburn, M. N., Smith, R. L., Sibley, C. C., and Johnson, V. A.,** Heparin binding and protease inhibitor activity of chemically modified antithrombin III, *Ann. N.Y. Acad. Sci.* 370, 700, 1981.
199. **Einarsson, R., Jahr, E., Stiber, E., Engman, L., Lundström, H., and Andersson, L.-O.,** Effects of the reduction and S-Carbamidomethylation on the conformation, activity and heparin-binding capactiy of human antithrombin III, *Biochim. Biophys. Acta,* 624, 386, 1980.
200. **Björk, I. and Nordling, K.,** Evidence by chemical modification for the ivolvement of one or more tryptophanyl residues of bovine antithrombin in the binding of high-affinity heparin, *Eur. J. Biochem.*, 102, 497, 1979.
201. **Jorgensen, A. M., Borders, C. L., Jr., and Fish, W. W.,** Arginine residues are critical for the heparin cofactor activity of antithrombin III, *Biochem. J.*, 231, 59, 1985.
202. **Danishefsky, I., Ahrens, M., and Klein, S.,** Effect of heparin modification on its activity in enhancing the inhibition of thrombin by antithrombin III, *Biochim. Biophys. Acta.* 498, 215, 1977.
203. **Machovich, R. and Arányi, P.,** Effect of heparin on thrombin inactivation by antithrombin-III, *Biochem. J.*, 173, 869, 1978.
204. **Longas, M. O., Ferguson, W. S., and Finlay, T. H.,** Studies on the interaction of heparin with thrombin, antithrombin and other plasma proteins, *Arch. Biochem. Biophys.*, 200, 595, 1980.
205. **O'Neal Speight, M. and Griffith, M. J.,** Calcium inhibits the heparin-catalyzed antithrombin-III/thrombin reaction by decreasing the apparent binding affinity of heparin for thrombin, *Arch. Biochem. Biophys.*, 225, 958, 1983.

206. **Olson, S.**, Heparin and ionic strength-dependent conversion of antithrombin III from an inhibitor to a substrate of α-thrombin, *J. Biol. Chem.*, 260, 10153, 1985.
207. **Ofosu, F. A., Blajchman, M. A., Modi, G., Cerskus, A. L., and Hirsh, J.**, Activation of Factor X and prothrombin in antithrombin-III-depleted plasma: the effects of heparin, *Thromb. Res.*, 23, 331, 1981.
208. **Holmer, E., Kurachi, K., and Söderström, G.**, The molecular weight dependence of the rate-enhancing effect of hepain on the inhibition of thrombin, Factor Xa, Factor IXa, Factor XIa, Factor XIIa and kallikrein by antithrombin III, *Biochem. J.*, 193, 395, 1981.
209. **Cerskus, A. L., Birchall, K. J., Ofosu, F. A., Hirsh, J., and Blajchman, M. A.**, Effects of heparin fractions of different affinities to antithrombin III and thrombin on the inactivation of thrombin and Factor Xa by antithrombin III, *Can. J. Biochem. Cell Biol.*, 62, 975, 1984.
210. **Scully, M. F. and Kakkar, V. V.**, Effect of pentosan polysulphate upon thrombin and Factor Xa inactivation by antithrombin III, *Biochem. J.*, 222, 571, 1984.
211. **Scott, C. F., Schapira, M., and Colman, R. W.**, Effect of heparin on the inactivation rate of human Factor XIa by antithrombin III, *Blood,* 60, 940, 1982.
212. **Machovich, R., Bauer, P., Arányi, P., Kecskés, É., Büki, K. G., and Horváth, I.**, Kinetic analysis of the heparin-enhanced plasmin-antithrombin III reaction. Apparent catalytic role of heparin, *Biochem. J.*, 199, 521, 1981.
213. **Owen, W. G.**, Effect of heparin on the extent of inhibition of thrombin by heparin cofactor, *Biochim. Biophys. Acta,* 494, 182, 1977.
214. **Griffith, M. J.**, Measurement of the heparin enhanced-antithrombin III/thrombin reaction rate in the presence of synthetic substrate, *Thromb. Res.*, 25, 245, 1982.
215. **Carlström, A.-S., Liedén, K., and Björk, I.**, Decreased binding of heparin to antithrombin following the interaction between antithrombin and thrombin, *Thromb. Res.*, 11, 785, 1977.
216. **Kowalski, S. and Finlay, T. H.**, Heparin and the inactivation of thrombin by antithrombin III, *Thromb. Res.*, 14, 387, 1979.
217. **Buchanan, M. R., Boneu, B., Ofosu, F., and Hirsh, J.**, The relative importance of thrombin inhibition and Factor Xa inhibition to the antithrombotic effects of heparin, *Blood,* 65, 198, 1985.
218. **Machovich, R., Regocxzi, E., and Hatton, M. W. C.**, The influence of heparin, NaCl, and $CaCl_2$ on the rate of the inactivation of the thrombin-antithrombin III reaction, *Thromb. Res.*, 15, 821, 1979.
219. **Griffith, M. J., Beavers, G., Kingdon, H. S., and Lundblad, R. L.**, Effect of monovalent cations on the heparin-enhanced antithrombin III/thrombin reaction, *Thromb. Res.*, 17, 29, 1980.
220. **Oshima, G. and Nagasawa, K.**, Effect of NaCl on inactivation of bovine thrombin by antithrombin III in the presence of low-affinity-heparin or dextran sulfate, *Thromb. Res.*, 37, 361, 1986.
221. **Carrell, R. W., Christey, P. B., and Boswell, D. R.**, Serpins: antithrombin and other inhibitors of coagulation and fibrinolysis. Evidence from amino acid sequences, in Thrombosis and Haemostasis, Verstraete, M., Vermylen, J., Lijnen, R., and Arnout, J., Eds., University Press, Leuven, Belgium, 1987, 1.
222. **Preissner, K. T., Zwicker, L., and Müller-Berghaus, G.**, Formation, characterization and detection of a ternary complex between S protein, thrombin and antithrombin III in serum, *Biochem. J.*, 243, 105, 1987.
223. **Ofosu, F., Blajchman, M. A., and Hirsh, J.**, The inhibition by heparin of the intrinsic pathway activation of Factor X in the absence of antithrombin III, *Thromb. Res.*, 20, 391, 1980.
224. **Vijaya Mohan Rao, I. and Rapaport, S. I.**, Studies of a mechanism inhibiting the initiation of the extrinsic pathway of coagulation, *Blood,* 69, 645, 1987.
225. **Hemker, H. C.**, The mode of action of heparin in plasma, in Thrombosis and Haemostasis, Verstraete, M., Vermylen, J., Lijnen, R., and Arnout, J., Eds., University Press, Leuven, Belgium, 1987, 17.
226. **Marciniak, E. and Gora-Maslak, G.**, Enhancement by heparin of thrombin-induced antithrombin III proteolysis: its relation to the molecular weight and anticoagulant activity of heparin, *Thromb. Res.*, 28, 411, 1982.
227. **Marciniak, E.**, Differential role of fractionated heparin in antithrombin III proteolysis, *Blood,* 59, 576, 1982.
228. **Hatton, M. W. C. and Moar, S. L.**, A role for pericellular proteoglycan in the binding of thrombin or antithrombin III by the blood vessel endothelium — The effects of proteoglycan-degrading enzymes and glycosaminoglycan-binding proteins on ^{125}I-thrombin binding by the rabbit thoracic sorts *in vitro, Thromb. Haemost.*, 54, 228, 1985.
229. **Buonassisi, V. and Root, M.**, Enzymetic degradation of heparin-related mucopolysacchrides from the surface of endothelial cell cultures, *Biochim. Biophys. Acta,* 385, 1, 1975.
230. **Hatton, M. W. C., Moar, S. L., and Richardson, M.**, On the interaction of rabbit antithrombin III with the luminal surface of the normal and deendothelialized rabbit thoracic aorta *in vitro, Blood,* 67, 878, 1986.
231. **Awbrey, B. J., Hoak, J. C., and Owen, W. G.**, Binding of human thrombin to cultured human andotheial cells, *J. Biol. Chem.*, 254, 4092, 1979.

232. **Delvos, U., Meusel, P., Preissner, T., and Müller-Berghaus, G.,** Formation of activated Protein C and inactivation of cell-bound thrombin by antithrombin III at the surface of cultured vascular endothelial cells — A comparative study of two anticoagulant mechanism, *Thromb. Haemost.*, 57, 87, 1987.
233. **Miura, Y., Aoyagi, S., Ikeda, F., and Miyamoto, K.,** Anticoagulant activity of artificial biomedical materials with co-immobilized antithrombin and heparin, *Biochimie*, 62, 595, 1980.
234. **Goosen, M. F. A., Sefton, M. V., and Hatton, M. W. C.,** Inactivation of thrombin by antithrombin III on a heparinized biomaterial, *Thromb. Res.*, 20, 543, 1980.
235. **Hatton, M. W. C., Rollason, G., and Sefton, M. V.,** Fate of thrombin and thrombin-antithrombin III complex absorbed to a heparinized biomaterial: analysis of the enzyme-inhibitor complexes displaced by plasma, *Thromb. Haemost.*, 50, 873, 1983.
236. **Chuang, H. Y. K., Crowther, P. E., Mohammad, S. F., and Mason, R. G.,** Interactions of thrombin and antithrombin III with artificial surfaces, *Thromb. Res.*, 14, 273, 1979.
237. **Crassous, G., Jozefowitz, M., and Sledz, J.,** Preparation of an assymetric semipermeable membrane with anticoagulant activity, *Biomaterials*, 5, 153, 1984.
238. **Fougnot, C., Jozefowitz, M., and Rosenberg, R. D.,** Affinity of purified thrombin or antithrombin III for two insoluble anticoagulant polystyrene derivatives. I. *In vitro* adsorption studies, *Biomaterials*, 4, 294, 1983.
239. **Machovich, R. and Horváth, I.,** Heparin-like effect of polymethacrylic acid on the reaction between thrombin and antithrombin III, *Thromb. Res.*, 11, 765, 1977.
240. **Ito, Y., Sisido, M., and Imanishi, Y.,** Synthesis and antithrombogenicity of polyetherurethane containing quaternary ammonium groups in the side chains and of the polymer/heparin complex, *J. Biomed. Mater. Res.*, 20, 1017, 1986.

Chapter 2

CLINICAL SIGNIFICANCE AND LABORATORY DIAGNOSIS OF ANTITHROMBIN III DEFICIENCIES

Géza Sas

TABLE OF CONTENTS

I. DETERMINATION OF AT-III

A. CLASSIFICATION, GENERAL CONSIDERATIONS

1. Introduction

In principle, the determination of antithrombin III (AT-III) is based on some of its specific biological characteristics. The majority of methods makes a quantitative measurement of one of the particular characteristics of AT-III possible, but some of them give useful information on the quality of this molecule.

For the quantitative determination of AT-III, two main groups of assays are available. In the first group, with the help of the specific antigen structure of AT-III, the immunological assays render it possible to measure the concentration of the AT-III antigen. In the second group of assays, the inhibitory activity of AT-III towards thrombin and factor Xa (F Xa) is measured quantitatively, and these methods are considered functional assays.

Obviously, these two groups of quantitative methods measure different characteristics of the AT-III molecule. Hence, the results of these two kinds of methods are not identical in many cases. When the AT-III level is mentioned, it is not specified whether the AT-III antigen concentration or thrombin (F Xa)-inhibiting activity was measured. This fact may explain many controversies in clinical investigations.

Qualitative assays of AT-III determination are mainly used to characterize qualitatively abnormal AT-III molecules, and as such, they cannot be sharply differentiated from the usual methods of protein chemistry.

The immunological assays of AT-III determination use monospecific, precipitating antibodies against human AT-III raised in rabbits or goats. The most rapid determination is the nephelometric quantitation of immunoprecipitation.[1,2] The rocket electroimmunoassay of Laurell appears to be the most widely applied method on account of its accuracy and relative simplicity.[3] The method most easy to perform is the radial immunodiffusion of Mancini et al.,[4] but accurate results are hardly obtained before 48 to 76 h.

Radioimmunoassay can measure smaller concentrations of AT-III than of the usual immunological methods mentioned above (detection limit: 25 μg/dl).[5] However, this advantage is counterbalanced by its laborious and time-consuming performance. The sandwich enzyme immunoassay has been also proposed.[6] Due to its high sensitivity (detection limit: 30 ng/dl), an AT-III determination in urine is possible.

Immunoassays are valuable research tools and may be useful in screening large numbers of plasma samples. But for most other purposes and particularly in urgent cases, functional assays are superior.

Functional assays of AT-III determination are based on measuring the thrombin or factor Xa inactivating activity of the sample tested. Two main groups of functional assays can be distinguished.

In the first main group of methods, the characteristic slow or "progressive" inactivation of thrombin or F Xa is measured. In these systems, heparin is not added to the reaction mixture and the "natural" inactivating activity of the blood is determined. This progressive antithrombin (antifactor Xa) activity has been measured in two different ways. In the first type of assays, the tested material is incubated with an excess of enzyme and the remaining activity is determined after equilibration.[7,8,9] These tests reflect the total thrombin- or F Xa-binding capacity of plasma. (These methods have only historical interest now.) The second type of assays reflects the initial rate of thrombin (or F Xa) inactivation. The incubation period is short and the amount of enzyme relatively small. The majority of these methods applies a two-stage system. In the first stage, the AT-III-containing sample is incubated with definied amount of the enzyme (thrombin or F Xa) and after a standard incubation time in stage two, the residual enzyme activity is measured by means of a suitable substrate. In clotting assays, fibrinogen is used as a substrate for thrombin and F X deficient plasma for F Xa activity.[10,11,12,13] In the amidolytic assay, synthetic substrates with high enzyme specificity are applied.[14]

The second main group of functional assays is characterized by the application of heparin in the incubation mixture. Heparin accelerates the inactivation of the enzyme (thrombin or F Xa) by AT-III. The incubation time is short and reliable measurements may be obtained in plasma samples of heparinized patients. As in the case of assays measuring the initial rate of progressive thrombin (or F Xa) inactivation, a two-stage system is applied in these "heparin cofactor assays." Heparin is mixed to the first incubation system and the residual enzyme activity is measured by means of a natural or synthetic substrate for thrombin or F Xa. Heparin cofactor assays measure either the initial rate of inactivation or the total enzyme neutralizing capacity of the test sample.[15,16,17,18]

In general, methods investigating the quality of AT-III are applied in research. The crossed immunoelectrophoresis with and without heparin in the first run makes it possible to investigate the abnormal AT-III molecules and AT-III-enzyme complexes.[19,20] Isoelectrofocusing and crossed-immunoelectrofocusing serve similar purposes.[21,22]

Table 1 demonstrates the classification of assays applied in the determination of AT-III.

In the following sections, we discuss the general problems of AT-III assays, separating the immunoassays and the functional methods. Then we shortly describe the AT-III assays which are used in our laboratory.

2. Problems with Immunoassays

The immunological assays of AT-III determination tacitly assume a perfect structural identity of all the AT-III molecules to be determined. In the case of this homogeneity, the number and sterical position of the immunologic epitops of AT-III are the same. Being in abundance of the monospecific, precipitating antibodies, the number of binding antigen-antibodies depends only on the concentration of the antigen, i.e., AT-III.

TABLE 1
Antithrombin III Assays

- I. Quantitative assays
  - A. Immunological assays
    - 1. Simple radial immunodiffusion
    - 2. Rocket electroimmunoassay
    - 3. Nephelometric assays
    - 4. Radioimmunoassay
    - 5. Sandwich enzyme immunoassay
  - B. Functional assays
    - 1. Methods measuring the progressive inactivation of the enzyme (without heparin)
      - a. Measurement of the total enzyme inactivating capacity of the test sample
        - Determination of thrombin-neutralizing capacity
        - Determination of F Xa-neutralizing capacity
      - b. Determination of the initial rate of inactivation of enzyme
        - Measurement of the rate of thrombin inactivation
        - Measurement of the rate of F Xa inactivation
    - 2. Assays measuring heparin cofactor activity
      - a. Measurement of the total enzyme inactivating capacity
        - Determination of thrombin-neutralizing capacity
        - Determination of F Xa-neutralizing capacity
      - b. Determination of the initial rate of enzyme inactivation
        - Measurement of the rate of thrombin inactivation
        - Measurement of the rate of F Xa inactivation
- II. Qualitative assays
  - 1. Crossed immunoelectrophoresis (with and without heparin)
  - 2. Isoelectrofocusing
  - 3. Crossed immunoelectrophocusing

In the vast majority of cases, the falsehood of this assumption causes no problem. Many clinical investigations have found a good correlation between immunological and functional AT-III assays.[23,24,25]

However, in specific conditions, the immunological difference of variant antigen structures gives rise to significant alterations. First of all, in part of the qualitative congenital AT-III deficiencies, such AT-III molecules are produced which display significant structural differences from that of "normal" AT-III molecules.[26] In these cases, the concentration of the pathologic AT-III cannot be measured accurately by the commercial antisera produced with normal AT-III. In the case of AT-III "Budapest", Lane[27] demonstrated a qualitative difference between two commercial AT-III antisera regarding abnormal AT-III.

In the course of a thrombin-AT-III reaction, AT-III binds to thrombin and a part of the AT-III molecule is not available for the antibody. It means that the AT-III of plasma is not identical with the AT-III of serum. In serum, a heterogeneity of the proteins with AT-III-like structures is detectable.[28] The results of the measurement of the AT-III antigen concentration in serum depend not only on the residual plasma AT-III concentration, but in a variable manner, on these complexed or degraded AT-III molecules as well. The practical consequence of this fact is that AT-III antigen concentration has to be measured in the plasma and not in the serum of the patients if we want to compare functional activities with antigen concentrations.

However, the problem of immunological methods is also complicated by the heterogeneity of antibodies against AT-III, as it was shown by Barrowcliffe and McKay.[29,30] In the course of the production of antiserum against AT-III, generally, at least two populations of AT-III antibodies are raised. One is against the native, biologically active AT-III molecule and the other against the AT-III-protease complex. A part of human AT-III complexes *in vivo* with proteases of the immunized animal (rabbit or goat). Thus, not only antibodies against AT-III, but antibodies against this complex are produced. Another cause of the heterogeneity of immunsera is ascribable to the heterogeneity of AT-III injected in animals. In the course of the purification of AT-III, a proportion of the molecules is denaturated and cannot bind heparin. Consequently, a part of the antibodies is directed against these non-binding AT-III molecules.

The heterogeneity of antibodies against AT-III has theoretical and practical significance as well. It must be taken into account in investigating variant AT-III molecules or AT-III complexes because various commercially available antisera differ not only in titre, but in this respect, too.

Modified crossed immunoelectrophoresis (heparin in agarose) was introduced by us in 1975.[20] During that time, we carried out investigations on coagulation factor concentrates produced by the Scottish National Blood Transfusion Service. In the course of this work, we wanted to detect AT-III in these concentrates by crossed immunoelectrophoresis. To prevent an artefactual activation of the coagulation factors, heparin was added to the agarose in the first run. Compared with the original AT-III peak, the electrophoretic mobility of AT-III increased. On the basis of this observation, which was serendepity, we started systematical investigations to clarify this phenomenon and the results were subsequently described.[31] Mixing various quantities of heparin with agarose in the first phase of the electrophoresis, AT-III from normal human plasma and serum revealed a heterogeneity which depended on the heparin concentration in the agarose gel. At heparin concentrations higher than 16 μ/ml, AT-III displayed three components with different electrophoretic mobilities. The component with the highest mobility (designated immunoantithrombin III_1) dominated in the plasma. In normal serum, however, the quantity of this component was decreased and the two other peaks with a slower electrophoretic mobility (IAT-III_2 and IAT-III_3) became more evident. The different mobilities of the particular AT-III components can be explained by their different affinities to heparin. Subsequent studies clarified that IAT-III_2 corresponds to the complexed form of AT-III, which may exist in a polymer form in serum, and that IAT-III_3 was identical with the low molecular weight AT-III, devoid of biological activity.[28,32] This method was applied soon in the studies on abnormal AT-III. On the basis of the decreased heparin-affinity of the pathological AT-III molecule, the existence of AT-III "Budapest" was directly proved.[26]

Although many other investigations supported our original observation, Andersson et al.[33] thought that multicomponent patterns sometimes arose because of the heparin "overtaking" the AT-III sample near the edge of the plate. This can be avoided by placing the sample in the middle of the plate or by also incorporating heparin in the electrophoretic buffer. However, these variations did not alter the AT-III patterns, as it was demonstrated by Barrowcliffe.[30] Investigating various AT-III concentrates, he concluded that having the sample in the middle of the gel could be misleading. Unfortunately, some authors did not realize the results of Barrowcliffe and performed the modified crossed immunoelectrophoresis as it was suggested by Andersson et al.[33] The data derived from these publications can be evaluated only cautiously. An important methodological observation was derived from the work of Chan and Chan.[34] They found that venous occlusion to the forearm before taking the blood resulted in the appearance of a slow second peak in the plasma. Hence, in the course of blood taking, a prolonged venous occlusion has to be avoided.

Although by the modified crossed immunoelectrophoresis technique (heparin in agarose) the AT-III complexes produced "*in vivo*" can be demonstrated, this method has not proved to be as useful as it was originally expected.[35,36] The explanation may be given partly in the different antigen structures of the complexes, or in their very short biological half-lives. Both forms of crossed immunoelectrophoresis (with and without heparin) were applied with more success in the investigations of variant AT-III molecules.

3. Problems with Functional Assays

By means of functional assays, we measure the thrombin- or F Xa-inhibiting activity of the sample. In most cases, the sample is the plasma of a patient or, rarely, a plasma fraction. Earlier, for avoiding the disturbing effect of fibrinogen of plasma, the inhibiting activity of serum was measured. However, the serum contained only a proportion (about 70%) of the original AT-III activity of the plasma. The residual thrombin- or F Xa-inhibiting activity of the serum depends on many conditions (e.g., the quantity of the procoagulants before the coagulation, the rate of prothrombin consumption in the serum, the time elapsed after the coagulation, etc.) which practically cannot be standardized. Consequently, functional AT-III assays should be performed with the plasma of the patients, instead of the serum.

In connection with functional assays, the following general problems arise:

1. Assays measuring the progressive thrombin inactivation are not entirely specific for AT-III because inhibitors other than AT-III take part in the inactivation of thrombin in plasma. According to Abildgaard, about 25% of the thrombin is neutralized by alfa$_2$-macroglobulin in these assays.[37] Alfa$_1$-antitrypsin also has some antithrombin activity.
2. As was discussed before, these assays must be performed with plasma instead of serum. However, when we incubate thrombin or F Xa with plasma, coagulation takes place and this renders it impossible to obtain the sample to be measured. In addition to this technical problem, a proportion of the thrombin molecules is adsorbed to fibrin (antithrombin I activity of Seegers), which also disturbs the quantification of the residual enzyme activity. To overcome this problem, a part of the assays uses heat to remove fibrinogen from the plasma to be tested. Heat defibrination at 56 C° for 3 min removes not only fibrinogen, but about 10 to 25% of the original AT-III activity. Defibrination can be performed with proteins which also coagulate fibrin. For this purpose, arvin (Ancrod) or reptilase is used in some assays. According to Howie et al.,[38] this method of defibrination causes less inaccuracy than heat defibrination. In amidolytic methods, defibrination can be omitted since plasma is largely diluted and pH and ionic strength are increased.
3. In the course of the incubation of the enzyme (thrombin or F Xa) with the sample, in addition to the specific inactivation, a proportion of the enzymes is inactivated nonspecifically. In the case of thrombin, two major reasons for this nonspecific loss of activity have been identified. One is the proteolytic degradation of alfa-thrombin, which leads to the formation of beta and gamma forms and is reflected in a loss of clotting activity, but only a small change in the ability of the enzyme to hydrolyze synthetic chromogenic substrates. The other loss is due to the adsorbtion of the enzyme to surface. Several measures for minimizing such losses have been advised. Some investigators made corrections for loss of the enzyme by controlling its activity parallel in time with the experiment performed or preadsorbing the tubes and pipettes with the enzyme waiting until the decrease in activity became acceptably small. Others used less adsorbing laboratory ware (siliconized glass or plastics) or added stabilizing agents. Recently, Latallo and Hall pointed out that glass, siliconized glass, polypropylene, and polystyrene surfaces adsorb thrombin in a similar manner.[39] The use of synthetic chromogenic substrates allows measurements of thrombin activity at enzyme concentrations approximately 100 times lower than in a clotting assay. When such a sensitive assay is applied to measure AT-III activity, elimination of adsorbtion loss is of crucial importance. In these cases, a complete and long-term prevention of adsorbtion loss of thrombin activity is achieved by the addition of 0.1% polyethylenglycoll (PEG) 6000 to the buffer and the use of tubes precoated with PEG 20,000, as it was demonstrated by Latallo and Hall.[39]

4. Mixing an appropriate quantity of heparin to the incubation system containing AT-III, the inactivation rate of thrombin increases about two-thousandfold. Thus, the heparin cofactor assays are more rapid than the methods based on the measuring of progressive thrombin inactivation. Heparin in test plasma has no influence on the results. Apart from these practical advantages, the heparin cofactor assays are more specific because the thrombin inhibiting effect of alfa$_2$-macroglobulin and alfa$_1$-antitrypsin is not increased by heparin. However, the thrombin inactivating effect of another proteinase inhibitor, heparin cofactor II, is also increased by heparin, which has to be taken into account, especially at low AT-III activities and high heparin concentrations. AT-III deficient, heparinized patients were found to have AT-III antigen levels in the 15 to 20% range of normal, while AT-III activities measured with amidolytic heparin cofactor assay were 35 to 40%. This difference can be experienced with methods using human thrombin.[40] When amidolytic methods were introduced to measure heparin cofactor activity, the amidolysis of some of these early synthetic substrates, for example S-1260, was influenced by heparin. Consequently, the presence of a heparin neutralizer (polybrene) was necessary in stage II. The amidolysis of the most recent thrombin substrates seems not to be influenced by heparin and with these substrates, polybrene may be omitted.
5. Functional assays use the determination of residual thrombin activity as an indirect measure of antithrombin activity. The measurement of the clotting time of fibrinogen, the natural substrate of thrombin, is used as a characteristic of the thrombin activity which is a part of these assays. The coagulant actions of thrombin, however, vary depending on the type of fibrinogen used in the assay procedure.[41] Thus, the type of fibrinogen in the assay may contribute to errors in the functional methods. With the advent of synthetic peptide substrates, great interest centered on assays using these compounds instead of fibrinogen. A synthetic substrate for a proteolytic enzyme has many advantages compared to a natural substrate: it can have better solubility, its enzymatic cleavage can be easily followed by photometric or fluorometric methods, and it can easily be standardized. Synthetic chromogenic (fluorogenic) peptid substrates have been modeled after the structure of natural substrates of enzymes. The structure preceding the scissile bond seems to be of prime importance for enzyme-substrate interaction, and the knowledge of the amino acid sequence immediately preceding this scissile bond of the natural substrate has been particularly useful for the construction of synthetic peptide substrates for serine proteases. The determining factor of substrate-enzyme specificity is not the size of the substrate molecule, but rather the steric configuration in the neighborhood of the bond which undergoes hydrolysis. The short amino acid sequence of a synthetic substrate may have the proper configuration, but this short amino acid sequence will contain a limited specificity. Good sensitivity and high specificity are important features for a synthetic substrate. One has, however, to remember that the substrates are not completely specific. The substrates S-2238 (H-D-Phe-Pip-Arg-pNA, KabiVitrum, Sweden), Chromozym TH (Tos-Gly-Pro-Arg-pNA, Pentapharm, Switzerland), and S-2222 (Bz-Ile-Glu-Arg-pNA, KabiVitrum, Sweden), are relatively specific for thrombin and F Xa, respectively. At equimolar enzyme concentrations, thrombin splits S-2238 about a hundred times faster than does F Xa, whereas F Xa splits S-2222 about fourteen times faster than thrombin does.[42]

In recent years, several other thrombin-specific chromogenic substrates have been synthesized and applied for the determination of AT-III activity, such as Spectrozyme TH (D-cyclo-hexyl-tyrosyl-alanyl-arginyl-paranitroanilide-dihydrochloride, American Diagnostica, U.S.), CBS 34.47 (D-cyclohexylglycylbutyl-arginyl-paranitroanilide-dihydrochloride, Diagnostica Stago, France), TH-I (D-cyclohexylglycyl-alanyl-arginyl-paranitronilide-dihydrochloride, Immuno, Austria), and Bz-Leu-Ala-Arg-NE (Benzoyl-L-leucyl-L-alanyl-L-arginine-α-naphthylester, Torii Co., Japan). In the case of chromogenic substrates, enzymatic hydrolysis leads to the release of chromophore (p-nitroaniline, amino-methylcoumarinamide, α-naphtol, etc.) and production of a color that may be easily quantified in a spectrophotometer. The functional AT-III assays, using a fluorescent substrate such as D-phenyl-alanine-proline-arginine-5-amidoso-phtalic acid dimethyl ester (American Dade, USA) or carbobenzoxy-glycine-proline-arginine-4-methoxy-β-naphtylamide (Enzyme Systems Products, Inc. U.S.), measure the rate of fluorescent tag release, which results from thrombin proteolysis of a synthetic substrate that mimics fibrinogen.[43,44]

Amidolytic assays may use two methods: kinetic measurement, which involves monitoring the formation of chromophore (fluorophore), or by an end-point measurement, where the reaction is stopped after a fixed incubation time. The most precise method for quantitative analysis is the measurement of the initial rate (kinetic assay). The kinetic measurement is to be preferred in research work. It consists of following adsorbancy changes during the first few minutes of a reaction. The temperature should be kept constant, and optimal pH and ionic strength are maintained with a correct buffer. An excess of substrate is of primary importance.

Alternatively, the end-point method can be employed. It is perhaps most popular in routine work when considerable numbers of assaies are performed. Usually, the reaction is carried out for a short, exactly determined time and stopped by the addition of concentrated acetic acid.

6. During the last decade, automation of AT-III assays has been developed, owing to the increasing number of tests performed and the need for accurate techniques. Clotting, amidolytic, and even immunologic methods have been automated or semiautomated. However, AT-III determination by the amidolytic assay is the most commonly automated procedure. Chromogenic methods are easily automated by the kinetic rate technique, and most of the instruments used in clinical chemistry laboratories are appropriate. Results obtained with the following instruments have been published: GEMSAEC centrifugal analyzer,[45,46] Multistat microcentrifugal analyzer,[47] ABA-100 Abbott,[48,49] Vitatron Automated Kinetic Enzyme and Substrate Analyzer,[48,50] Gilford 3500,[47,51,52] Isamat Isabiologie,[53] Kem-O-Mat 2T Coultronics,[54] LKB,[55] Eppendorf 5020,[48] Cobas Bio,[56] and aca Du Pont.[57] Since incubation times, volumes, reaction times, substrates, and thrombin differ from one automated technique to the other, it is important to include lyophilized or frozen human plasma controls in the normal and low ranges.[58]
7. Thrombin can be converted by proteolysis and autolysis to β and γ forms, which exhibit esterolytic and amidolytic activities, but possess relatively weaker coagulant properties than the α form. It is known that commercially available preparations of thrombin may contain varying proportions of α, β, and γ forms and, therefore, may differ in their relative amidolytic and coagulant properties. Thus, a thrombin solution containing these various molecular forms may bring about great differences in the results of AT-III functional assays depending on the substrate applied.[59] In addition to this disturbing effect of molecular heterogeneity, the species origin of the enzyme (human or bovine) may influence the results in the assays.[60,61] The rate of thrombin inhibition by AT-III alone differs depending upon the origin and form of the enzyme used, and these differences can be augmented when heparin is present. This point is overlooked in many publications discussing the superiority of the amidolytic methods to the clotting assays. Ionic strength also highly influences the results. These differences clearly indicate that the thrombin used in the assay has to be well-defined in terms of origin, molecular form, and specific activity. Without this, AT-III activities obtained in various laboratories are not likely to be informative.

4. Which AT-III Assay to Choose?

In previous paragraphs, we discussed the theoretical and methodological problems of AT-III determinations. A good deal of controversial opinions have been described on the values of the particular tests.[62,63,64] However, they can be easily explained by the differences regarding the quality of immunsera, the source of AT-III (plasma, serum, or plasma-fraction), the substrate applied (fibrinogen or synthetic substrate), and the heterogeneous composition of the enzyme (α, β, and γ thrombin), not mentioning other variables (pH, ionic strength, etc.). All the methods have their advantages and disadvantages as far as their specificity, sensitivity, cost, etc. are concerned. Therefore, when we choose an assay for the determination of AT-III, several circumstances have to be taken into account.

For screening purposes in the case of a thrombophilic patient, a heparin cofactor assay seems to be preferable because both quantitative and qualitative abnormalities of AT-III can be detected by it. If the heparin cofactor activity is reduced, the performance of additonal tests is necessary. The immunochemical determination of AT-III antigen concentration and the measurement of the progressive thrombin inactivation can provide further information. In the majority of AT-III deficient patients, all three methods reveal a similar reduction of activities and antigen concentration (Type I AT-III deficiency).

Normal AT-III antigen concentration and reduced heparin cofactor activity suggest a qualitative (Type II) AT-III deficiency. Decreased progressive thrombin inactivation indicates the disturbance of the active center of the molecule. Crossed immunoelectrophoresis with and without heparin, heparin affinity chromatography, and measurement of the inactivation of F Xa in the presence and absence of heparin make the characterization of the particular disorder possible.

In the cases of acquired AT-III deficiency, such as in chronic liver diseases, nephrotic syndrome or DIC, a simple quantitative functional test, is the most valuable. The simultaneous performance of an immunoassay may provide supportive or additional information to the result of the functional method. A moderately reduced antigen level with a low functional activity suggests the presence of an inactive form of AT-III, such as the thrombin-AT-III complex.

B. IMMUNOLOGICAL ASSAYS

1. Radial Immunodiffusion

This method was independently introduced in 1965 by two groups of investigators.[4,65] We will describe the method shortly as we use it in our laboratory for the determination of the AT-III concentration of a sample.

We prepare an agarose gel in a concentration of 1% (Agarose, Reanal Institute, Budapest, Hungary). The agarose is dissolved in a TRIS buffer (0.1 *M* TRIS-HCl, pH 7.3). The agarose gel (10 ml) is mixed with 0.1 ml of anti-AT-III immune serum (Behringwerke, Marburg, West Germany). The two substances are thoroughly mixed at 56°C and poured onto a horizontal glass plate (8 × 8 cm). After cooling, wells with a diameter of 2.5 mm are prepared by a standard pattern and 0.005 ml of the sample is measured into each well. The plate is put into a moist chamber and left for 48 h at room temperature. Then, the plate is rinsed in saline for 24 h and, at the end, for 1 h in distilled water. After drying at room temperature for 12 h, Coomassie Brillant Blue staining is used (Figure 1).

2. Rocket Immunoelectrophoresis

This method was described by Laurell in 1966.[3] For the determination of the AT-III concentration of a sample, we perform the assay as follows: A mixture of 12 ml, 1% agarose (Reanal Institute, Budapest, Hungary) and 0.1 ml anti-AT-III immune serum (Behringwerke, Marburg, West Germany) is poured onto a glass plate (8 × 8 cm) at 56°C. Eighteen wells (3 mm in diameter) are prepared in the agarose layer by a standard pattern. Also placed in

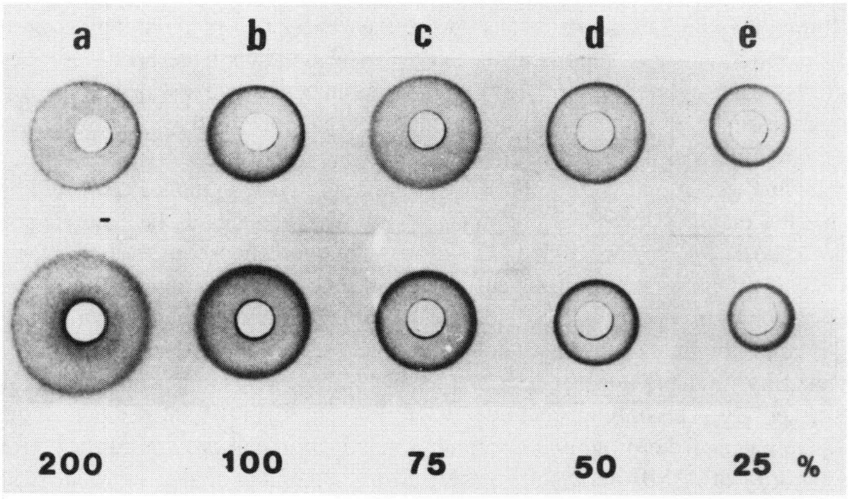

FIGURE 1. Measurement of AT-III concentration by radial immunodiffusion. In the upper row, *a, b, c,* and *d* represent the plasma samples of a thrombophilic family with a qualitative abnormality of AT-III (AT-III "Budapest"). *e* shows the decreased AT-III concentration of the plasma of a patient with DIC. In the lower row, the precipitation rings of the various dilutions of normal plasma can be seen. The higher the AT-III concentrations of the sample, the bigger the diameter of the precipitation ring. (From *Thromb. Diath. Haemorrh.*, 32, 105, 1975. With permission.)

each well is 10 μl of AT-III-containing solutions. Electrophoresis is carried out at 20 V/cm for 4 h. Barbitone buffer (pH 8.6, 0.05 *M*) is used in the agarose gel and buffer tanks. After 1 h rinsing in distilled water, the plates are covered with filter paper (Whatman No. 1) and left overnight to dry. Coomassie Brillant Blue staining is used. The length of the "rockets" is measured and the AT-III concentration of the sample is expressed as a percent of normal plasma from a calibration curve which is prepared from the dilutions of normal plasma on each plate (Figure 2).

3. Crossed Immunoelectrophoresis

This method was described by Laurell in 1965.[19] The original procedure and modification of it (using heparin in the agarose for the first electrophoresis as it was described by Sas et al.[20]) proved to be very useful in the investigation of AT-III. For the investigation of AT-III in a sample, we perform the procedure as follows: Poured onto a glass plate (8 × 8 cm) is 12 ml of a 1% agarose (Reanal Institute, Budapest, Hungary) solution. On one plate, the agarose does not contain heparin, while on the other plate it does (20 units per ml agarose, Heparin, Richter Gedeon Pharmaceutical Company, Budapest, Hungary). After solidification of the agarose, a well of 3 mm diameter is prepared in one corner of the plate (15 mm from both edges) and 5 μl of the sample is measured into the well. Electrophoresis is carried out at 4°C. Barbitone buffer (pH 8.6, 0.05 *M*) is used in the agarose gel and buffer tanks. After the first electrophoresis (at 20 V/cm for 2 h), the agarose gel is cut in two parts, the direction of the cut is parallel with that of the elctrophoresis and is located 20 mm from the edge of the plate. The smaller part of the agarose layer, which contains the proteins separated by the first electrophoresis, is kept, while the wider part is removed. Then, 10 ml of 1% agarose is mixed with 0.1 ml anti-AT-III immune serum (Behringwerke, Marburg, West Germany) at 56°C, poured into the site of the discarded gel, the plate rotates through 90°, and electrophoresis continues at 20 V/cm for 4 h at 4°C. After electrophoresis, the plates remain in a moist chamber overnight and are rinsed in saline three times for 2 h. After a final 1 h

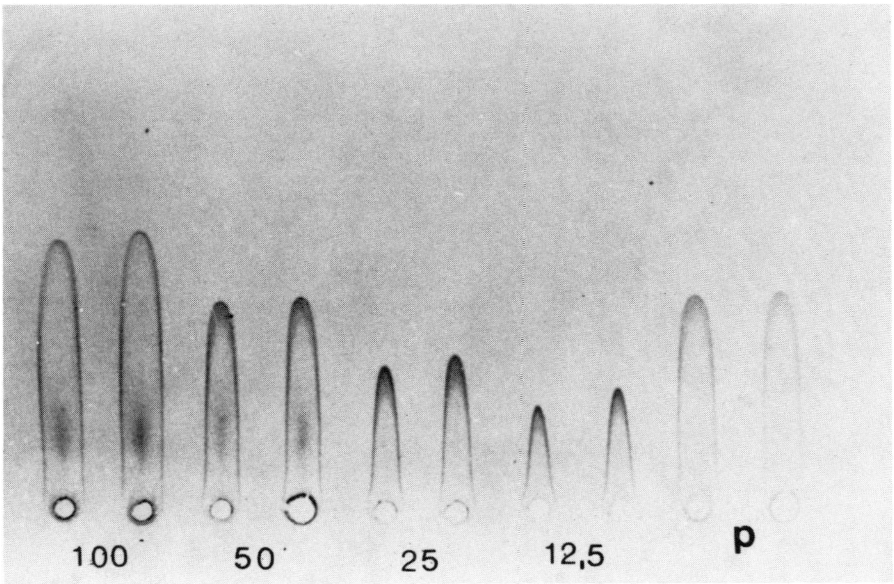

FIGURE 2. Measurement of AT-III concentration by rocket immunoelectrophoresis. The "rockets" of the patient's plasma can be seen in the right side of the figure. The other rockets represent the dilution series of normal plasma (100, 50, 25, and 12.5%) in duplicates. The higher the AT-III concentration of the sample, the bigger the distance of the top of the "rocket" from the well.

rinse in distilled water, the plates are covered with filter paper (Whatman No. 1) and left to dry overnight. Coomassie Brillant Blue staining is used. The electrophoretic mobility of AT-III is expressed as the distance between the center of the well and the projected point on to the base line (Figure 3).

C. FUNCTIONAL ASSAYS

1. Methods Measuring the Progressive Inactivation Of the Enzyme (Without Heparin

a. Inactivation of Thrombin in Plasma (Clotting Assay, Gerendás' Method)

This method was described originally for the determination of the inactivation of thrombin in serum.[10] It reflects the initial rate of thrombin-inactivation. In our laboratory, we have applied this method for more than 20 years, mainly for screening purposes. However, in the course of time, several modifications (or more accurately, "modernizations") have been performed on it. We will describe this method shortly as we use it in our laboratory at present.

Citrated plasma of the patient is defibrinated with reptilase. One vial of Reptilase-Reagent (Boehringer Mannheim GmbH, West Germany) is solved in 10 ml distilled water and 0.1 ml of this diluted reptilase is added to 0.9 ml plasma. The mixture is incubated for 20 min at 37°C. Then, the fibrin is removed by centrifugation (2000 g for 10 min.) In the assay, 0.3 ml defibrinated plasma is mixed with 0.2 ml Tris-saline buffer (pH 7.4, containing 0.05 *M* tris and 0.15 *M* saline, titrated to pH 7.4 with 1 *M* HCl) and incubated for 30 sec in a clotting tube at 37°C. Then, 0.3 ml thrombin solution (30 NIH unit per ml) is added to and mixed with the buffered defibrinated plasma. After 1, 2, 3, 4, and 5 min, 0.1 ml samples are taken and mixed with 0.1 ml fibrinogen solution at 37°C. (The fibrinogen solution contains 4 mg fibrinogen per ml.) The clotting times of the second incubation mixture are measured. Using a semilogarithmic paper for the plotting, a straight line can be obtained (Figure 4).

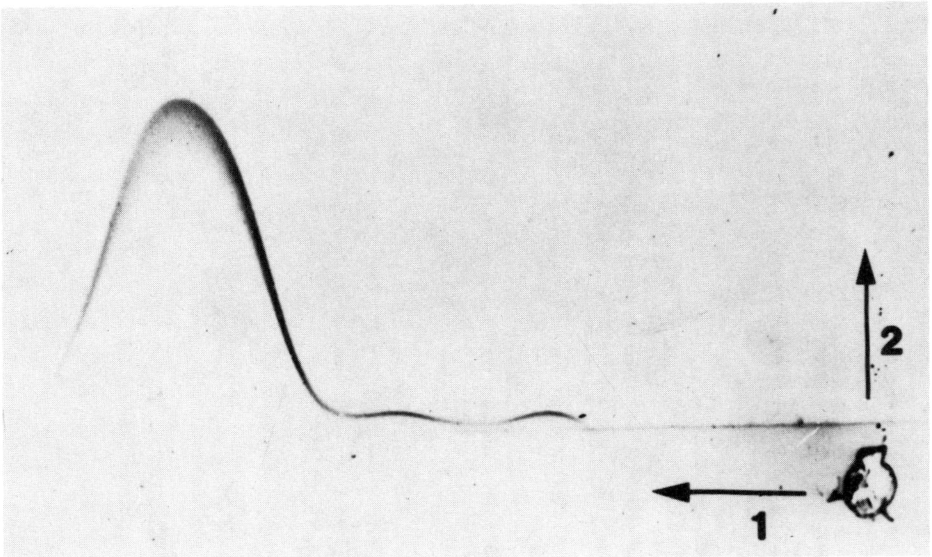

FIGURE 3. AT-III pattern of normal plasma obtained by the modified crossed immunoelectrophoresis method (heparin in agarose). In the presence of heparin, the electrophoretic mobility of normal AT-III increases in the first dimension ($\leftarrow_1$). In the course of the second electrophoresis ($\uparrow_2$), AT-III migrates into the gel containing the AT-III specific antibody. The height and localization of the precipitation arches depend on the concentration and electrophoretic mobility of AT-III, respectively.

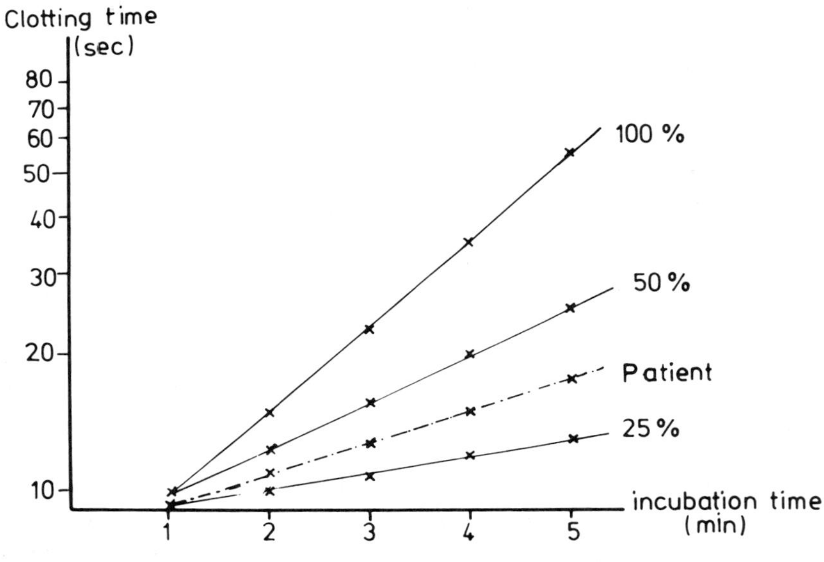

FIGURE 4. Inactivation of thrombin in defibrinated plasma. Incubating thrombin with defibrinated plasma, samples are taken at various times (1, 2, 3, 4, and 5 min), and their thrombin activities are measured by the clotting of the fibrinogen solution. Depending on the AT-III activity of the plasma, the clotting times increase progressively. The higher the AT-III activity of the sample, the faster the increase of the clotting time, i.e., the less the residual thrombin activity. Preparing a dilution series of normal plasma (100, 50, and 25%), the AT-III activity of the patient's plasma can be determined by interpolation. (From *Thromb. Diath. Haemorrh.*, 32, 105, 1975. With permission.)

Preparing a dilution series of defibrinated pooled normal human plasma with a citrated buffer (citrated tris-saline buffer is made from one part 3.8% sodium citrate and nine parts tris-saline buffer), the thrombin-inactivating activity of the patient's plasma can be expressed in percent of the normal value. The mixed plasma of at least eight healthy donors is defibrinated by Reptilase (see earlier), and the thrombin-inactivation of the particular dilutions has to be measured as it is described here.

b. Inactivation of Thrombin in Plasma (Clotting Assay, Abildgaard's Method)

This assay also measures the initial rate of thrombin inactivation.[12] Defibrinated plasma is diluted and incubated with thrombin in the first stage. After a standard incubation time, the residual thrombin activity is proportional with the AT-III activity of the tested plasma. The thrombin activity is measured in the second stage by clotting diluted bovine plasma. This assay is sometimes used in our laboratory as an alternative to the Gerendás method.

For removing fibrinogen from the test plasma, heat defibrination is applied. In a stoppered glass tube, 1 ml of test plasma is immersed in a waterbath of 56°C for exactly 5 min with occasional tiltings, immersed in ice water for 5 min, and centrifuged at 2000 g for 7 min. The defibrinated plasma is pipetted off and 1/10 dilution is prepared with a phosphate buffer (0.053 *M* pH 8.0). Then, 0.4 ml diluted defibrinated plasma is mixed with 0.1 ml thrombin solution (30 NIH units/ml). After exactly 3 min incubation at 37°C, a 0.1 ml sample is transferred from this incubation mixture to 0.3 ml diluted bovine plasma. (Diluted bovine plasma, pH 7.1 to 7.3, ionic strength: 0.12. One volume of bovine plasma is mixed with 2 volumes of veronal buffer, pH 7.35 and 2 volumes of 0.03 *M* phosphate buffer, pH 7.0.) For the determination of AT-III activity of the patient's plasma, serial dilutions of normal plasma are prepared (1:8, 1:10, 1:13, 1:20), and their thrombin-inactivating activity is measured as described earlier. A standard curve can be prepared by the clotting times obtained with the various dilutions, and the AT-III activity of the patients' plasma can be determined by interpolation.

c. Inactivation of Thrombin in Plasma (Amidolytic Assay, Abildgaard's Method)

This method is used mainly for research purposes in cases of qualitative abnormalities of AT-III. We use this assay to measure the rate of inactivation of thrombin in the absence of heparin, i.e., the function of the active center of the AT-III molecule can be investigated independently from the heparin-sensitive site by this method. The original assay of Abildgaard et al.[14] was adapted to our laboratory and later, instead of S-2160, the more specific and sensitive chromogenic substrate, S-2238, was applied. We describe this assay shortly as we use it in our laboratory.

In essence, defibrinated plasma is incubated with thrombin, and at various times, samples are taken from this mixture and added to the solution of the chromogenic substrate. The residual thrombin activity, which can be measured spectrophotometrically by the production of p-nitroaniline (pNA) is inversely proportionate to the AT-III activity of the plasma tested.

In stage I, 0.10 ml buffer (Phosphate buffer, 0.1 *M*, pH 7.4), 0.10 ml saline, 0.2 ml defibrinated plasma, and 0.10 ml thrombin (25 NIH units per ml) are mixed and incubated at 37°C. In stage II, 0.1 ml sample is taken from the first incubation mixture at various times (0.5, 4, 8, and 11 min) and added to and mixed with 0.4 ml S-2238 solution (S-2238 solution: 1 vial, Kabi Diagnostica Sweden, is solved in 8.5 ml distilled water at 60°C and diluted with phosphate buffer in a proportion of 1:9. Before use, the solution is prewarmed at 37°C). The adsorbance of the substrate sample mixture is measured every 30 sec at 37°C. The thrombin-inactivating activity of the patient's plasma can be expressed in percent of the normal value if we carry out the assay with different dilutions of pooled normal plasma.

d. Inactivation of Activated Factor X (F Xa) in Plasma (Clotting Assay, Biggs' Method)

This assay is applied mainly for the investigations of qualitative AT-III deficiencies. In our laboratory, the method of Biggs et al.[13] is used with some modifications.

In essence, F Xa is incubated with plasma and samples are taken after various intervals to measure the residual F Xa activity of the incubation mixture. The higher the F Xa inactivating activity of the plasma tested, the longer the clotting time of the detector system which consists of factor X deficient plasma, phospholipid, and calcium.

Placed and mixed in a plastic tube are 0.2 ml F Xa (Factor Xa, Sigma Chemical Co., U.S.) 0.1 ml saline and 0.2 ml diluted plasma. (The test plasma is diluted with citrated saline in a proportion of 1:2). The incubation tube is covered by Parafilm. After 5, 10, and 20 min of incubation, the 0.1 ml sample is taken from this mixture and transferred to a 0.1 ml volume of 0.05 *M* $CaCl_2$ solution. Immediately afterwards, 0.2 ml of the mixture (1:1) of factor X-deficient substrate plasma and platelet substitute (Asolectin, Associated Conc. U.S.). A stock solution of 3.8% concentration is prepared with saline. From this stock solution, a 1:10 dilution is prepared with saline, is added and the clotting time recorded. By means of a dilution series of normal pooled plasma (1:2, 1:3, 1:4 dilutions with citrated saline) and of measuring the F Xa inactivation of the various dilutions as it was described earlier, a calibration curve can be prepared. Plotting the clotting times obtained with the patient's plasma, the F Xa inactivating activity can be interpolated by the calibration curve.

e. Inactivation of Activated Factor X (F Xa) in Plasma (Amidolytic Assay, Ødegard's Method)

This method is used mainly for research purposes in cases of the qualitative abnormalities of AT-III. The rate of inactivation of F Xa can be measured with this assay independently from the heparin cofactor activity of the AT-III molecule. The original assay of Ødegard et al.[18] has been adapted to our laboratory and we perform it as follows: In essence, defibrinated plasma is incubated with F Xa and, at various times, samples are taken from this mixture and added to the solution of the chromogenic substrate. The residual F Xa activity, which can be measured spectrophotometrically by the production of pNA, is inversely proportionate to the AT-III activity of the plasma tested.

In stage I, 0.05 ml buffer (phosphate buffer, 0.1 *M*, pH 7.4), 0.05 ml saline, 0.1 ml defibrinated plasma, and 0.05 ml F Xa solution (F Xa: Sigma Chemical Co., U.S.) (reconsituted in 0.5 ml distilled water and kept in an ice water bath) are mixed and incubated at 37°C. In stage II, a 0.1 ml sample is taken from the first incubation mixture at various times (0.5, 4, 8, and 11 min) and added to and mixed with 0.4 ml S-2222 solution (S-2222 solution: 1 vial, KabiDiagnostica, Sweden) is solved in 8.5 ml distilled water at 60°C and diluted with phosphate buffer in a proportion of 1:9. Before use, the solution is prewarmed at 37°C. The adsorbance of the substrate-sample mixture is measured in every 30 sec at 37°C. The F Xa inactivating activity of the patient's plasma can be expressed in percent of the normal value if we perform the assay with different dilutions of pooled normal plasma as well.

2. Methods Measuring the Inactivation of the Enzyme in the Presence of Heparin (Heparin Cofactor Assays)

a. Heparin Cofactor Activity of Plasma (Using Thrombin and Fibrinogen)

We introduced this assay in our laboratory in 1966, as it was described by Hensen and Loeliger.[11] Since that time, several modifications ("modernizations") of the method have been performed. We describe this assay here as we perform it in our laboratory at present.

In essence, diluted defibrinated plasma is mixed with heparin and a standard quantity of fibrinogen. Thrombin is added to this mixture: the clotting time depends on the heparin cofactor activity of the plasma tested. By a dilution series of normal plasma, the heparin cofactor activity of the patient can be expressed in percent of the normal value.

Citrated plasma of the patient and citrated pooled normal human plasma are defibrinated with reptilase. One vial of Reptilase-Reagent (Boehringer Mannheim Gmbh, West Germany) is solved in 10 ml distilled water, and 0.1 ml of this diluted reptilase solution is added to 0.9 ml plasma (the patient's and normal plasma). The mixture is incubated for 20 min at 37°C. Then, the fibrin is removed by centrifugation (2000 g for 10 min).

From the defibrinated plasma of the patient, a 1:9 dilution is prepared with citrated tris-saline buffer (citrated tris-saline buffer is made of one part 3.8% sodium citrate and nine parts tris-saline buffer). From the defibrinated normal plasma, a dilution series of 1:5, 1:9, 1:14, 1:19, and 1:24 are prepared with citrated saline.

Diluted defibrinated plasma (0.1 ml) is mixed with 0.1 ml heparin (5 U/ml, Richter Gedeon Pharmaceuticals, Hungary) and with fibrinogen solution (0.2 ml, 4 mg/ml, KabiVitrum AB, Sweden). The mixture is prewarmed at 37°C for 1 min and clotted with 0.1 ml thrombin (10 NIH U/ml). The clotting times are measured at least in duplicate. A calibration curve can be prepared by the clotting times obtained with the various dilutions of defibrinated normal plasma, and the heparin cofactor activity of the patient's plasma can be determined by interpolation.

b. Heparin Cofactor Activity of Plasma (Using Thrombin and Chromogenic Substrate)

At present, this method is used most frequently for the determination of AT-III activity.[67] Both quantitative and qualitative AT-III deficiencies give abnormal (low) AT-III values with this assay. Hence, this method is advised for screening purposes. In our laboratory, we use the COATEST Antithrombin (Kabi Diagnostica, Sweden) reagent kit, which contains all the reagents required (chromogenic substrate S-2238, heparin, thrombin, and polybren).

Rationale of the assay: test plasma, not defibrinated, is diluted in buffer containing EDTA and heparin. Thrombin is added in excess, and the mixture is incubated at 37°C for a certain period of time. An amount of thrombin is inhibited by the AT-III-heparin complex in proportion to the amount of AT-III. After neutralizing the heparin with Polybrene, the remaining amount of thrombin catalyzes the splitting of pNA from the substrate. The release of pNA is allowed to proceed for a certain period of time and is stopped with acetic acid. The adsorbance of free pNA, measured at 405 nm, decreases linearly with increasing concentrations of AT-III. The concentration of AT-III is calculated from a standard curve prepared from human normal plasma dilutions.

Procedure: To construct a reference curve, 300 μl of pooled normal human plasma is diluted with 3.25 ml of buffer with heparin (buffer with heparin: Tris 50 mmol/l, EDTA 7.5 mm/l, and 3 IU heparin per ml, pH 8.4, I 0.2) and than further diluted as follows:

Standards AT-III activity(%)	Buffer with heparin (μl)	Diluted normal plasma (μl)
25	2300	100
50	2200	200
75	2100	300
100	2000	400
125	1900	500

The test plasma is prepared for assay by diluting 50 μl with 3.5 ml buffer with heparin. A sample (400 μl) of the diluted test plasma or standard is incubated at 37°C for 3 to 6 min, and thrombin (100 μl, 30 nkat/ml) is added with mixing. Exactly 30 sec later, 300 μl of prewarmed S-2238 solution (S-2238 with Polybrene, 7 mg S-2238, and 5 mg Polybrene, lyophilized and reconstituted with 15 ml distilled water) is added with vigorous mixing at

37°C. After an additional 30 sec, 300 μl of 50% acetic acid is added to stop the reaction. Absorbance at 405 nm is measured against its blank (Blank: 400 μl of the diluted test plasma, diluted pooled normal plasma, 300 μl of 50% acetic acid, and 400 μl distilled water).

The AT-III concentration can be read from the standard curve.

c. Heparin Cofactor Activity of Plasma (Using Activated Factor X in the Clotting Assay)

This method is based originally on the assay of Biggs et al.,[13] but it was modified to measure the accelerating effect of heparin in the reaction of F Xa and AT-III. In general, we perform this assay simultaneously with the measurement of the progressive inactivation of F Xa (clotting assay, in absence of heparin).

In essence, F Xa is incubated with plasma in the presence of heparin, and samples are taken after various intervals to measure the residual F Xa activity of the incubation mixture. The higher the F Xa inactivation activity of the plasma tested in the presence of heparin, the longer the clotting time of the detector system which consists of factor X deficient plasma, phospholipid, and calcium.

Placed and mixed in a plastic tube are 0.2 ml F Xa, (Factor Xa, Sigma Chemical Co., U.S.) 0.1 ml heparin solution (0.5 U/ml of activity) and 0.1 ml diluted plasma. (The test plasma is diluted with citrate saline in a proportion of 1:2.) The incubation tube is covered by Parafilm. After 1, 3, and 5 min, incubation, a 0.1 ml sample is taken from this mixture and transferred to 0.1 ml volume of 0.05 *M* $CaCl_2$ solution. Immediately afterwards, 0.2 ml of mixture (1:1) of factor X deficient substrate plasma and platelet substitute (Asolectin, Associated Conc., U.S.), stock solution of 3.8 concentration, is prepared with saline. From this stock solution, a 1:10 dilution is prepared with saline, and the clotting time recorded. By means of a dilution series of normal pooled plasma (1:2, 1:3, 1:4 dilutions with citrated saline) and of measuring the F Xa inactivation of the various dilutions as it was described earlier, a calibration curve can be prepared. Plotting the clotting times obtained with the patient's plasma, the heparin cofactor activity can be interpolated by the calibration curve.

d. Heparin Cofactor Activity of Plasma (Using Activated Factor X in the Amidolytic Assay)

We use this method mainly for research purposes and perform it in the course of investigations of variant AT-III molecules. A kinetic variant of the original method of Ødegard et al.[16] has been developed in our laboratory and generally, we perform it simultaneously with the measurement of the progressive inactivation of activated factor X (the amidolytic method, in the absence of heparin).

Defibrinated plasma is incubated with F Xa in the presence of heparin. At various times, samples are taken from this incubation mixture and added to the solution of the chromogenic substrate. The residual F Xa activity, which can be measured spectrophotometrically by the production of pNA, is inversely proportionate to the heparin cofactor activity of the plasma tested.

In stage I, 0.05 ml buffer (phosphate buffer, 0.1 *M*, pH 7.4) 0.05 ml heparin in saline (0.1 and 0.05 unit heparin per ml) 0.1 ml defibrinated plasma, and 0.05 ml activated factor X (F Xa) solution (F Xa: Sigma Chemical Co., U.S.), reconstituted in 0.5 ml distilled water and kept in an ice water bath) are mixed and incubated at 37°C. In stage II, a 0.1 ml sample is taken from the first incubation mixture at various times (0.5, 1.0, 1.5, and 2.0 min) and added to and mixed with 0.4 ml S-2222 solution (S-2222 solution: one vial, KabiDiagnostica, Sweden, is solved in 8.5 ml distilled water at 60°C and diluted with a phosphate buffer in a proportion of 1:9. Before use, the solution is prewarmed at 37°C). The adsorbance of the substrate-sample mixture is measured every 30 sec at 37°C. The heparin cofactor activity of the patient's plasma can be expressed in percent of the normal value if we perform the assay with different dilutions of pooled normal plasma.

D. HEPARIN-AFFINITY CHROMATOGRAPHY

This method is used mainly for the separation of AT-III and, in the course of investigations of various qualitative AT-III deficiencies, to characterize the heparin-affinity of a particular AT-III variant.

In our laboratory, we use the method of Miller-Andersson et al.,[15] using Heparin-Sepharose CL-6B (Pharmacia, Sweden) instead of preparing heparin-agarose from cyanogen bromide-activated agarose gel. The Heparin-Sepharose CL-6B column (2.54 × 30 cm, V_c = 190 ml) is equilibrated with a 25 m*M* morpholinopropane-sulfonic acid (MOPS Sigma, U.S.) buffer (pH 7.4) containing 0.15 *M* NaCl. Applied and washed with the buffer (4 to 5 volumes of total column) is 10 ml of plasma. A linear NaCl gradient (from 0.15 to 1.2 *M*) is introduced in 4 h with a flow rate of 45 ml/h using LKB Ultragrad Gradient Mixer and collecting 5 ml fractions. AT-III is detected by the Uvicord II system and measured by the Mancini technique.

E. EXPRESSION OF THE RESULTS, STANDARDIZATION

As it was mentioned in the introduction of this chapter, the AT-III level can be expressed in different ways. In the case of immunological assays, the AT-III concentration of a sample can be expressed simply in weight units, i.e., g/l (earlier mg/100 ml). However, the concentration of AT-III in many cases, such as congenital qualitative AT-III deficiencies or DIC, is not parallel with functional activity.

Hence, in the case of functional assays, the expression of the AT-III activity of a sample in units seems to be preferable. Most often, one AT-III unit is defined as the AT-III activity of 1 ml of normal pooled human plasma. The results of immunoassays can also be expressed in units (defining 1 unit as the AT-III antigen concentration of normal pooled human plasma). This method proved to be reliable in practice on account of the relatively constant AT-III activity and concentration of healthy individuals (not taking oral contraceptives, etc.). An international collaborative study, establishing a reference preparation for AT-III, used this approach for standardization.[68] As a reference preparation, the freeze-dried pooled normal plasma proved to be superior compared with purified AT-III preparations. Later, in accordance with the endeavors of the international standardization of laboratory data, Conard et al.[69] proposed to express the AT-III level in molar concentration. However, this method also seems not to be flawless. First, the basic assumption is a 1:1 stoichiometry in the thrombin-AT-III reaction, which is not perfectly correct because inhibitors other than AT-III take part in the inactivation of thrombin in plasma. Second, in the case of qualitatively abnormal AT-III molecules, the stoichiometry of the thrombin-AT-III reaction is uncertain. In some variants, even the molecular weight of AT-III is different from that of normal. Therefore, the expression of a AT-III level in molar concentration seems to be theoretically inaccurate, practically complicated, like in the cases of other proteins.

F. DETERMINATION OF THROMBIN-AT-III COMPLEXES

The clinical significance of the determination of thrombin-AT-III complexes lies in the diagnoses of thrombotic events. Patients disposed to thrombosis and disseminated intravascular coagulation are found to have elevated concentrations of this complex.

Collen and De Cock first presented evidence that antisera may be raised in rabbits with a purified thrombin-AT-III complex.[289,290] After purification, these antisera form precipitation lines with serum containing the complex, but not with plasma containing the precursor molecule. A latex agglutination technique was developed using polystyrene particles coated with specific antibodies for the quantitation of thrombin-AT-III complex in human blood.[291] In patients with coagulation tests suggestive of disseminated intravascular coagulation, elevated titers of the complex were found.[292]

Lau and Rosenberg described a radioimmunoassay for the determination of thrombin-

AT-III complex.[293] They raised antisera against human thrombin-AT-III complex and purified the respective immunoglobulin fractions. The specific antibody population obtained was utilized to construct a double antibody radioimmunoassay capable of measuring as little as 30 ng/ml of the complex. The immunoreactivities of prothrombin and AT-III were negligible. The factor Xa-AT-III complex was about 320 times less reactive than the thrombin-AT-III complex on a molar basis. The same group of investigators used this method for the determination of the concentration of thrombin-AT-III complexes in patients with disseminated intravascular coagulation.[294,295] As expected, the level of thrombin-AT-III complexes was significantly elevated during the *in vivo* activation of the hemostatic mechanism.

The investigators of the Behring Institute, West Germany, developed a method for the determination of thrombin-AT-III complexes by the sandwich principle.[296] The reagents for this method are now commercially available (''Enzygnost-TAT'') and the first clinical experiences seem to prove the usefulness of this reagent kit. During the first incubation, the thrombin-AT-III complex present in the plasma sample is bound to the thrombin antibodies fixed to the surface of plastic tubes. After washing, peroxidase-conjugated antibodies to human AT-III are bound to the free AT-III determinants in a second reaction. The excess enzyme-conjugated antibodies are washed out, and the bound enzyme activity is subsequently determined. The enzymatic reaction of hydrogen peroxide with chromogen is stopped by the addition of dilute sulfuric acid. The color intensity is proportional to the concentration of the thrombin-AT-III complexes.

II. AT-III DEFICIENT STATES

A. INTRODUCTION

Before discussing AT-III deficient states, we have to clarify some notions.

First, we have to define the concept of ''AT-III deficiency'' itself. At first glance, it seems to be very easy to do, because in a deficient state, the AT-III level is lower than the normal value. However, in this definition, the normal value of AT-III is critically important because the AT-III level (concentration and functional activity) even in healthy persons, may depend on many conditions (e.g., race, age, sex, the assay system applied etc.). Furthermore, we have to know the normal distribution of the AT-III level in the particular section of the population before declaring an AT-III deficient state. Hence, we first have to discuss the problem of ''normal value of AT-III.''

Second, having encountered an AT-III deficient state, we have to classify it for theoretical and practical reasons as well. In principle, the AT-III deficient state can be the result of either the decrease (or qualitatively abnormal) production of this protein or increased consumption (catabolism). A third possibility of a low AT-III level is an increased transcapillary flux. Although this approach is correct for the theoretical point of view, it is almost useless in practice. On the one hand, we cannot easily determine a particular patient's metabolic characteristics of AT-III. On the other hand, the simultaneous decrease of production and increased loss of AT-III experienced in many cases, makes this classification inappropriate. Therefore, the principles of classification of AT-III deficient states need a separate discussion.

B. NORMAL VALUE OF AT-III

Earlier reported estimates of the AT-III concentration in normal human plasma vary between 0.10 and 0.42 g/l. The lowest level was described by Abildgaard,[70] while the highest one was described by Heimburger.[71] These measurements were based on the determination of the protein concentration of purified AT-III preparation having the same inhibitor activity and/or antigen amount taken as reference plasma. The main sources of error in such measurements are the presence of inactive protein in the purified preparation and errors related to the determination of protein. The very high AT-III concentration reported by Heimburger

TABLE 2
Classification of AT-III Deficient States

I. Congenital AT-III deficiencies
  A. Type 1 (quantitative deficiency of AT-III)
  B. Type 2 (qualitative AT-III deficiency of AT-III)
    1. Type 2a (combined functional deficiency
    2. Type 2b (isolated disorder of serpin activity)
    3. Type 2c (isolated disorder of the heparin-AT-III reaction)
  C. Type 3 (quantitative and qualitative deficiency of AT-III)

II. Acquired AT-III deficiencies
  (caused by reduced synthesis and/or increased catabolism and/or increased transcapillary flux)

probably reflects the presence of inactive protein in his preparation.[71] Murano et al.[72] reported a doubling of the specific activity of their AT-III preparations after removing inactive material. The very low AT-III concentration reported by Abildgaard can be explained by the use of an inappropriate extinction coefficient.[70] Further investigations with more sophisticated, and accurate methods measured the AT-III concentration of normal human plasma to be 0.19 ± 0.02 g/l.[5,72,73] Conard et al.,[69] using a purified bovine thrombin preparation in the thrombin-AT-III reaction, reported a 0.15 g/l (2.57 μmol/l) value for AT-III level in normal human plasma.

In clinical practice, we compare the AT-III level of a particular plasma sample to the normal human plasma and express the results in units or percent, taking 1 unit or 100 percent value for the normal human plasma. Different pooled reference plasma preparations may differ as to their contents of AT-III. This source of error is slight when care is taken to exclude donors using contraceptive pills or other drugs influencing AT-III levels (e.g., heparin, metabolic steroids, etc.) because the variation with age and sex is slight. Ødegard et al.[74] measured the heparin cofactor activity with an amidolytic method and AT-III concentration with simple radial immundiffusion in plasma from 219 men and 177 women. Narrow ranges for AT-III activity and AT-III concentration were found. The standard deviation for the heparin cofactor activities in men and women were 8.6 and 10.1, respectively, for AT-III concentrations of 10.4 and 12.5 (percent). In men, mean AT-III levels (both activity and concentration) decreased significantly with increasing age. In women, mean heparin cofactor activities and mean AT-III concentrations tended to be lower in fertile age. Similar observations were published by Panicucci et al.[75]

Taking these data into consideration, reference plasma (pooled normal plasma) for AT-III determinations can be prepared from the blood of 20 normal human donors of both sexes, aged 18 to 40, not on medication. Blood is collected in a 1:9 volume of 0.106 *M* sodium citrate and centrifuged at 3000 g for 30 min. Equal amounts of citrated plasma from the donors are mixed and the aliquot kept frozen at −20°C. The activity of the various pools differ less than 2%.[69]

C. PRINCIPLE OF THE CLASSIFICATION OF AT-III DEFICIENT STATES

In the clinical practice, the AT-III deficient states are divided into two main groups (Table 2).

The AT-III deficiencies, characterized by an inherited, congenital deficiency of AT-III, belong to the first group. In these cases, the production of AT-III is impaired quantitatively or, rarely, qualitatively. The first reports on congenital AT-III deficiency-described thrombophilic families characterized by low AT-III functional activities and antigen concentrations.[76,77,78] Therefore, this type of AT-III deficiency is called Type 1 quantitative or sometimes, "classical" type of AT-III deficiency. Generally, the AT-III concentration is about half of the normal value in the plasma of these patients. Later, thrombophilic families have been reported, characterized by diminished functional activities but normal AT-III concentrations.[79,80,81] These cases belong to the qualitative disorders of AT-III production, designated qualitative, of Type 2 AT-III deficiencies or, sometimes, "dysantithrombinemias." In cases of qualitative AT-III deficiencies, only a proportion (generally 50%) of the AT-III molecules is abnormal, the other part is normal. In Type 2 AT-III deficiency, various subtypes have also been differentiated.[83] In one subgroup, Type 2a, a profound disorder of AT-III molecules can be detected. Cases belonging to this subgroup are characterized by at least two independently detectable pathological changes of AT-III molecules. In a Type 2b abnormality, the active center of a AT-III molecule is impaired. In these patients, an isolated deficiency of thrombin and F Xa inactivation can be found. In a Type 2c AT-III deficiency, only the heparin cofactor activity is decreased; the active center of the AT-III molecule functions well, shown by normal progressive thrombin and F Xa inactivation. The heterogeneity of even this subgroup is obvious and will be discussed in details later on.

The third main group of congenital AT-III deficiencies (Type 3) is characterized by the combined quantitative and qualitative disturbance of AT-III production.

This classification of the congenital AT-III deficiencies is based mainly on the laboratory methods available at present and it serves practical diagnostic and therapeutic purposes. From the theoretical point of view, a classification based on the molecular basis of the particular variants seems to be more preferable. At present, however, only in a slight minority of the cases is the molecular defect definied precisely.

Sometimes it is not an easy task to prove that an AT-III abnormality is congenital or not. In the majority of cases, patients with quantitative or qualitative AT-III abnormalities have characteristic clinical features and laboratory signs which can be detected in other family members as well. However, it may occur that there is no other available member of the family for investigations. In these cases, only family history can give some information demonstrating the frequent thromboembolic complications at the other family members in young age. However, in the case of Type 2c AT-III deficiency, a part of the patients is not affected by thromboembolic complications and the disorder turns out by chance. In lack of other family members, the congenital or acquired type of the disorder can hardly be differentiated.

The other main group of AT-III deficiency is acquired, that is, it develops only in a later stage of life; it is generally connected with some basic disease. This group of AT-III deficiencies is also very inhomogenous. In a part of this disorder, the AT-III production is diminished, while in others, the low AT-III level is connected with increased consumption. Not infrequently, the combination of decreased production and increased consumption is in the background of the AT-III deficiency. Earlier, it was thought that in severe liver disease subnormal AT-III production in DIC increased consumption are responsible for a low AT-III-level. But further studies suggest that low production may occur in DIC and increased consumption in liver failure.[84,85] Making the situation even more complicated, an increased transcapillary flux of AT-III may contribute to a low AT-III level in liver disease.[86] Therefore, the acquired AT-III deficiencies are discussed according to the basic diseases.

D. CONGENITAL AT-III DEFICIENCIES

1. Prevalence of AT-III Deficiencies

Since the discovery of familial AT-III deficiency by Egeberg, the disorder has been reported in all parts of the world.[76] Such cases were found in Europe, America, Africa, Asia, and Australia.[77,78,82,87,96-108] Clearly, AT-III deficiency is involved in the pathogenesis of thromboembolic diseases all over the world. However, the frequency of this disorder has not been firmly established yet; we have only rough estimations.

Ødegard and Abildgaard studied the prevalence of AT-III deficiencies in a Norwegian population of 25,000 women and established it to be one per 5000,[109] whereas the estimate for the Massachusetts population by Rosenberg is one per 2000.[110] Winter suggests a lower frequency in Scotland.[111] Another approach to studying the frequency of AT-III deficiencies is to measure the AT-III level in patients with deep venous thrombosis and/or pulmonary embolism. Lechner et al.[89] measured the plasma AT-III levels in 290 patients with thromboembolic manifestations and found nine families with AT-III deficiencies. Juillet et al.[112] studied 86 patients admitted to a hospital for recurrent or extensive venous thrombosis and found two families with AT-III deficiencies. Rosenberg estimates a frequency of 2% in such patients.[110] These data suggest a frequency of 2 to 3% in patients presenting deep venous thrombosis or pulmonary embolism.

The prevalence of AT-III deficiencies probably is different in various populations of the world. However, when we compare data from various sources, we have to consider many circumstances establishing real differences. An important factor is the method applied for screening purposes. Only heparin cofactor assays can reveal all types of AT-III deficiencies (quantitative + qualitative) because other methods can only detect a proportion of them. By immunological methods, we cannot detect qualitative disorders, although there are some very rare exceptions. Similarly, assays measuring progressive thrombin or F Xa inactivation cannot furnish information about isolated heparin cofactor (Type 2c AT-III) deficiencies.

When we study the frequency of AT-III deficencies in patients with thromboembolic symptoms, further factors of uncertainty come to effect. It is a well-known fact that the diagnoses of thromboembolic diseases is rather vague on the basis of clinical symptoms. In some cases, there are no symptoms at all, while in others, the "typical" thromboembolic symptoms are brought about by other diseases. Thus, the real frequency of AT-III deficiencies depends not only on the real prevalence of the disorder, but on the objective methods applied as well. Another disturbing factor is the lack of thromboembolic manifestations in the majority of patients with isolated heparin cofactor deficiencies (Type 2c AT-III deficiencies). This abnormality is discovered sometimes by chance in healthy persons.

2. Various Forms of Congenital AT-III Deficiencies

The first reports on congenital AT-III deficiencies described thrombophilic families with a low (about half the normal value) activity and concentration of AT-III in the affected members.[76,77,78] The parallel decrease of progressive thrombin inactivation and heparin cofactor activity in these cases supported the notion about the identity of the plasma protein responsible for the progressive inactivation of both thrombin and activated F X in blood with the protein connected with the anticoagulant action of heparin. Because of the precedence of these reports and of the high frequency of this type of AT-III deficiency, compared with the later discovered types, the parallel decrease of functional activity and concentration of AT-III are the main characteristics of the quantitative or "classical" type (Type 1) of AT-III deficiency. It was thought that in a Type 1 AT-III deficiency a normal AT-III molecule was synthesized at about half the normal rate. This notion was supported by the investigations of Ambruso et al.[113] More recently, Knot et al.[114] also proved the reduced absolute catabolic rate (synthesis) of AT-III in congenital AT-III-deficient patients, using highly purified radiolabeled AT-III in a three-compartment model. Gomperts et al.[105] were the first in 1976 to demonstrate that in a thrombophilic family belonging to the "classical" type of AT-III deficiency, AT-III molecules migrated slower in the heparinized agarose gel than that of the normal AT-III. Later, having the opportunity to compare two AT-III deficient families, we demonstrated directly the heterogeneity of a Type 1 AT-III deficiency.[82] In both families, the affected members had about half the activity and concentration of AT-III compared with normal plasma, but the patterns of the precipitaion arches were different in the modified crossed immunoelectrophoresis system (heparin in agarose), as demonstrated by Figure 5.

In one family, the electrophoretic mobility of AT-III was identical with that of normal AT-III. In the other, the AT-III displayed a decreased electrophoretic mobility in the hep-

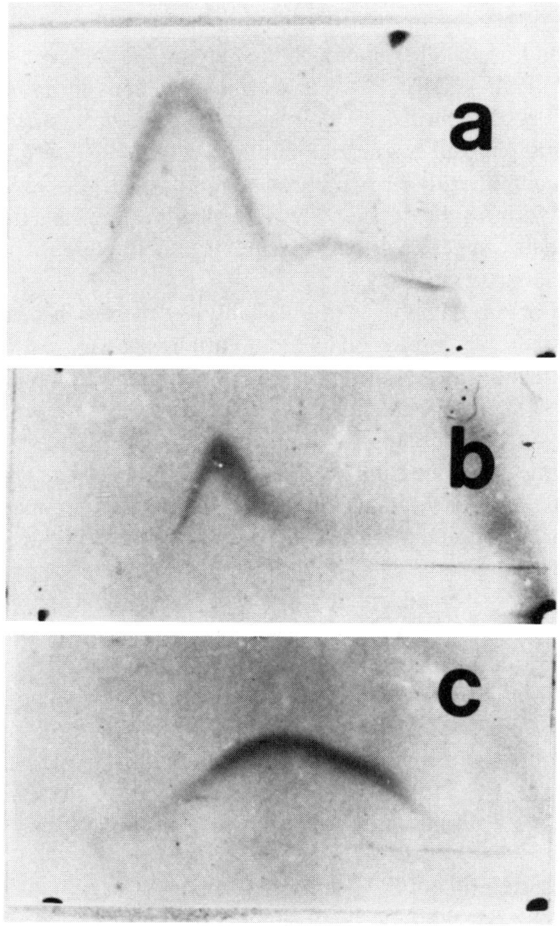

FIGURE 5. Various AT-III patterns of different plasma samples obtained by the modified crossed immunoelectrophoresis method (heparin in agarose): (a) normal plasma, (b) Type 1 (quantitative) AT-III deficiency, (c) Type 3 (quantitative + qualitative) AT-III deficiency (previously designated as Type 1b AT-III deficiency).

arinized agarose gel. The relatively low affinity of this AT-III to heparin could be directly proven by heparin-agarose affinity chromatography, too. On the basis of these findings, we differentiated Type 1a and Type 1b AT-III deficiencies. AT-III deficiencies belonging to the Type 1a subclass were thought to be characterized by a ''pure'' quantitative deficiency, i.e., the AT-III molecules were qualitatively normal in the blood of these patients, but their amounts were decreased. Cases belonging to the Type 1b AT-III deficiency were characterized by a low level of AT-III (both activity and concentration) and a low affinity to heparin of the AT-III molecules. These data were confirmed by Williams and Murano.[116] Further investigations of Abildgaard revealed that even in the first AT-III deficient family described by Egeberg, the AT-III molecules were different from normal concerning their heparin affinity and immunological characteristics.[118] However, by applying more and more sensitive techniques, various forms of quantitative AT-III deficiencies have been described in which other qualitative abnormalities of AT-III molecules have also been detected. Hence, the Type 1b subclass proved to be too narrow to include all variants characterized by quantitative and qualitative abnormality of AT-III production. Consequently, these combined forms of AT-III deficiencies are classified now into a separate main group (Type 3 AT-III deficiency, vide infra).

In some families with Type 1 AT-III deficiencies, treatment with oral anticoagulants results in considerably elevated AT-III [78,80] This has not been found in other AT-III deficient families.[90,94] According to our observations, this heterogeneity of Type 1 AT-III deficiencies is independent from the heterogeneity experienced with the heparin affinity of AT-III molecules.

Prochownik et al.,[119] using a recombinant DNA technique, also demonstrated the heterogeneity of the quantitative AT-III deficiency. In one family, the deficiency is the result of a complete gene deletion, while in the other, probably a mutation gives rise to a AT-III deficiency which cannot be detected by the resolution afforded by conventional Southern blot analysis.

As it was discussed earlier, the second main group of congenital AT-III deficiences (Type 2) is characterized by reduced functional activity, but normal or nearly normal concentrations of AT-III in the plasma of these patients. In these cases, qualitatively abnormal-AT-III molecules are produced which display different degrees of deviation from normal AT-III.

AT-III abnormalities belonging to the Type 2a subclass are characterized by profound structural changes of molecules, reflected in different low thrombin and F Xa inactivations, abnormal heparin-AT-III reactions, and aberrant immunochemical structures. The heterogeneity of this subgroup is evident: in some cases, the degree of the abnormality is so high that in addition to the defect of the active center and the heparin binding site(s) of the molecule, the immunological determinants and size of the AT-III molecule are different from that of the normal. In others, the pathological change is milder, but at least two different abnormalities of the AT-III molecule have to be assumed (e.g., disturbance of the active center + abnormal immunochemical structure). The first reported family with an abnormal AT-III, AT-III "Budapest" belongs to this subgroup.[79] A middle-aged man, B.J., a member of a consanguineous family with a high prevalence of thromboembolic episodes, was admitted to our clinic in 1972 with recurrent deep venous thrombosis. He was given heparin intravenously (10,000 units) intermittently, but the clotting time remained almost unchanged. Taking this observation and the family history into account, the suspicion of AT-III deficiency arose. The very low thrombin and F Xa inactivating activities of the defibrinated plasma and of the serum, and the reduced *in vitro* activity of heparin supported this assumption. However, we were perplexed by the fact that the AT-III concentration measured by simple radial immunodiffusion was only slightly decreased repeatedly. Then, we performed these investigations on the family members available and found reduced functional activities with quite normal AT-III antigen concentrations at them. To exclude the failure (e.g., nonspecificity) of the commercial immunserum applied, we measured the AT-III concentration of one of our patients' plasma (who had typical clinical and laboratory signs of disseminated intravascular coagulation) together with the thrombophilic family. Figure 1 demonstrates that the AT-III concentration of B.J. and of his family was normal, but the patient with DIC displayed a low level of AT-III.

On the basis of these data, we hypothesized the existence of an abnormal AT-III molecule, designated AT-III "Budapest," in the plasma of the affected patients, which explained the discrepant results of the functional and immunochemical methods.

A direct proof of the existence of this abnormal AT-III was derived from our experiments with crossed immunoelectrophoresis. We found that in the presence of heparin in the first phase of crossed immunoelectrophoresis, the electrophoretic mobility of plasma AT-III increases.[20] When we investigated the proband's plasma in this system, we found that two different populations of AT-III molecules were present. A minor part of the AT-III molecules migrated to the position corresponding to normal AT-III, while the bulk of the proteins with AT-III antigenicity displayed a reduced electrophoretic mobility in the heparinized agarose gel.[26] In the original crossed immunoelectrophoresis system of Laurell,[19] in which no heparin was added to the agarose, no difference could be established comparing normal plasma with our patient's plasma. The AT-III pattern of the proband's plasma is demonstrated in Figure 6.

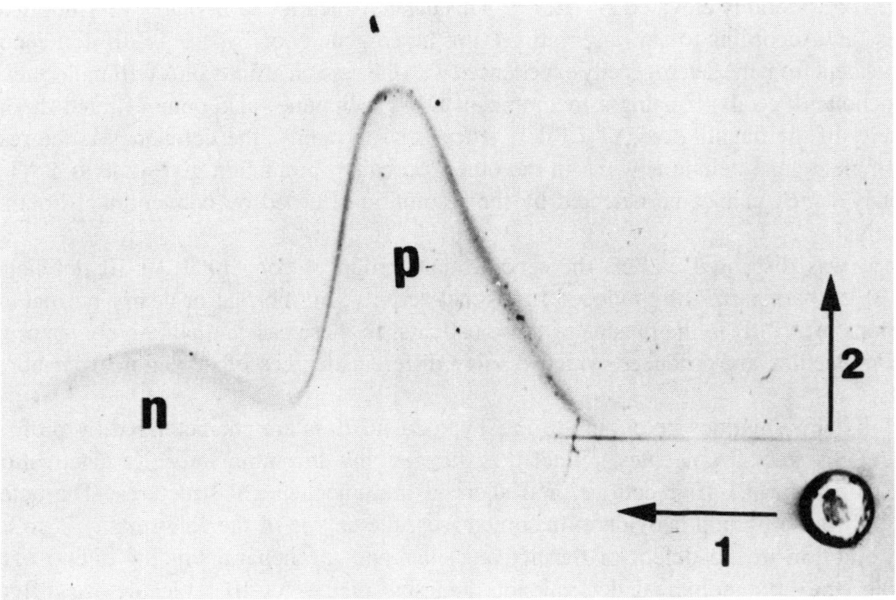

FIGURE 6. AT-III pattern of the proband's plasma with the abnormality of AT-III "Budapest" obtained by the modified crossed immunoelectrophoresis method (heparin in agarose): (n) precipitation arch of the AT-III molecules with normal electrophoretic mobility, (p) precipitation arch of the abnormal AT-III molecules with a decreased electrophoretic mobility in the heparinized agarose gel. (From *Thromb. Diath. Haemorrh.*, 33, 564, 1975. With permission.)

The abnormal AT-III pattern was demonstrated in the affected members of the family as well. In the plasma of his son and his daughter, pathological AT-III molecules could be detected, although in a lower amount. His brother and both his sisters had abnormal AT-III in their blood with a moderate decrease of normal AT-III activity. The direct detection and measurement of the abnormal AT-III made it possible to determine more accurately the type of inheritance of this possible abnormality. Analyzing the AT-III pattern of the various members of this consanguinuous family, the data indicated an autosomal codominant type of inheritance.[120]

The molecular size of abnormal AT-III (AT-III Budapest) was apparently larger than normal. Experiments with gel filtration showed that the pathological AT-III molecules were eluted earlier from the Sephadex G-200 column than that of normal AT-III.[25] The reduced heparin-affinity of AT-III Budapest was demonstrated directly later, comparig AT-III "Budapest" with AT-III "Aalborg."[121]

A very similar abnormality of AT-III was reported by Tengborn et al.[122] Values for heparin cofactor activity (S-2238) and for anti-Xa activity (S-2222) both determined in the presence of heparin, were about 50% the normal. In the absence of heparin, values for progressive AT-III and anti-Xa activity showed a slightly higher — although distinctly lower than the lower normal — limit. Crossed immunoelectrophoresis in the presence of heparin revealed an abnormal (slower) AT-III peak in addition to the normal (fast) peak. This abnormality seems to be a mutation which is transmitted in an autosomal dominant way. No data are provided about the molecular size (or weight) of this abnormality reported in Malmö. Further investigations are needed to prove or exclude the identity of AT-III "Budapest" and AT-III "Malmö."

Another variant, designated AT-III "Tokyo," was reported by Murayama and Matsuda.[123] This variant exerted no inhibition against thrombin and factor Xa; a greatly reduced affinity to heparin was demonstrated by crossed immunoelectrophoresis and heparin-Sepharose affinity chromatography. Partial immunological identity was noted with the normal AT-III molecule by double immundiffusion. The abnormal AT-III molecule, however, preserved a single chain structure and an apparently identical molecular weight with that of the normal molecule. In a further report, the same authors considered the possibility that this abnormality may be acquired rather than genetically determined.[124]

AT-III "Chicago" was reported by Bauer et al.[125] This abnormality was found in a thrombophilic family. Medical histories of 46 family members revealed 12 individuals with previous thromboembolic episodes. The subjects, investigated in detail, were found to have normal plasma concentrations of immunoreactive AT-III, decreased plasma levels of progressive AT-III activity, and reduced amounts of plasma heparin cofactor activity. A normal AT-III pattern was obtained when the plasma of the propositus was run in the crossed immunoelectrophoresis system, with or without the incorporation of heparin in the first gel dimension. By heparin-Sepharose chromatography, two populations of AT-III molecules could be differentiated: one with normal heparin-affinity and another with increased heparin affinity. These features of AT-III "Chicago" differentiate it from other AT-III variants reported up to now.

The first abnormality to show an abnormal crossed-immunoelectrophoresis in the absence of heparin was AT-III "Trento."[126] The disorder was observed in a 38-year-old female who had several episodes of deep vein thromboses of both legs. Thrombin and factor Xa inactivation was reduced regardless of the presence or absence of heparin in the assay system. The AT-III antigen concentration was normal. The most conspicuous feature of this disorder was an abnormal peak in the crossed immunoelectrophoretic system (without heparin). The abnormal peak was more anodal than the normal counterpart. The AT-III pattern was normal in the crossed immunoelectrophoretic system containing heparin in the agarose. The heparin affinity of this variant was apparently normal. Four other females were affected with this abnormality. (They were asymptomatic at the time of the publication.) Recently, the same group of investigators have demonstrated that in this family, the AT-III "Trento" abnormality was associated with von Willebrand disease.[127] The two defects seemed to segregate independently. None of the patients with a double defect showed thrombotic disease, indicating a possible protective action of the von Willebrand defect against thrombotic manifestations. No data are available for us in connection with further biochemical characterization of AT-III "Trento."

Another AT-III variant belonging to Type 2a abnormalities is AT-III "Northwick Park." In this family, the possibility of a qualitative AT-III disorder was first raised by Brozovic et al.[128] Further investigations showed reduced levels of heparin cofactor (41 to 67%) and of progressive AT-III activity (44 to 62%), but normal levels of immunoreactive AT-III. Crossed immunoelectrophoresis of AT-III in the absence of heparin revealed an abnormal, fast-moving (anodal) peak in addition to the normal peak, but the AT-III peak appeared normal in the presence of heparin. A mutation affecting the binding site of thrombin was hypothesized.[129] However, recent investigations on this abnormality detected a slightly higher affinity for heparin of the abnormal AT-III than that of the normal AT-III.[130] Variant AT-III is present in about 120,000 mol wt inactive AT-III complex that can be reduced with dithiotreitol to a molecular weight of about 60,000, indicating disulphide bridging. Using ion exchange chromatography, the inactive complex has been isolated and shown to migrate in the same position as the anodal peak on crossed immunoelectrophoresis.

A very similar variant, AT-III "Milano 1" was described by Wolf et al.[131] In eight members of an Italian thrombophilic family, a descrepancy between a normal amount of antigen and a decreased inactivation of thrombin and factor Xa (in the presence and absence of heparin) was found. By crossed immunoelectrophoresis in the absence of heparin, two peaks of AT-III were present in all the patients' plasma. Using heparin affinity chromatography, two populations of AT-III molecules were detected. The first fraction (normal AT-

TABLE 3
Type 2a AT-III Deficiencies[a]

AT-III	"Budapest" (Sas et al.,[26] Sas et al.[79])
AT-III	"Malmö" (Tengborn et al.[122])
AT-III	"Tokyo" (Murayama and Matsuda.[123])
AT-III	"Chicago" (Bauer et al.[125])
AT-III	"Trento" (Girolami et al.[126])
AT-III	"Northwick Park" (Brozovic et al.,[128] Howarth et al.,[129] Lane et al.[130])
AT-III	"Milano 1" (Wolf et al.[131])
AT-III	"Glasgow" (Lane et al.[184])

[a] Characterized by combined functional deficiencies and/or immunochemical alterations.

III) contained AT-III activity, migrated as a single peak by crossed immunoelectrophoresis, and sodium dodecyl sulphate-polyacrylamide gel electrophoresis (SDS-PAGE) demonstrated a single band with a molecular weight identical to that of normal AT-III. Conversely, the last fraction, devoid of AT-III activity, migrated as a single abnormal peak by crossed immunoelectrophoresis (in the absence of heparin). By SDS-PAGE, two bands with AT-III antigenicity were observed: one with a molecular weight of 60,000 and a second one with a molecular weight of 120,000. Reduction of the 120,000 molecular weight band by beta-mercaptoethanol converted it to a single 60,000 band, suggesting the presence of an abnormal dimeric form of AT-III. The authors assumed a single mutation involving a cystein residue of AT-III molecule in the case of AT-III "Milano." Further investigations by the same group of authors showed that no thrombin-AT-III complexes could be demonstrated with either the monomeric or dimeric forms of purified variant AT-III and thrombin. Similarly, no binding to thrombin-Sepharose was observed, thus indicating that the molecular defect of AT-III Milano is related to its absence of reactivity with thrombin.[297]

Another variant belonging to the Type 2a AT-III deficiency was reported by Lane et al.[184,254] This disorder was identified in three generations of a family with a high incidence of deep venous thrombosis. AT-III "Glasgow" is characterized by an increased affinity for heparin, but reduced ability to inactivate thrombin (50%). This variant can be differentiated from two other AT-III variants with high heparin affinities ("Milano 1" and "Northwick Park"), but has similar features to those of AT-III "Chicago." Table 3 shows the AT-III abnormalities belonging to the Type 2a subgroup.

In the Type 2b AT-III abnormality, only the derangement of the active center of the molecule can be detected. The first variant of this type was reported by Sørensen et al.[132] In a thrombophilic family, seven members displayed decreased thrombin inactivating activity, four of whom had previous thrombotic episodes. Immunochemical investigations revealed normal AT-III antigen concentrations. Further investigations, partly in our laboratory, showed that this abnormal AT-III (AT-III "Aalborg") has normal affinity to heparin and the AT-III pattern in the crossed immunoelectrophoresis system is normal both in the absence and in the presence of heparin.[121] On the basis of these observations, an isolated disturbance of the active center of the molecule was assumed. However, the inactivation of factor Xa took place normally in the plasma of the patient, showing a very selective derangement of AT-III molecule.

AT-III "Vicenza" was reported by Barbui and Rodeghiero in 1981.[133] In the affected members of an Italian thrombophilic family, the thrombin inactivating activity was decreased (62 to 68% the normal activity), but the AT-III antigen concentration was normal. The AT-III pattern of the plasma was normal in the absence and in the presence of heparin in the crossed immunoelectrophoresis system, but in the serum, an abnormal pattern was found.[134] Further investigations showed a normal affinity to heparin of the abnormal AT-III, and the abnormal AT-III did not form a complex with thrombin. The abnormal AT-III pattern of the serum in the crossed immunoelectrophoresis system is brought about by the fact that AT-III ''Vicenza'' loses its heparin affinity upon thrombin treatment.[135]

AT-III ''Hvidovre'' was described by Jørgensen et al.[136] This abnormality was found in a thrombophilic family in Denmark. The thrombin inactivating capacity of plasma was reduced approximateely 50%, but the AT-III antigen concentration was normal. Two populations of AT-III molecules could be distinguished in the plasma of the affected members of the family: one was normal as far as its thrombin inactivating activity was concerned, while the other was nonreactive. SDS-PAGE and crossed immunoelectrophoresis showed that only approximately half of the purified AT-III was capable of forming a complex with thrombin. The AT-III pattern of the patients' plasma was normal in the crossed immunoelectrophoresis system with and without heparin. Heparin affinity chromatography also demonstrated a normal affinity to heparin. The factor Xa inactivating activity of the patients' plasma was not investigated. The affected family members appeared to be heterozygous with two autosomal codominant alleles that encode a normal and an abnormal AT-III protein, respectively.

AT-III ''Denver'' was described and characterized by Sambrano et al. in 1986.[137] According to our classification system, this abnormality, too, belongs to the Type 2b subclass of AT-III deficiencies. This abnormality is characterized by reduced (50%) thrombin and factor Xa inactivation. When thrombin-AT-III complexes were formed by incubating excess thrombin, SDS-PAGE analysis revealed that half the patient's AT-III formed complexes with thrombin, while the remainder migrated as free AT-III. The heparin affinity of abnormal AT-III is normal. Turnover studies suggested that AT-III ''Denver'' is removed from the plasma slightly more rapidly than normal. According to Stephens et al., the structural abnormality in AT-III ''Denver'' is a replacement of serine 394 (near the target arginine) by leucine.[138]

Another AT-III variant, AT-III ''Charleville,'' is also characterized by the isolated derangement of the active center of the molecule. This abnormality was described by Aiach et al. about a French family with a possible inclination to thrombosis.[139] Both thrombin and factor Xa inactivating activities were decreased in the absence and in the presence of heparin, while the AT-III antigen concentration was normal. Abnormal AT-III was copurified with functional AT-III using heparin affinity chromatography. The AT-III pattern was normal in the crossed immunoelectrophoresis system with and without heparin, but in the presence of heparin, a small proportion of an abnormal component was found. As in normal plasma, the bulk of the AT-III had the most anodic migration. However, besides a small peak which appears in all the plasma samples in cathodic position, the patients' plasma displayed a third intermediate component. It is very difficult to evaluate this finding, partly because crossed immunoelectrophoresis (with heparin) always displays three peaks in our hands and partly because some technical manipulations can modify the AT-III pattern as it was demonstrated by Chan and Chan.[34] No abnormality was found in the molecular mass. AT-III ''Charleville'', as with AT-III ''Vicenza'', after contact with thrombin, is no longer able to bind heparin.

AT-III ''Milano 2'' was described by Tripodi et al.[140] Four members of an Italian thrombophilic family had qualitative defects of AT-III reflected by normal antigen concentrations and half-normal thrombin inactivating activities. Anti-factor Xa activities were borderline low (about 70% normal). For the propositus' plasma and serum, the patterns of AT-III in crossed immunoelectrophoresis, with or without heparin, were indistinguishable from those of normal plasma or serum. A normal affinity of AT-III ''Milano 2'' for heparin was documented by heparin-Sepharose chromatography. Affinity adsorbtion of the propositus' plasma to human alfa-thrombin immobilized on sepharose beads revealed a defective binding of the AT-III to thrombin-sepharose. AT-III ''Milano 2'' is very similar to the other AT-III variants belonging to the Type 2b AT-III deficiency, but the borderline anti-Xa activity differentiates this AT-III variant from AT-III ''Aalborg'' (no impairment of anti-Xa activity)

TABLE 4
Type 2b AT-III Deficiencies[a]

AT-III	"Aalborg" (Sørensen et al.[132])
AT-III	"Vicenza" (Barbui and Rodeghiero[133])
AT-III	"Hvidovre" (Jørgensen et al.[136])
AT-III	"Denver" (Sambrano et al.,[137] Stephens et al.[138])
AT-III	"Charleville" (Aiach et al.[139])
AT-III	"Milano 2" (Tripodi et al.[140])
AT-III	"Pescara" (Leone et al.[141])
AT-III	"Hamilton" (Carter et al.[177])
AT-III	"Avranches" (Aiach et al.[188])

[a] Characterized by isolated deficiencies of serpin activity.

and from AT-III "Vicenza," AT-III "Denver," and AT-III "Charleville" (low anti-Xa activities).

AT-III "Pescara" was reported by Leone et al.[141] This variant was found in a thrombophilic Italian family. In all the affected subjects, AT-III antigen concentrations were normal, whereas the thrombin and factor Xa inactivating activities, as well as heparin cofactor activities were low. Crossed immunoelectrophoresis, performed either in the absence or in the presence of heparin, showed a normal plasma pattern. A normal affinity to heparin was found. An abnormal plasma pattern was established by crossed immunoelectrofocusing. AT-III "Pescara" is characterized by a defective binding to serine proteases and is clearly identifiable only by crossed immunoelectrofocusing.

AT-III "Hamilton" was described by Carter et al.[177] AT-III functional activities in the propositus' plasma, using both thrombin and factor Xa substrates, were reduced by approximately 50%, whereas immunoreactive AT-III levels were within the normal range. The same functional abnormalities of AT-III were detected in the propositus' two children.

Recently, a new AT-III variant (AT-III "Avranches") was described by Aiach et al.[188] A decreased plasma AT-III activity, in the presence or in the absence of heparin, was found in a patient with recurrent venous thromboembolism. Laboratory investigations demonstrated the isolated disturbance of the protease binding site of the AT-III molecule. The same abnormalities were found in the patient's two relatives, indicating the hereditary feature of the disorder. Half of the patients' AT-III molecules were normal, but the others had a defective protease binding site. Table 4 summarizes the AT-III variants belonging to Type 2b AT-III deficiencies.

Another subclass of qualitative AT-III disorders, Type 2c abnormalities, is characterized by the isolated derangement of the AT-III molecule at the heparin-reactive site(s). As a consequence, both the heparin cofactor activity and heparin affinity of the AT-III molecule are reduced or lacking in the majority of cases. Nagy et al.[80] and Penner et al.[142] were the first to report such cases in 1979. They observed patients with normal progressive thrombin inactivations and normal AT-III antigen concentrations, but with decreased heparin cofactor activities. However, no detailed characterization of their cases were presented.

A more thoroughly investigated isolated disorder of the heparin cofactor activity was published by Tran et al.[143,144] This abnormality was found in a 28-year-old male patient who had suffered from recurrent superficial thrombophlebitis of the leg. No other member of his family suffered thromboembolic events. A low heparin cofactor activity (0.6 U/ml) was observed with a normal AT-III antigen concentration, and the progressive thrombin inactivation was also normal. The crossed immunoelectrophoresis, in the presence of heparin in the agarose gel, separated the patient's AT-III antigen into two fractions with different mobilities. With the help of heparin-agarose chromatography, the separation and purification of the two AT-III populations (normal and abnormal) was performed. Both AT-IIIs shared several identical properties, such as molecular weight, ability to form complexes with thrombin, and inactivate activated factor X. At low heparin concentrations, the abnormal AT-III inactivated both thrombin and factor Xa more slowly than normal AT-III. At high heparin concentrations, the difference between abnormal AT-III and normal AT-III became very small. Further investigation of the pathological AT-III molecule (AT-III "Basel") showed that the amino acid sequence of the peptide, comprising residues 40 to 46, had a single substitution of proline (normal) by leucine (abnormal) at position 41. This substitution is close to an Arg (residue 47) and Trp (residue 49), which have been shown to be critical for heparin binding by AT-III. This replacement could cause a conformational change by increasing both the helical structure and the hydrophobicity around residue 41.[145]

AT-III "Paris" is also characterized by the isolated partial deficiency of the heparin cofactor activity.[146] This abnormality was found in a woman, who had her first thrombosis at the age of 30. The AT-III abnormality was present in seven female members of the family over four generations. All the other affected members were asymptomatic. In the patients' plasma, normal progressive thrombin and factor Xa inactivations were found, but in the presence of heparin, these inactivations were reduced compared with normal plasma (with heparin). The heparin cofactor activity of the patient was about 50% the normal value. The qualitative abnormality of AT-III was confirmed by crossed immunoelectrophoresis. In the absence of heparin, a single peak was obtained, but in the presence of heparin, two peaks of AT-III were observed; the abnormal one showed a decreased mobility. The two populations of AT-III molecules (normal and abnormal) could be separated by affinity chromatography on heparin-agarose. Of the patient's AT-III, 50% was bound to the agarose beads. The remainder, recovered in the supernatant, migrated in crossed immunoelectrophoresis as a single peak with the same mobility in the presence or absence of heparin and was devoid of heparin cofactor activity.

A AT-III "Padua 1" abnormality was found in a 38-year-old female patient with a negative family history as far as thromboembolic diseases were concerned.[147] Although the proposita had also a carcinoma of the ovary, another condition known to be frequently associated with thrombosis, and in spite of that, no thrombotic phenomenons ever occured. Thrombin inactivation was normal, both in the absence and in the presence of heparin. AT-III antigen concentration was normal. By crossed immunoelectrophoresis (heparin in the agarose), a major abnormal peak, less anodal than the normal counterpart, and a smaller, apparently normal peak were demonstrated. AT-III Padua 1 seems to be unique in respect of the reaction with heparin because in spite of the reduced reaction with heparin in the crossed immunoelectrophoresis system, the enhancing effect of heparin seems to be retained.

AT-III "Padua 2" was also described by Girolami et al.[148] This abnormality was found in five members of a family. None of the affected members showed thrombotic manifestations. AT-III assays measuring progressive thrombin and factor Xa inactivation and AT-III antigen concentration displayed normal values. However, slightly decreased AT-III activities were found in all assays carried out in the presence of heparin. Crossed immunoelectrophoresis in the absence of heparin showed a normal pattern both in plasma and in serum. However, in the presence of heparin, a major, less anodal abnormal peak and a smaller normal peak were demonstrated in the propositi's plasma.

AT-III "Toyama" was reported by Sakuragawa et al.[149] The abnormality was found in a 23-year-old female, who had suffered from recurrent thrombophlebitis involving her lower extremities. Her plasma AT-III antigen concentration was higher than normal, and progressive thrombin and factor Xa inhibitory activities were at normal levels. However, the heparin cofactor activity of her plasma was as low as 26% of normal control. On crossed immunoelectrophoresis, containing heparin in the first dimension agarose, the patient's AT-III showed no increase in electrophoresis mobility compared to that in the absence of heparin. From the pattern of AT-III in the crossed immunoelectrophoresis, the patient was found to be a homozygote; the parents and one of her younger sisters were heterozygotes. From the clinical point of view, it is noteworthy that no other (heterozygous) family member had thrombotic symptoms. On the other hand, the homozygous patient had not only thrombophlebitis, but cerebral thrombosis as well. The biochemical characterization of the abnormal AT-III showed that AT-III "Toyama" has the same molecular size, molecular weight, aminoterminal sequence, and carboxyterminal amino acid as normal AT-III.[150] Amino acid sequence analysis of the abnormal AT-III indicated that the arginine-47 of normal AT-III had been replaced by cystein in AT-III "Toyama."[151]

An abnormal AT-III was described in 1983 by Fischer et al.[152] For the sake of avoiding confusion, it seems to be useful to designate this abnormality as AT-III "Paris 2" in accordance with the convention of toponyms. In the proposita, a 46-year-old female, more than 30 thromboembolic accidents (arterial and venous) occured. The qualitative abnormality was suggested by the disprepancy between a normal level of AT-III antigen and a decreased heparin cofactor activity (64%). One of the two patient's sons had the same abnormality, but was asymptomatic. Crossed immunoelectrophoresis revealed a normal pattern in the absence of heparin, but two peaks were obtained in the presence of heparin: one with the same fast mobility as the control, and the other with a slower migration. Only about 50% of the AT-III molecules was bound to heparin agarose.

AT-III "Tours" was described by Chasse et al.[153] An abnormal AT-III was found in nine members of a French family. No history of thrombotic episodes was associated with this abnormality; AT-III antigen concentrations and progressive thrombin inactivations were normal, but heparin cofactor activities were decreased by about 50% in the plasma of the affected patients. Crossed immunoelectrophoresis in the presence of heparin demonstrated two peaks of AT-III; the slower one was not influenced by heparin at all. The abnormal AT-III did not bind to heparin-Sepharose. Only the heparin-binding site seemed to be affected by molecular alteration. Molecular characterization of AT-III "Tours" was performed by a recombinant gene technique.[154] A single nucleotid variation, CGT → TGT, was found in exon 2, corresponding to the replacement of Arg-47 by Cys. The same amino acid change was described for AT-III "Toyama" by Koide et al.[151] Therefore, AT-III "Toyama" and AT-III "Tours" seem to be identical pathological variants of the AT-III molecule.

Another homozygous AT-III variant, AT-III "Alger," belonging to the Type 2c AT-III abnormality was described by Fischer et al.[155] This qualitative abnormality of AT-III was found in the plasma of a 41-year-old Algerian man from a consanguinous family. The propositus suffered from recurrent episodes of thromboembolism: left and right reversible hemiplegia attributed to cerebral arterial thrombosis, and thrombosis of both the right and left femoral arteries. The functional defect is characterized by the inability of heparin to enhance the inactivation of thrombin and factor Xa, whereas normal AT-III antigen level and normal progressive AT-III activity were found. This abnormal AT-III does not bind to heparin as evidenced by crossed immunoelectrophoresis in the presence of heparin and by affinity chromatography on heparin-Sepharose gel. Fourteen relatives were investigated. In five subjects, AT-III levels were normal, whatever tests used, but in nine other subjects, the AT-III study revealed abnormalities that could be explained by a heterozygous state of the same defect, i.e., intermediate results between normal values and the propositus. Except for the propositus, no members of the family suffered thromboembolism, including his parents, who were deceased.

AT-III "Fontainebleau," another homozygous variant of AT-III belonging to Type 2c AT-III deficiencies, was reported by Boyer et al.[156] This qualitative defect of AT-III was demonstrated in four members of a large Tunisian family by a discrepancy between a normal amount of antigen and a decreased or absent heparin cofactor activity. The proposita, a 3-year-old girl, died from massive intracardiac thrombosis. Heparin cofactor activity, measured with thrombin or factor X2, was undetectable in her plasma. The lack of affinity of the propositus' AT-III for heparin was demonstrated by crossed immunoelectrophoresis and chromatography on heparin-Sepharose. The parents, first cousins, and the sister of the propositus also demonstrated a qualitative abnormality of AT-III, with levels of heparin cofactor activity close to 50% the normal range. These data suggest that the abnormal AT-III was present at the heterozygous state in the parents and the sister, and at the homozygous state in the proposita. None of the affected family members had thrombotic episodes, except for the proposita.

Recently, a new AT-III variant, AT-III "Geneve," was described by de Moerloose et al.[157] This abnormal AT-III is characterized by an isolated decrease of heparin cofactor activity, a characteristic of Type 2c AT-III deficiencies. The progressive inactivation of thrombin and factor Xa was normal in the propositus' plasma, but the heparin cofactor activity was 50% the normal value. Crossed immunoelectrophoresis in the absence of heparin showed a normal pattern, but in the presence of heparin, an abnormal peak was found as compared to the controls. Affinity chromatography on heparin-Sepharose revealed two populations of AT-III, one of which was devoid of heparin cofactor activity.

Although the abnormality was found in a 43-year-old man with a pulmonary embolism, the link between the predisposition of thrombosis and the molecular abnormality was questioned by the authors themselves. The pulmonary embolism developed in the propositus after trauma and prolonged bed rest, which might give rise to thrombosis alone. Most of the family members with the molecular abnormality had no thromboses at all. There were two exceptions, where the thromboembolic episodes might have been connected with other predisposing factors (prostatic cancer in old age and heavy smoking).

AT-III "Rouen 1" was reported by Owen et al.[185] This abnormality was found in a 40-year-old woman with a sudden sensorineural hearing loss and balance impairment. A single cerebral occlusion was assumed, but there was no thrombotic history in her family. Laboratory investigations revealed a decreased heparin cofactor activity, but with normal progressive thrombin and F Xa inactivation. A heterozygous form of a Type 2c AT-III abnormality was established. The disorder seems to be inherited because one of the patient's daughters showed the same biochemical abnormality. By heparin-Sepharose chromatography, AT-III Rouen 1 was separated from the normal AT-III. The amino acid analysis and sequence studies demonstrated a substitution of an arginine at residue 47 for a histidine. Results of this investigation suggest that replacement of Arg 47 by a partially positively charged histidine has less effect on heparin binding than does replacing it with a neutral cystein as in AT-III "Toyama," in which no heparin binding was observed. Because of the 55% heparin cofactor activity of the patient's plasma and of the partial disturbance of the heparin binding, heparin binding per se is not a sufficient condition to activate AT-III.

AT-III "Rouen 2" was described by Borg et al.[186] in a 40-year-old patient with a myocardial infarction, but no other history of thrombosis was found. This variant also displayed an isolated reduction of heparin cofactor activity, and a heterozygous disorder of the heparin-AT-III reaction was demonstrated. Amino acid and sequence analysis revealed the replacement of Arg 47 by serine.

AT-III "Amiens" was found in an asymptomatic woman in the course of a routine laboratory examination by Roussel et al.[187] This variant also belongs to the Type 2c AT-III abnormality because of the reduced heparin cofactor activity and of normal progressive thrombin and FXa inactivation. Crossed immunoelectrophoresis (heparin in agarose) demonstrated the presence of the abnormal AT-III molecules directly in the patient's plasma. AT-III "Amiens" seems to be a hereditary abnormality because the daughter of the proposita was carrying the same molecular abnormality.

Aiach et al.[253] identified an inherited qualitative deficiency of (AT-III AT-III "Clichy") in an asymptomatic family. Thrombin and F X a inactivations were normal, but the interaction with heparin, hepain sulphate, and low molecular weight heparin was uniformly decreased.

TABLE 5
Type 2c AT-III Deficiencies

AT-III	"Basel" (Tran et al.,[143] Chang and Tran[145])
AT-III	"Paris 1" (Wolf et al.[146])
AT-III	"Pauda 1" (Girolami et al.[147])
AT-III	"Pauda 2" (Girolami et al.[148])
AT-III	"Toyama" (Sakuragawa et al.,[149] Koide et al.[151])
AT-III	"Paris 2" (Fischer et al.[152])
AT-III	"Tours" (Chasse et al.,[153] Duchange et al.[154])
AT-III	"Alger" (Fischer et al.[155])
AT-III	"Fontainebleau" (Boyer et al.[156])
AT-III	"Geneve" (de Moerloose et al.[157])
AT-III	"Rouen 1" (Owen et al.[185])
AT-III	"Rouen 2" (Borg et al.[186])
AT-III	"Amiens" (Roussel et al.[187])
AT-III	"Clichy" (Aiach et al.[253])

An immunoblotting technique performed in plasma showed a normal complex formation with thrombin. By using heparin-Sepharose affinity chromatography and crossed immunoelectrophoresis, two fractions of the low affinity AT-III were obtained. A minor one had no antiprotease activity; the other one was further purified to homogeneity and found to have normal specific activity in the absence of heparin and a 50% decreased activity in the presence of heparin. On the basis of the isolated disturbance of the heparin-AT-III reaction, AT-III "Clichy" belongs to Type 2c AT-III deficiencies, but the heterogeneity of the abnormal AT-III is a distinctive feature of this variant compared with other forms of Type 2c AT-III deficiencies. Table 5 summarizes the AT-III deficiencies belonging to Type 2c.

The third main group of congenital AT-III deficiencies, Type 3, is characterized by the quantitative and qualitative disorder of AT-III production. In these variants, the functional and immunochemical AT-III assays show decreased AT-III activities and antigenic levels. Furthermore, by various methods, qualitative abnormalities of the AT-III molecules can be demonstrated. As it was discussed before, first an abnormal heparin-affinity of the AT-III molecules was found in several AT-III deficient families.[82,105]

Leone et al.,[117] using crossed immunoelectrophoresis and crossed immunoelectrophocusing, also demonstrated abnormal AT-III molecules in a family with decreased AT-III levels. In the crossed immunoelectrophocusing system, two additional peaks were found in the anodal position. Furthermore, a double peak, higher than the cathodal peaks, was located in the position of the normal anodal peak. On the basis of the qualitative disorder, they designated this variant as AT-III "Roma."

The difficulties of the classification of congenital AT-III deficiencies are demonstrated by the AT-III deficiency found in a Utah pedigree. In the first report, it seemed to be an example of the "pure" quantitative (Type 1) deficiency.[115] In deficient family members, decreased AT-III activities were associated with decreased AT-III antigenic levels. Crossed immunoelectrophoresis (with and without heparin) of plasma and serum from deficient family members revealed no qualitative abnormalities of the AT-III antigen. However, subsequent studies, applying more sensitive techniques, detected the presence of electrophoretically abnormal inhibitor molecules in the plasma of the affected patients.[233] Hence, the "pure" quantitative AT-III deficiency of the "Utah" family proved to be a quantitative-qualitative type in reality.

The thrombophilic family reported by Matsuo et al.[106] probably belongs to this subclass. The AT-III was depressed in both functional and immunological tests, but the functional defect was milder than the reduction of the antigen concentration. In the absence of a detailed biochemical analysis, only assumptions can be made in connection with this AT-III deficient family. The authors hypothesized a "reversed type of AT-III Budapest" abnormality, but a quantitative-qualitative disorder seems to be more probable in which the abnormality is expressed mainly in the immunochemical structure.

The reductions in both functional activity and antigen in a Type 3 AT-III deficiency can be explained by two mutations or by one single mutation which brings about a profound structural alteration of the AT-III. In the latter case, the alteration not only disrupts the binding of thrombin or heparin to the AT-III molecule, but might also cause enough denaturation of the protein so as to significantly alter its half-life.

Clearly, further investigations are needed for a more precise characterization of the AT-III molecules of patients with quantitative-qualitative AT-III deficiencies. The comparison of the particular variants by advanced methods could furnish information about the identities or diversities of the particular variants.

Another perplexing factor in the classification of congenital AT-III deficiencies is the existence of various isoforms of AT-III.

Isoelectrophocusing investigations on the AT-III of a normal population revealed different isoforms.[21,298,299] In some cases, the differences of the patterns obtained by isoelectrophocusing could be eliminated by previous neuraminidase treatment, i.e., these differences could be explained by unequal contents of sialic residues of the particular variants. About 10% of the AT-III from normal human plasma can be isolated on the basis of its higher affinity for heparin. This AT-III beta is also less negatively charged and has a lower molecular weight than normal AT-III alpha. The absence of carbohydrate at Asn 135 explains these characteristic features of AT-III beta.[232] In other cases, the differences may be due to the difference in polypeptide structure. Unfortunately, some of these isoforms have been designated with toponyms, although these variants do not represent pathological forms of AT-III molecules, they are probably identical with isoforms described by others. In cases of other proteinase inhibitors, such as alfa$_1$-proteinase inhibitor, the isoforms are not designated by toponyms, but they are characterized by the anodal (or cathodal) distance and specified by letters.[300] Thus, the designation of the various AT-III isoforms with toponyms, in cases of normal variants, seems to be confusing and illogical.

There are only few reports on the platelet functions in congenital AT-III deficiencies. Tullis and Watanabe[158] reported a case of platelet antithrombin deficiency, but this may be totally unrelated to an AT-III deficiency. Carvalho and Ellman[159] studied the platelet functions in an AT-III deficient family (Type 1) and found them to be normal. Following gel filtration, the platelets were very sensitive to thrombin. In an AT-III variant, which was described by Matsuo et al.[106] and characterized by the quantitative and qualitative disturbance of AT-III production, displayed the hyperaggregability of both gel-filtered platelets and platelet-rich plasma. When we compared the aggregability of the platelets in the plasma of our patients with different types of AT-III deficiencies, we found that in Type 1 AT-III deficiencies, the platelet aggregation induced by ADP, collagen, and arachidonic acid were normal. In the proposita of a Type 3 deficiency, we observed a slightly reduced aggregability induced by ADP and collagen. In the patient with the AT-III "Budapest" abnormality, only a moderately reduced aggregability of platelets induced by ADP was observed; the aggregation of the thrombocytes induced by collagen, adrenalin, and arachidonic acid were similar to the control.[160] Because these changes were observed only in single cases of different types of AT-III abnormality, these slight alterations could not be considered as typical changes for a particular variant. At present, the data on platelet functions in congenital AT-III deficiency seem to be insufficient to draw any conclusions in this respect.

3. Clinical Features of Congenital AT-III Deficiencies

Heterozygous patients with the most frequent ("classical" or type 1) form of AT-III deficiency have a high risk of venous thrombosis and pulmonary embolism. The homozygous form of this disorder seems to be incompatible with life, because such a case has not been reported. However, in a qualitative variant of the AT-III deficiency, Type 2c, which is characterized by the isolated deficiency of heparin cofactor activity, patients display a slight, if any, predisposition to thrombosis.

The analytical studies, which are based on more than 100 published AT-III-deficient families, characterize amply the most important clinical features of the "classical" form of this disorder.[103,161,162,163] About 55% of the reported patients had at least one thrombotic episode. The frequency of the thromboembolic episodes increases with age. Thrombosis occurred in only 10% of the children (under age 15) with an AT-III deficiency. In the neonatal period, AT-III deficiency (Type 1) may predispose to aortic thrombosis.[164] Two cases with thromboses of the inferior vena cava have been reported in childhood.[165,166] The onset of thrombotic events occurred between the ages of 10 and 35 in two-thirds of the patients, with median age of 24 years. More than 85% of the patients older than 50 had at least one thrombotic episode. Exceptionally old patients with AT-III deficiencies and a good deal of other predisposing factors may remain asymptomatic. In one case, reported by Halal et al.[103] an obligate female carrier was still asymptomatic at 83 years, after bearing nine children. Rarely, the inherited AT-III deficiency may be accompanied by a hereditary haemorrhagic disorder, and in such cases, thrombotic events occur only infrequently. The two defects may segregate independently, as was the case with AT-III "Trento" and von Willebrand disease, reported by Girolami et al.[127]

The increasing number of clinical manifestations with age may be explained by observations that in the majority of AT-III-deficient patients, the first thrombotic event occurred in conjunction with a condition known to trigger thrombosis, such as surgery, delivery, pregnancy, major trauma, and the use of oral contraceptives. In females with AT-III deficiencies and thrombosis, in about a third of the cases, pregnancy and delivery were the triggering events. It is interesting that thrombosis develops more frequently in early pregnancy than in late pregnancy. This early occurance is uncommon in women without AT-III deficiencies. In another third of the female patients, no triggering event can be detected. In the remaining third, operations (appendectomy, Cesarean section, hysterectomy, cardiac catheterization, pacemaker implantation, trauma, oral contraceptives, and respiratory-tract infection) were the triggering events. Oral contraceptives apparently play a quite different role in the induction of thrombosis in AT-III-deficient females in different populations. The thrombosis copromoting effect of oral contraceptives may depend on many circumstances in these situations, such as the amount of estrogen in the pill, the relative frequency of taking oral contraceptives in a particular population, etc. These differences may explain that in some statistics, the triggering role of oral contraceptives is surprisingly low. In AT-III-deficient males and in about only half of the cases are the thromboses connected with some triggering event. Thromboembolic episodes develop generally with pneumonia, trauma, and an operation.

The most common sites of thrombosis were the deep leg and iliac veins; about 90% of the thromboses developed in these veins of the AT-III-deficient patients. As a consequence of the localization of the thromboses, leg ulceration and varicose veins are frequent complications of AT-III deficiencies. Superficial leg vein thrombosis was much less common and usually associated with deep vein thrombosis. In about 60% of the patients, thrombosis was recurrent. Clinical signs of pulmonary embolisms were present in about 40% of the patients. Thrombosis of the mesenteric veins was reported in nearly 10% of the cases with thrombosis and AT-III deficiencies.[88,98,101,167,168] In rare cases, thrombosis was reported in the inferior caval vein; the brachial and axillary veins; the renal, liver, portal and retinal veins; and in the cerebral sinus.

A Type 1 AT-III deficiency does not appear to increase the risk of arterial thrombosis. Although in some cases peripherial arterial occlusive disease, myocardial infarction, and thrombosis of cerebral arteries were described in older patients, but the frequency of these events was not higher than in patients without AT-III deficiencies at the same age.

The number of patients with qualitative disorders of AT-III (Type 2 AT-III deficiencies) is much lower than that of patients with quantitative AT-III deficiencies. Hence, the clinical characteristics of the former group are much less well-defined.

However, in the heterozygous forms of Type 2a and 2b AT-III deficiencies, the clinical symptoms seem to be very similar to the "classical" AT-III deficiency, i.e., both of them are characterized by a high risk of venous thrombosis. The isolated disorder of heparin cofactor activity, i.e., Type 2c AT-III deficiency, predisposes to thrombosis far less, if at all, in its heterozygous form. In four families, no thromboembolic episodes occured even in the propositi.[142,147,148,153] In one case, the thrombosis developed after trauma and bed rest.[157] In three other families, although the propositi had recurrent venous thromboses, no other family members suffered thrombosis.[143,146,152] Homozygous patients with Type 2c AT-III deficiencies, suffered severe thromboses in venous, arterial, or intracardiac localization, but the heterozygous relatives were free of symptoms.[149,155,156]

The clinical analysis of the various AT-III deficiencies suggest that two different antithrombotic mechanisms are encoded in the AT-III molecule.[169] A partial deficiency (about 50% the normal value) of the progressive thrombin and factor Xa inactivation, either a quantitative or qualitative disorder of the active center of the AT-III molecule, predisposes to thrombosis, mainly in the veins. The relative lack of thrombin-inactivating activity brings about excessive thrombin generation, and subtreshold thrombin activities may give rise to thrombosis in such conditions.[170,171] In fact, Borg et al.[172] detected the markers of intravascular coagulation in Type 1 AT-III deficiencies, while in isolated heparin cofactor deficiencies (Type 2c AT-III deficiencies), no derivatives of intravascular thrombin generation were present in the plasma of the patients. The importance of the progressive thrombin and factor Xa inactivation is underlined by the fact that no patient was reported with a homozygous defect of this activity, suggesting that a severe defect of thrombin and factor Xa inactivation is incompatible with life.

At first glance, the lack of obvious predisposition to thrombosis in heterozygous patients with Type 2c AT-III deficiencies and the lack of intravascular coagulation in the blood of such patients seem to contradict the importance of the heparin-like molecules along the vascular endothelium. It has been claimed that AT-III inactivates the activated serine proteases, mainly at the surface of the endothelial cells, due to the accelerating effect of these heparin-like molecules.[173,174] If the heparin-AT-III binding had an exclusive importance in the physiological inactivation of thrombin and other serine proteases, the Type 2c AT-III deficiency would be accompanied by a similar frequency of thromboembolic manifestations, as with other types of AT-III deficiencies. Clinical and experimental data do not support this assumption.

On the other hand, homozygous patients with Type 2c AT-III deficiencies had severe thromboses in large vessels (veins, arteries, and intracardially). This fact shows that the physiological importance of the heparin-binding site of the AT-III molecule cannot be neglected. The situation with the defect of heparin cofactor activity seems to be somewhat similar to the deficiency of the procoagulants (prothrombin, factor VIII, etc.). In cases of congenital coagulopathies, bleeding symptoms appear only at very low factor levels, and a moderate (50% the normal value) decrease of the procoagulants does not cause coagulopathy. The appearance of thrombosis in the veins, arteries, and heart of young patients with homozygous Type 2c deficiencies suggests two things. First, the heparin cofactor II activity of the blood cannot compensate for the lack of heparin cofactor activity of AT-III. Second, the very low heparin cofactor activity of the AT-III molecule predisposes to thrombosis not only in the veins (as in the other forms of AT-III deficiencies), but in the arteries and intracardially as well. The importance of a critical level of heparin cofactor activity may explain why a Type 1 AT-III deficiency may give rise to thrombosis in the aorta of neonates.[164] Physiologically, the AT-III level is an about 50% the normal (adult) value in neonates, but a similar low level of procoagulants compensates this deficiency and neither thromboses nor bleeding disorders occur.[176] However, in the case of a hereditary AT-III deficiency (Type 1), the heparin cofactor activity decreases to or below 25% the normal value in neonates, which may predispose to thrombosis in the large vessels.

In one part of the patients with congenital AT-III deficiencies, oral anticoagulant treatment can increase the AT-III level.[78,99] In other cases, such improvement was not observed.[95,115] This different response seems to be not only a methodological, but a real one because in a few cases, the same authors observed both the increased and unchanged AT-III levels after introduction of coumarin therapy.[89,90,175] This different response was observed mainly in patients with Type 1 AT-III deficiencies, which also suggest the heterogeneity of the "classical" AT-III deficiency. However, this heterogeneity is apparently independent from the heterogeneity experienced on heparinized agarose gel in the crossed immunoelectropohoresis system because we observed no increase of AT-III levels in both Type 1a and Type 1b AT-III-deficient patients.

The genetic aspects of AT-III deficiencies are discussed in detail in a separate chapter of this book. Only the main features of the inheritance are summarized here, which belong to the clinical symptomatology of AT-III deficiency.

The autosomal-dominant type of inheritance of an AT-III deficiency was already pointed out in the first description of this disease.[76] Subsequent studies reporting other thrombophilic families with AT-III deficiencies supported this notion.[77,78,89] Halal et al.[103] reviewed the clinical data on 120 individuals with Type 1 AT-III deficiencies (from four personally studied families and 14 families from literature). The data indicate that autosomal-dominant (clinically symptomatic) AT-III deficiency is an age-dependent trait with full penetrance and quite variable expressivity.

The inheritance of Type 2 AT-III deficiencies is less well-studied. In the case of AT-III "Budapest," autosomal codominant type of inheritance was suggested, and in addition to the codominant alleles, the possible existence of some modifying gene was assumed.[120] In the majority of cases, the inheritance mode of Type 2 AT-III deficiencies is autosomal dominant because both sexes are equally affected; the trait appears in every generation, and unaffected persons do not transmit the trait to their children. In the case of AT-III "Paris," too, an autosomal-dominant mode of inheritance was suggested, although all the patients affected (seven members over four generations) were female.[146] In consanguineous families with Type 2c AT-III deficiencies, homozygous patients were found. In these cases, both parents were in a heterozygous state with the same abnormality.[149,155,156]

4. Laboratory Diagnosis of Congenital AT-III Deficiencies

On the basis of clinical symptoms (recurrent thromboembolic episodes in a member of a thrombophilic family), the suspicion of an inherited AT-III deficiency may arise soon. To verify this assumption, laboratory tests should be performed. In a previous part of this chapter, we discussed the various problems of laboratory tests including the methodological details. Here we summarize only the principles of the laboratory diagnosis of the congenital AT-III deficiency.

For screening purposes, a heparin cofactor assay should be performed first.[178] With a reliable and simple method, such as the heparin cofactor assay of Abildgaard et al.,[67] all types of congenital AT-III deficiencies can be detected. The heparin cofactor activity is reduced in both quantitative or qualitative deficiencies of AT-III. In general, an activity of lower than 70% of normal pooled plasma is measured in the plasma of the AT-III deficient patients. A reduction of about 50% of the normal activity was observed in the majority of the cases. At borderline values (60 to 75% of the normal value), various conditions should be considered, such as the age and sex of the patient, use of oral contraceptives, etc. Furthermore, the possibility of an acquired AT-III deficiency also should be taken into account, such as DIC, chronic liver disease, nephrotic syndrome, etc. In these uncertain cases, the investigation of other family members and/or a more detailed analysis of the patient's plasma (performance of other AT-III assays and coagulation tests), measurement of enzyme activities connected with liver function, etc.) may be required.

In a typical case with an unambiguous reduction of heparin cofactor activity and with the absence of other causes of the reduced heparin cofactor activity, the determination of the AT-III antigen concentration is required by an immunochemical method. Both the simple radial immunodiffusion method of Mancini et al.[4] and the electroimmunodiffusion method of Laurell are suitable for this purpose.[3] If a parallel decrease of heparin cofactor activity and AT-III antigen concentration is found, the diagnosis of a Type 1 AT-III deficiency can be set up. By the modified crossed immunoelectrophoresis method of Sas et al.,[20] the distinction of Type 1 and some Type 3 deficiencies can be achieved. In the case of Type 1 AT-III deficiencies, AT-III molecules migrate in the heparinized agarose with the same speed as normal AT-III molecules. However, in some cases of Type 3 AT-III deficiencies, the electrophoretic mobility of the AT-III molecules is decreased.

If reduced heparin cofactor activity is accompanied with a normal AT-III antigen concentration, a functional disturbance of AT-III production, i.e., Type 2b AT-III deficiency, can be assumed. In this case, further detailed analysis is required, but before performing this, to avoid frustration, the repetition of basic tests (heparin cofactor assay and immunochemical determination of AT-III antigen concentration) is recommended. If the divergence of heparin cofactor activity and the AT-III antigen concentration is real, the determination of progressive thrombin and factor Xa inactivation, the performance of crossed immunoelectrophoresis with and without heparin, are required. By means of these relatively simple methods, the classification of the particular functional AT-III deficiency can be achieved. In Type 2a AT-III deficiencies, a combined defect is found (e.g., abnormal pattern in crossed immunoelectrophoresis with decreased thrombin inactivation, etc.) suggesting a profound abnormality of the AT-III molecule. In Type 2b AT-III deficiencies, only a low progressive thrombin and/or factor Xa inactivation is characteristic; the crossed immunoelectrophoresis with and without heparin does not reveal abnormality. In these cases, the abnormality of the active center of the molecule can be assumed. In Type 2c AT-III deficiencies, the progressive inactivation of thrombin and factor Xa is normal, but the crossed immunoelectrophoresis with heparin displays an abnormality of heparin-AT-III binding. In these cases, the abnormality of the heparin binding site(s) of the AT-III molecule can be hypothesized.

For further characterization of the variant AT-III molecules, their isolation is required and the determination of the sequence of amino acids may define the abnormal AT-III molecule, as it was carried out with AT-III "Toyama" and AT-III "Basel."[151,145] Using a recombinant gene technique, the molecular defect can be determined by the analysis of the DNA sequence coding the AT-III molecule, as it was performed in the case of AT-III "Tours."[154]

5. Prevention and Therapy of the Thrombosis in Patients with Congenital AT-III Deficiencies

In AT-III-deficient patients, the prevention and therapy of thrombosis have some special features.

Thrombosis prophylaxis is absolutely indicated at patients with known AT-III deficiencies who had thrombosis previously. As we pointed out, even in the absence of an AT-III deficiency, continuous oral anticoagulant (coumarin) therapy is indicated in patients with thrombosis of the deep (femoral or iliac) veins.[179] In the course of deep vein thrombosis, the valvular system of the affected vein becomes incompetent, the intima is damaged, and the collateral veins dilate. These alterations without an AT-III deficiency enormously increase the risk of the recurrence of thrombosis. Hence, in our opinion, the necessity of a continuous thrombosis prophylaxis is undisputable in AT-III-deficient patients with previous thrombosis. The development of the control of oral anticoagulant (coumarin) therapy tremendously increased the safety of this treatment. Furthermore, such level of anticoagulation is efficient for the prevention of venous thrombosis, which does not increase the risk of bleeding complications significantly. However, in some circumstances, the oral anticoagulant therapy must be abandoned in AT-III-deficient patients with previous thrombosis.

First, coumarin therapy is contraindicated in pregnancy. The patient may become pregnant during the oral anticoagulant therapy and, in this case, the cessation of the pregnancy is indicated on account of the danger of fetal damage. It may occur that young females with known AT-III deficiencies and previous thrombosis want to be pregnant and to deliver children. In our practice, we first call the patient's attention to the risks connected with pregnancy (recurrence of thrombosis, 50% probability of giving birth of a child with an AT-III deficiency, etc.) If the woman insists on the baby, the anticoagulant therapy is abandoned before conception and heparin prophylaxis is initiated (2 × 10,000 IU calcium-heparin daily, subcutaneously). Undoubtedly, the value of heparin-prophylaxis in a AT-III deficiency is limited, partly because of the reduced effectivity of heparin on account of the low AT-III level and partly because the heparin administration may even further reduce the AT-III level. Despite these fears, the effectivity of this measure has been proved.[180] Bolwerk et al.[181] found that the 4 × 5000 IU doses of heparin (per day) are more effective than the 2 × 5000 IU doses (per day) in thrombosis prophylaxis of an AT-III-deficient patient, but the former doses of heparin further decrease the AT-III level. We found that even higher doses of heparin did not reduce the AT-III levels in some Type 3 AT-III-deficient patients. This observation may be explained by the reduced affinity of the AT-III molecules to heparin in this group of patients.

Second, oral anticoagulant therapy has to be suspended when a major surgical operation is needed. Although bleeding complications are rare at a prophylactic level of anticoagulation with coumarins, a safer thrombosis prophylaxis can be achieved by the transient restoration of the AT-III level by an AT-III concentrate. Mannucci et al.[182] applied AT-III concentrates for thrombosis prophylaxis without the simultaneous administration of heparin. Supranormal AT-III activities (120 to 180% the normal) were achieved by high doses of AT-III concentrates. They observed that a 0.74 units/kg of AT-III resulted in 1% increase of AT-III level after concentrate infusion. The half-life of AT-III was about 66 h. Hence, the AT-III concentrate was administered every other day. The AT-III antigen concentration was consistently higher than the heparin cofactor activity, especially immediately after the infusion. This discrepancy was associated with the presence in the patient's plasma of an AT-III fraction showing a slower mobility than the main AT-III peak on the two-dimensional immunoelectrophoresis in the presence of heparin. Thus, a biological assay (such as a heparin cofactor assay) is preferred to an immunological assay in monitoring replacement therapy with AT-III concentrate.

On account of the high cost of an AT-III concentrate, a substitution for the normal or near-normal AT-III levels plus a low dose of heparin prophylaxis seem to be more meaningful. An AT-III concentrate (1500 to 2000 U) is administered daily in infusion with 2 × 5000 IU heparin subcutaneously. The details of the application of the AT-III concentrate are described in Chapter 5.

More controversial is the question of thrombosis prophylaxis of patients who have not suffered thrombosis yet. In these cases, the deficiency turns out either by chance or in the course of investigation of the family having a member with thromboembolism. As we discussed before, the probability of the manifestation of the thromboembolic episodes increases with age, but the patient may remain asymptomatic even at old age. Some authors suggest long-term prophylaxis as soon as the diagnosis of the AT-III deficiency is made.[80] Others suggest starting only after the first thrombotic episode or advocate only short-term prophylaxis when known risk factors are present.[99,108] However, the latter suggestion does not help prevent the occurance of spontaneous thromboembolic episodes. Obviously, all these suggestions are disputable: in one case, the oral anticoagulants may be unnecessary or even harmful, while in others, the withholding of the anticoagulants may give rise to thrombosis.

Thrombosis prophylaxis starts with good counseling of the affected individuals (without previous thrombosis, but with an AT-III deficiency) about various risk factors, such as obesity, immobility, trauma, infection, surgery, and pregnancy. An AT-III-deficient woman should not take oral contraceptives because it further decreases the plasma AT-III level and increases the risk of thrombosis.[162] Whenever the patient is exposed to predisposing factors, some preventive measures should be made. If the predisposition lasts a shorter time (e.g., a few weeks), an AT-III concentrate plus heparin-prophylaxis is preferred. Excellent results were reported on the "adjusted" heparin-prophylaxis.[180] If the predisposition period lasts a longer time (e.g., a few months), oral anticoagulant therapy is indicated. However, in the case of pregnancy, subcutaneous heparin prophylaxis should be indicated for avoiding the teratogenic effect of coumarin-compounds.

Acute deep venous thrombosis or pulmonary embolism of an AT-III-deficient patient should be treated with either some thrombolytic agent (streptokinase, urokinase, etc.) or with heparin as soon as possible. In the case of heparin therapy, however, one must keep in mind that heparin further reduces the AT-III level.[183] Because of the low AT-III level, the usual doses of heparin are not effective enough, hence, higher doses of heparin must be administered, such as 500 to 800 units/kg daily, by intravenous infusion or subcutaneously. However, the higher the dose of the heparin, the more pronounced the further reduction of the AT-III level. Therefore, AT-III concentrates are indispensable in this situation. Administering a safe (virus-free) AT-III concentrate (2000 units daily) the heparin may be administered in coventional doses with full effect. During the combined AT-III concentrate + heparin therapy, the AT-III level of the plasma should be measured daily. Those AT-III assays are preferred which are not influenced by the presence of heparin in the plasma to be tested, such as the method of Abilgaard et al.[67] with the chromogenic substrate S-2238. In addition to the AT-III level, the activated partial thromboplastin time should also be measured twice a day for monitoring the efficency of the heparin therapy.

E. ACQUIRED DEFICIENCIES AND ALTERATIONS OF AT-III

As we discussed it in a previous paragraph in connection with the principle of classification of AT-III-deficient states, acquired AT-III deficiencies generally occurred in connection with some basic disease. In some cases, the production of AT-III is diminished, while in others, an increased consumption is responsible for the low AT-III level. Furthermore, an increased transcapillary flux of AT-III may also bring about the acquired AT-III-deficient state. However, for the classification of acquired AT-III deficiencies, these three mechanisms seem to be unsuited because in many cases their combination gives rise to a low AT-III level. In the majority of cases, a reduced level of plasma AT-III is brought about by various diseases and conditions, but sometimes an increase of AT-III level may occur. Hence, mainly for practical reasons, acquired AT-III deficiencies and alterations will be discussed according to the basic diseases or conditions.

1. AT-III in Liver Diseases

For many years, the production site of AT-III has been inferred from patients with chronic liver diseases who have decreased plasma AT-III levels.[11,189,190] However, synthesis of AT-III has also been observed in endothelial cells.[191] A more direct evidence of the hepatic synthesis of AT-III has derived from the work of Fair and Bahnak, who detected the synthesis of AT-III in a hepatoma cell line.[192] Therefore, there are two possible production sites of AT-III, i.e., the hepatocytes and the vascular endothelium, but the clinical experience support the importance of the hepatic synthesis. It was observed that the decrease of AT-III is correlated with the degree of parenchymal injury of the liver. In cases of steatosis hepatitis or chronic, persisting hepatitis, no decrease of AT-III concentration was observed. A moderately reduced AT-III level was found in chronic aggressive hepatitis, while low AT-III activities were measured in cirrhosis hepatis.[193,194] In acute hepatic failure, extremely low AT-III levels were measured.[196] In acute hepatitis, AT-III activity is usually found to be normal.[195] Measuring AT-III activities in patients with liver cirrhosis, one has to keep in mind that progressive antithrombin activity does not give an exact evaluation of AT-III because a normal or increased α_2-macroglobulin level may influence the results.[197]

The mechanism of the diminution of AT-III in liver disease is complex: insufficient hepatic synthesis, altered transcapillary flux ratio, and low-grade diffuse intravascular coagulation may take part in it.[86] Although the contributing role of the various mechanisms are different, patients with liver cirrhosis or liver failure have no increased risk of thrombosis. This may be explained by a simultaneous and proportional decrease in procoagulants. This procoagulant-inhibitor balance at a low level may easily be upset if either an intravascular activation of the clotting system occurs or procoagulants, e.g., prothrombin concentrates, are administered. Increased fibrinogen turnover and a low AT-III level were observed in patients with liver cirrhosis and this was considered as a consequence of DIC.[212] The selective correction of AT-III activity with an AT-III concentrate completely reversed the increased turnover of radio-labeled fibrinogen to normal. These observations indicate that decreased AT-III activity contributes a major part to the occurance of intravascular coagulation in liver cirrhosis.

Decompensated disseminated intravascular coagulation may arise following the introduction of a LeVeen shunt, which drains ascitic fluid from the peritoneal cavity into the systemic circulation. Ascitic fluid contains procoagulants and coagulation activators which may give rise to fibrin formation in the circulation. Human AT-III concentrates have been trasfused prior to LeVeen shunt surgery, followed by continuous infusion, but these prophylactic measures could not or could only slightly influence the development of DIC.[198,199]

2. AT-III in Renal Diseases

Although renal diseases are very often associated with bleeding complications, sometimes thrombotic events may occur. Thromboembolic episodes of nephrotic patients, intravascular coagulation processes in acute renal failure, and thrombosis of the extracorporeal system during dialysis are such examples, and AT-III plays a more or less role in the pathogenesis of these events.

The inclinaton of nephrotic patients to thrombosis has been a well-known fact for about 40 years. During a mean observaton time of 2 to 3 years, thrombotic complications in nephrotic syndromes occur early in 30% of the patients. The incidence of thromboembolism is especially high in patients with AT-III values below 75%.[200,201,202,203] The inverse correlation of AT-III level and the frequency of thromboembolic events suggest a causative role of decreased AT-III concentration of plasma in the pathogenesis of thromboembolism. Undoubtedly, other factors, such as diminished fibrinolytic activity, increased platelet count and aggregation, hypercoagulability, hyperlipidemia, increased plasma viscosity, and decreased plasma volume, contribute to the development of thrombosis. The selective proteinuria, i.e., the increased loss of proteins with low molecular weight such as AT-III, changes the balance of procoagulants and inhibitors because of the higher molecular weights of procoagulants. However, many patients are able to enhance AT-III synthesis to compensate renal AT-III loss and some patients have even slightly increased levels. AT-III deficiency occurs when the synthesis fails to compensate the AT-III loss. In general, AT-III values are correlated to proteinuria and, because of its similar molecular weight, to serum albumin.[200,205,206] AT-III deficiencies are often found in patients with proteinuria above 5 g per 24 h and usually in patients with serum albumin below 2 g%.[200,202,203] However, urinary and plasma AT-III levels are not correlated, suggesting that the increased consumption or turnover of AT-III is not simply related to increased filtration.[213] The correlation of AT-III levels and degree of proteinuria is valid only in patients without corticosteroid therapy because the administration of corticosteroids stimulates AT-III synthesis both in animal experiments and in patients.[203,204] Recently, Drijfhout et al.[288] concluded that the AT-III catabolism was increased in nephrotic syndrome, not only due to urinary protein loss, but also to other mechanisms such as changes in flux ratio and increased consumption in the central compartment.

In nephrosis syndrome, about a third of the thromboses develops in the renal veins, and this preferred localization could also be explained by a loss of AT-III because renal protein loss may cause an AT-III deficiency in the renal veins, possibly without low systemic AT-III values. The risk of thrombosis is probably not so high in children as in adults.[206] This observation may explain why thromboembolic episodes are more often seen in nephrotic patients with membranous or membranoproliferative glomerulonephritis.

Because of the high risk of thrombosis, some authors recommend chronic oral anticoagulant prophylaxis in nephrotic patients, especially if the serum albumin is under 2 g%.[200]

In acute renal failure, depending on the basic disease, low AT-III levels develop. Disseminated intravascular coagulation plays a pathogenetic role in these cases. Septicaemia, multiple trauma, and abdominal surgery are the most frequent causes of acute renal failure, accompanied by a low AT-III level, a consequence of the intravascular activation and inactivation of blood coagulation. This acquired AT-III deficiency leads to diminished protection against intravascular coagulation processes and, therefore, possibly to the progression of the illness. Indeed, a massive increase of fibrin monomers indicates thrombin generation in patients with acute renal failure. As a morphological proof of this mechanism, fibrin deposits and hyaline thrombi were demonstrated in the kidneys in a part of the patients with acute renal failure.[207,208,209,210]

In chronic renal failure, no significant changes of AT-III were observed. In patients undergoing dialysis procedures with necessary heparin therapy (hemodialysis, hemofiltration), the AT-III levels are slightly lower than in patients treated by peritoneal dialysis, which does not require heparin therapy. The difference between these groups may partly be due to the heparin therapy. A decrease in AT-III concentrations could only be found in dialysis patients who suffered from additional complications (septicaemia, operations, etc.).[211]

3. AT-III and DIC

Normal haemostasis depends upon a delicate balance between the procoagulant system and associated inhibitors as well as the fibrino(geno)lytic system and associated inhibitors. When the hemostasis system is driven in the procoagulant direction with generation of serine proteases (IIa, IXa, Xa, and XIa factors), AT-III consumption would be expected to occur as it combines irreversibly with these activated clotting factors. In a condition or disease, associated with the pathologic generation of activated coagulation enzymes, such as occurs in disseminated intravascular coagulation, one should see the increased consumption of AT-III.

Unfortunately, the definition of DIC is far from being accomplished. It is beyond the scope of this chapter to discuss the pathophysiology, diagnostics, and therapy of DIC. We'll restrict our interest only on the problems of DIC connected with AT-III. However, the difficulties of the definition of DIC render the discussion of AT-III in DIC more difficult because different conditions have been interpreted as DIC. Hence, comparing the results of the different studies, we have to be very cautious to avoid misinterpretations or unfounded generalizations. For demonstrating the terminological problems, I discuss briefly the post-surgical decrease of AT-III which has been described by several authors.[214,215,216] These investigations showed a post-operative fall of AT-III which may play a role in the occurence of deep venous thrombosis.[217,218] An increased consumption of AT-III is caused by local intravascular coagulation, induced by the liberation of tissue thromboplastin and exposure of subendothelial structures during the trauma of surgery. Can we interprete this low AT-III level as a sign of DIC? If we consider that *local* intravascular coagulation induced it, the answer is not. However, the consequences (e.g., the low AT-III level) are not restricted to the site of the surgical intervention, i.e., they are diffuse. Taking this into account, the answer may be yes. Instead of discussing these terminological problems, we describe those various diseases and conditions in which an intravascular hypercoagulability may play a role in the decrease of an AT-III level.

In earlier studies, low AT-III levels and increased turnovers of AT-III were found in patients who had DIC.[24,219,220] In a clinical study, Bick et al.[221] monitored AT-III before and during therapy in 38 patients who had acute or chronic DIC. Pathologically decreased levels of AT-III were found in 34 of 38 patients, suggesting a diagnostic role of the measurement of AT-III. In all 38 patients, there were significant increases in AT-III after the initiation of therapy for the intravascular clotting process. Hence, the rise of AT-III may serve as an indicator of the efficacy of therapy in stopping the clotting process. In the majority of cases, malignancy, sepsis, shock, and the combination of these conditions are in the background of DIC. A particular attention was directed to AT-III in patients with sepsis.[222,223,225] These studies demonstrated that persistently low values of AT-III in patients after surgery and trauma were strongly suggestive of complicating septicemia. Of particular practical importance is the finding that continuously low values for this parameter during surgical septicaemia is suggestive of a persistent focus, whereas AT-III values returned towards the normal range within the second week after successful drainage of the septic focus. In medical septicaemia, low functional AT-III activities indicate a poor prognosis. In meningococcal infections, AT-III was the only factor distinguishing patients who developed complications from those with an uneventful recovery.[224] Henny et al.[226] reported a patient with toxic shock syndrome after elective orthopaedic surgery in whom an acquired AT-III deficiency, severe thrombocytopenia, and low levels of several coagulation and fibrinolytic parameters suggested DIC. Because of the concurrent hypalbuminaemia, they suggested a multicasual pathogenesis of the AT-III deficiency, i.e., not only increased turnover through forming 1:1 complexes with activated clotting factors. But decreased synthesis due to hepatic damage and increased leakage into an expanded extravascular compartment may play a role in the low AT-III level. A treatment regimen of antibiotics and AT-III concentrates, low-dose heparin, fresh frozen plasma, packed cells, and multiple platelet concentrate infusions normalized the plasmatic coagulation system with a concurrent decreased severity of the concomitant respiration distress syndrome. A regimen of AT-III concentates plus low-dose heparin in addition to fresh frozen plasma, platelet concentrates, packed cells and, if necessary, coagulation factor concentrates to control DIC was applied by Schipper et al.[227] Thaler and Kleinberger demonstrated a low AT-III level and DIC in septicaemia whether of gram negative or gram positive origin.[228] Low AT-III activities and increased incidences of thrombosis were reported in patients with severe burns complicated by infections.[229]

Intravascular activation of the coagulation enzymes has been demonstrated in the course of acute pancreatitis.[235,236] As a consequence of this activation, AT-III activity is reduced, especially in the severe form of the disease. In several of the patients with severe conditions, very low values of AT-III, amounting to a 70 to 80% reduction of normal values, were found during the first week after admission.[237]

An acquired deficiency of AT-III was reported in malignancy, attributed to the hypercoagulability and DIC.[230,231] AT-III levels are diminished in these cases, especially if liver metastases are present.[220] However, occasionally, normal or elevated levels of AT-III were found in some patients with malignancy and DIC. This observation was explained either by an over compensatory increase in levels of AT-III or the increase of the acute-phase reactant proteins. AT-III as an alpha$_2$-globulin belongs to these proteins.[221] Because of the increased intravascular activation of coagulation enzymes (IIa, Xa, etc.), we tried to detect the complexes of AT-III with these activated enzymes in DIC with the help of the modified crossed immunoelectrophoresis system (heparin in the agarose).[35] However, only in some cases could these complexes be detected. Rodeghiero and Barbui[36] also used this method to detect thrombin-AT-III complexes in patients with acute leukemia and DIC. The case with the most severe clinical and laboratory picture of DIC showed a clear increase of IAT-III$_2$ (corresponding to the thrombin-AT-III complex). Nalli et al.[234] observed an increase of IAT-III$_2$ in half of the patients with DIC, but they found the same in the plasma of normal subjects. Because of the lack of both specificity and sensitivity, this method has been abandoned in the investigation of patients with DIC.

The gynecological aspects of AT-III and DIC are discussed in Chapter 3.

In some diseases, low AT-III levels are not connected only with the intravascular activation of coagulation enzymes. In inflammatory bowel disease, the pathogenetic role of the increased activation can be assumed because of the thrombotic tendency of these patients, and the reduced AT-III activity, at least in part, may be a consequence of it.[238] On the other hand, an increased leakage of AT-III may also play a role in the reduction of AT-III level. Indeed, a low AT-III level was demonstrated in protein losing enteropathy.[239] Extensive resection of the small bowel may also bring about the reduction of AT-III level.[240]

4. AT-III and Diabetes Mellitus

In diabetes, levels of AT-III have varied.[241,242,243,244,245,246] This may be realized to differences in functional and immunological assay methods, discrepancies between functional and immunological assays which these studies have employed, and due to a failure to distinguish between insulin-dependent (Type 1), insulin-treated, and noninsulin-dependent (Type 2) diabetic patients. Some studies of Type 2 diabetes have shown a reduction in functional activity.[242,243,247] Perez-Requejo et al.[247] suggested a low functional activity with a normal immunological level of AT-III in Type 2 diabetes. Small et al.,[248] studying Type 2 diabetic patients, found that glycosylated haemoglobin concentration showed significant correlations with AT-III antigen concentration and a negative trend with AT-III activity. Improved glycaemic control might lead to an improvement of AT-III function leading to a reversal of the "hypercoagulable state" found in Type 2 diabetes. They demonstrated a discrepancy between the functional and immunological concentration of AT-III. This discrepancy could be explained by a structurally modified protein which retains immunoreactivity but is functionally depressed, as it was previously suggested by Ceriello et al.[249] There is *in vitro* evidence that the glycosylation of AT-III leads to the reduction of its functional activity.[250] As was demonstrated by Small et al.[248] the discrepancy between the functional activity and antigen concentration of AT-III disappeared after 3 months of insulin treatment. Ceriello et al.[251] suggested that glucose, probably through a labile, nonenzymatic glycation process, might influence the biological activity of AT-III. Heparin treatment preserves the AT-III activity from glycaemia-induced alterations and, on the basis of this observation, they hypothesized that heparin and glucose competed *in vivo,* both against the same catalytic residue of AT-III. Hansen and Jørgensen also observed a discrepancy in insulin-dependent diabetic patients between the functional activity (measured by chromogenic substrate) and concentration (measured by electroimmunoassay) of AT-III.[252] However, the thrombin-neutralizing activity of their diabetic patients was higher than the antigen concentration. In the crossed immunoelectrophoresis system, with or without heparin in the first dimension, there was no difference in the mobility of AT-III of the diabetic patients when compared with control. However, in the presence of lectin, the patient's samples showed a slower mobility of AT-III in the crossed affinoimmunoelectrophoresis.

In conclusion, a qualitative change of the AT-III molecule seems to be proved in diabetes mellitus, but the exact characterization of this change has not been performed yet. The pathogenetic significance of this alteration has to be further investigated.

5. AT-III in Ischaemic Heart Disease

The results of the investigations on AT-III levels in ischaemic heart disease are rather controversial. The elevation of AT-III has been observed in myocardial infarction by several authors.[255,256] Others, on the contrary, reported low AT-III levels in myocardial infarction.[257,258] Innerfield et al.[259] found low AT-III levels in severe coronary artery disease. However, these latter authors performed the measurement of AT-III levels in serum, instead of plasma. Hence, the *in vivo* relevance of their findings is disputable. The differences of the various investigations may be explained partly by the methodological differences, but also by the heterogeneity of the patients. In the early phase of acute myocardial infarction, an AT-III level may be elevated as a consequence of the increase of the ''acute phase proteins'' which is absent in other stages of ischaemic heart disease. Taking into consideration the minor role of AT-III in the pathogenesis of the thrombosis of the arteries and the controversial reports, no decisive alterations of AT-III level seem to be probable in coronary artery disease.

6. Alterations of AT-III Levels Induced by Various Drugs

In 1973, Marciniak and Gockerman reported that heparin therapy reduced the plasma level of AT-III.[260] Rao et al.[261] found a uniform decrease of 30% in the plasma levels of AT-III antigens and activities in all patients with thromboembolic disorders receiving continuous intravenous heparin therapy (keeping the activated partial thromboplastin time in the therapeutic range). The lowest levels were recorded between 3 to 5 d after the discontinuation of heparin. Low-dose subcutaneous heparin given to patients without thrombotic problems did not affect AT-III levels.[262,263] However, at doses of 3×7500 I.U. per 24 h, the AT-III antigen concentration of plasma decreases.[265] The mechanism underlying the decrease in the AT-III levels during intravenous heparin therapy is unknown. There is evidence suggesting that heparin may alter the rate of turnover of AT-III in patients with thrombotic problems. Collen et al.[73] have studied the metabolism of labeled AT-III in patients with venous thrombosis and found the plasma radioactivity half-life was significantly shortened and the fractional catabolic rate increased in patients treated with heparin as compared to patients not treated with heparin. The clinical significance of the heparin-induced decrease of AT-III appears to be the recurrence of thrombosis in patients who were treated with heparin because of previous thrombosis, but the heparin was stopped abruptly. In this situation, the low AT-III level persists for a while and hypercoagulable state develops. It is especially true for patients with congenital or acquired AT-III deficiencies in whom the additional AT-III-reducing effect of heparin treatment produces very low AT-III levels. Bolwerk et al.[264] observed that in hereditary AT-III-deficient patients, even the subcutaneous heparin therapy decreased the AT-III levels in the plasma of the patients (4×5000 I.U. per 24 h, by approximately 0.20 U/ml). Nagy et al.[193] reported the heparin sensitivity of AT-III levels in patients with chronic liver diseases.

For avoiding a hypercoagulable state, adequate anticoagulation with vitamin K antagonists prior to the discontinuation of intravenous heparin therapy has to be achieved. In the case of an AT-III deficiency, the administration of an AT-III concentrate may be helpful to restore the AT-III level in the course of heparin therapy.

The effect of oral anticoagulant (vitamin K antagonists) treatment of the AT-III level of plasma is disputed. Several authors reported a rise of AT-III levels in patients on treatment with vitamin K antagonists.[266,267,268,269] However, this finding has not been confirmed by others.[270,271] The different degree of anticoagulation seems to be an improbable explanation for the conflicting opinions because De Stefano et al.[272] could not demonstrate any difference in the plasma AT-III levels of groups of patients anticoagulated intensely or moderately, or not anticoagulated at all. Hence, oral anticoagulant treatment has only a minor effect on an AT-III level if it has at all. Either the methodological differences or heterogeneity of anticoagulated patients may explain the different results. It is conceivable that oral anticoagulant therapy stops the hypercoagulable state with reduced AT-III levels in some patients. In these patients, coumarin therapy may undoubtedly influence plasma AT-III levels.

The functional activity and immunochemical concentration of AT-III are indisputably higher in the serum of anticoagulated patients than that of untreated subjects because of the reduced consumption of AT-III in the course of clotting.

Factor IX concentrates, too, can influence the plasma AT-III both quantitatively and qualitatively.[273,274] Factor IX concentrates contain or induce the production of some activated coagulation factors, which are complexed with AT-III in the plasma of the patient. Factor IX concentrate-treated hemophilic plasma contains a nonfunctional, high molecular weight form of AT-III associated with the presence of neonantigen, which may represent complexed and/or modified AT-III produced by the action of the concentrates *in vivo*.[275]

L-asparaginase, a chemotherapeutic agent employed in the treatment of acute lymphocytic leukemia (ALL) induces AT-III deficiency.[276,277,278] Several reports link this abnormality with thromboembolic phenomena.[277,279,280,284] The mechanism of the reduction of an AT-III level during L-asparaginase therapy is disputed. It has been hypothesized that L-asparaginase may regularly induce a hypercoagulable state. This view was challenged by Bauer et al.,[281] who could not demonstrate a hypercoagulable state after the administration of L-asparaginase. They explained the reduction of an AT-III level during L-asparaginase treatment with the depression of the synthesis of AT-III. L-asparaginase leads to a depression in the synthesis of a variety of proteins by the liver. In addition to AT-III, the concentration of several coagulation proteins, such as factor IX, XI, and fibrinogen, are greatly diminished by this enzyme.[282,283] However, Bauer et al.[281] studied the effect of L-asparaginase therapy only in children with ALL in remission, and these observations can be extrapolated only with caution to older patients with different types of malignancy.

A plasma AT-III level is influenced by steroid hormones as well. The majority of the data derives from investigations on progestational drugs, and this question is discussed in detail in another chapter of this book. Thus, we'll deal here only briefly with some general problems which are out of the scope of gynecology and neonatology.

According to Nagasawa et al.,[285] steroid hormones influence the AT-III activity of plasma by a direct effect, i.e., steroid hormones bind to AT-III, which is attended by a conformational change in the latter. As a consequence of this change, AT-III activity decreases. However, only therapeutic doses of steroid hormones can interact with AT-III *in vivo*. The hormonal influence of AT-III activity has a great importance in patients with prostatic carcinoma. Out of the three current therapeutic measures (estrogens, antiandrogens, and bilateral orchydectomy), only high-dose estrogen treatment is accompanied with a selective decrease in AT-III activity.[286] A significant decrease in AT-III activity of 27% (range 7 to 46%) was found in patients on initially high-dose estrogen (15 mg diethylstilbestrol daily) treatment regime. Patients with the lower end of the normal range of pretreatment plasma AT-III activity may suffer acquired AT-III deficiencies and, thus, a concomittantly increased risk of thromboembolic complication arises as a result of estrogen treatment. Hence, Büller et al.[287] suggested measuring the AT-III levels before and during estrogen therapy of patients with prostatic cancer and, in case of a significant decrease, a prophylactic low dose of heparin should be adminstered subcutaneously.

REFERENCES

1. **Schmitz-Huebner, U., Nachbar, J., and Asbeck, F.,** The determination of antithrombin-III, α_2-macroglobulin and α_2-antiplasmin in plasma by laser nephelometry, *J. Clin. Chem. Clin. Biochem.*, 18, 221, 1980.
2. **Balla, G., Misz, M., and Rák, K.,** Antithrombin III determination by rate (kinetic) nephelometry, *Thromb. Haemostas.*, 51, 9, 1984.
3. **Laurell, C. B.,** Quantitative estimation of proteins by electrophoresis in agarose gel containing antibodies, *Ann. Biochem.*, 15, 45, 1966.
4. **Mancini, G., Carbonara, A. O., and Heremans, J. F.,** Immunochemical quantitation of antigens by simple radial immunodiffusion, *Int. J. Immunochem.*, 2, 235, 1965.
5. **Chan, V., Chan, T. K., Wong, V., Tso, S. C., and Todd, D.,** The determination of antithrombin III by radioimmunoassay and its clinical application, *Br. J. Haematol.*, 41, 563, 1979.
6. **Tanaka, M. and Kato, K.,** Determination of antithrombin III by sandwich enzyme immunoassay technique, *Thromb. Res.*, 22, 67, 1981.
7. **Astrup, T. and Darling, S.,** Measurement and properties of antithrombin, *Acta Phys. Scand.*, 4, 293, 1942.
8. **Seegers, W. H., Miller, K. D., Andrews, E. B., and Murphy, R. C.,** Fundamental interactions and the effect of storage, ether, adsorbants and blood clotting on plasma antithrombin activity, *Am. J. Phys.*, 169, 700, 1952.
9. **Hallén, A.,** A method for measuring antithrombin, *Thromb. Diath. Haemorrh.*, 8, 56, 1962.
10. **Gerendás, M.,** Die Thrombininaktivierung als Enzymprozess, *Thromb. Diath. Haemorrh.*, 4, 56, 1960.
11. **Hensen, A. and Loeliger, E. A.,** Antithrombin III. Its metabolism and its function in blood coagulation, *Thromb. Diath. Haemorrh. Suppl.*, 1, 9, 1963.
12. **Abildgaard, U., Gravem, K., and Godal, H. C.,** Assay of progressive antithrombin in plasma, *Thromb. Diath. Haemorrh.*, 24, 224, 1970.
13. **Biggs, R., Denson, K. W. E., Akman, N., Borret, R., and Hadden, M.,** Antithrombin III, antifactor Xa and heparin, *Br. J. Haematol.*, 19, 283, 1970.
14. **Abildgaard, U., Lie, M. and Ødegard, O. R.,** A simple amidolytic method for the determination of functionally active antithrombin III, *Scand. J. Clin. Lab. Invest.*, 36, 109, 1976.
15. **Miller-Andersson, M., Borg, H., and Andersson, L. O.,** Purification of antithrombin III by affinity chromatography, *Thromb. Res.*, 5, 439, 1974.
16. **Ødegard, O. R., Lie, M., and Abildgaard, U.,** Heparin cofactor activity measured with an amidolytic method, *Thromb. Res.*, 6, 287, 1975.
17. **Gitel, S. N. and Wessler, S.,** Plasma antithrombin III: a quantitative assay of biological activity, *Thromb. Res.*, 1, 5, 1975.
18. **Ødegard, O. R., Lie, M., and Abildgaard, U.,** Antifactor Xa activity measured with amidolytic methods, *Haemostasis*, 5, 265, 1976.
19. **Laurell, C. B.,** Antigen-antibody crossed electrophoresis, *Anal. Biochem.*, 10, 358, 1965.
20. **Sas, G., Pepper, D. S., and Cash, J. D.,** Plasma and serum antithrombin III: differentiation by crossed immunoelectrophoresis, *Thromb. Res.*, 6, 87, 1975.
21. **Kera, Y., Yamasawa, K., and Komura, S.,** Phenotypic variation of human antithrombin III in normal plasma: detection by isoelectric focusing, *Jpn. J. Hum. Genet.*, 28, 249, 1983.
22. **Leone, G. Valori, V. M., Cotumaccio, R. and Massi, G.,** Human antithrombin III heterogeneity: a study by isoelectrofocusing and crossed immunoelectrofocusing, *Haemostasis*, 13, 369, 1983.
23. **Frigola, A.,** Standardization of a simple method for the determination of antithrombin activity, *J. Clin. Pathol.*, 30, 881, 1977.
24. **Abildgaard, U., Fagerhol, M. K., and Egeberg, O.,** Comparison of progressive antithrombin activity and the concentration of three thrombin inhibitors in human plasma, *Scand. J. Clin. Lab. Invest.*, 26, 349, 1970.
25. **McLellan, D. S., Devlin, J. D., Heyse-Moore, G. H., and Aronstam, A.,** Comparison of three methods for the estimation of plasma antithrombin, *J. Clin. Pathol.*, 33, 438, 1980.
26. **Sas, G., Pepper, D. S., and Cash, J. D.,** Further investigations on antithrombin III in the plasma of the patients with the abnormality of antithrombin III "Budapest", *Thromb. Diath. Haemorrh.*, 33, 564, 1975.
27. **Lane, J. L.,** Some immunological investigations on antithrombin III "Budapest", *Br. J. Haematol.*, 40, 459, 1978.
28. **Pepper, D. S., Bánhegyi, D., and Cash, J. D.,** The different forms of antithrombin III in serum, *Thromb. Haemostas.*, 38, 494, 1977.
29. **McKay, E. J.,** Immunochemical analysis of active and inactive antithrombin III, *Br. J. Haematol.*, 46, 277, 1980.
30. **Barrowcliffe, T. W.,** Studies of heparin binding to antithrombin III by crossed immunoelectrophoresis, *Thromb. Haemostas.*, 42, 1434, 1980.

31. **Sas, G., Pepper, D. S., and Cash, J. D.,** Investigations on antithrombin III in normal plasma and serum, *Br. J. Haematol.*, 30, 265, 1975.
32. **Sas, G. and Pepper, D. S.,** Detection of thrombin-antithrombin III complex by crossed immunoelectrophoresis, *Thromb. Res.*, 9, 95, 1976.
33. **Andersson, L-O., Engman, L., and Henningson, E.,** Crossed immunoelectrophoresis as applied to studies on complex formation. The binding of heparin to antithrombin III and the antithrombin III-thrombin complex, *J. Immunol. Methods*, 14, 271, 1977.
34. **Chan, V. and Chan, T. K.,** Heparin-Antithrombin III binding. *In vitro* and *in vivo* studies, *Haemostasis*, 8, 373, 1979.
35. **Sas, G., Köves, Á., and Petõ, I.,** Detection of antithrombin III (AT-III) complexes in "hypercoagulable" and hyperfibrinolytic states, *Thromb. Haemostas.*, 38, 164, 1977.
36. **Rodeghiero, F. and Barbui, T.,** Two dimensional immunoelectrophoresis of antithrombin III during disseminated intravascular coagulation in acute leukemia, *Thromb. Res.*, 12, 191, 1977.
37. **Abildgaard, U.,** Purification of two progressive antithrombins of human plasma, *Scand. J. Clin. Lab. Invest.*, 19, 190, 1967.
38. **Howie, P. W., Prentice, C. R. M., and McNicol, G. P.,** A method of antithrombin estimation using plasma defibrinated with ancrod, *Br. J. Haematol.*, 25, 101, 1973.
39. **Latallo, Z. S. and Hall, J. A.,** Reaction of thrombins with human antithrombin III. I. Enzyme activity losses unrelated to the inhibitory reaction and their prevention, *Thromb. Res.*, 43, 507, 1986.
40. **Frieberger, P., Egberg, N., Holmer, E., Hellgren, M., and Blomback, M.,** Antithrombin assay — the use of human or bovine thrombin and the observation of a "second" heparin cofactor, *Thromb. Res.*, 25, 433, 1982.
41. **Mihályi, E. and Williams, S. B.,** Mislabeling of commercial fibrinogen preparations: bovine or human? *Thromb. Res.*, 35, 725, 1984.
42. **Ødegard, O. R. and Lie, M.,** On use of chromogenic substrates for studies of coagulation inhibitors, *Haemostasis*, 7, 121, 1978.
43. **Mitchell, G. A., Hudson, P. M., Huseby, R. M., Pochron, S. P., and Gargiulo, R. J.,** Fluorescent substrate for antithrombin III, *Thromb. Res.*, 12, 219, 1978.
44. **Bishop, R. C., Hudson, P. M., Mitchell, G. A., and Pochron, S. P.,** Use of fluorogenic substrates for the assay of antithrombin III and heparin, *Ann. N.Y. Acad. Sci.*, 370, 720, 1981.
45. **Ødegard, O. R., Rosenlund, B., and Ervik, E.,** Automated antithrombin III assay with a centrifugal analyser, *Haemostasis*, 7, 202, 1978.
46. **Andreasen, T.,** Automated two-stage assay for determination of antithrombin III with a centrifugal analyzer, *Haemostasis*, 9, 65, 1980.
47. **Holmes, E. W., Fareed, J., and Bermes, E. W., Jr.,** Automation of plasma antithrombin III assays, *Clin. Chem.*, 27, 816, 1981.
48. **Bartl, K. and Lill, H.,** A versatile assay method of antithrombin III using thrombin and Tos-Gly-Pro-Arg-pNA, *Thromb. Res.*, 18, 267, 1980.
49. **Brandt, J. T. and Senhauser, D. A.,** Clinical laboratory determination of antithrombin III, *Am. J. Clin. Pathol.*, 73, 687, 1980.
50. **Kahle, L. H., Schipper, H. G., Jenkins, C. S. P., and ten Cate, J. W.,** Antithrombin III. I. Evaluation of an automated antithrombin III method, *Thromb. Res.*, 12, 1003, 1978.
51. **Conard, J., Barbier, P., and Samama, M.,** Automated amidolytic method for AT-III determination, *Thromb. Haemostas.*, 4, 1350, 1979.
52. **Cederholm-Williams, S. A.,** Automated enzyme assay of antithrombin, *Ann. Clin. Biochem.*, 17, 183, 1980.
53. **Aiach, M., Schreiber, N., Nussas, C., Angebault, M., and Leclerc, M.,** Dosage de l'antithrombine III a l'aide d'une methode chromogenique automatisee, *Pharmacol. Biol.*, 14, 103, 1980.
54. **Droulle, C., Caron, Y., Poignot, J. L., Lafurie, M., Remy, M. G., and Potron, G.,** Interet du dosage de l'antithrombine III (cofacteur de l'heparine) par methode automatique., *Rev. Fr.*, 93, 12, 1981.
55. **Scully, M. F. and Kakkar, V. V.,** Methods for semi-micro or automated determination of thrombin, antithrombin and heparin cofactor using the substrate H-D-Phe-Pip-Arg-P-Nitroanilide-2 HCL., *Clin. Chem. Acta*, 79, 595, 1977.
56. **Prellwitz, W., Schitt, K. F., Machner, M., Schuster, C. J., and Weilemann, L.,** Two automated methods for plasma antithrombin III compared, and the clinical relevance of the results. *Clin. Chem.*, 28, 2249, 1982.
57. **Fareed, J., Messmore, H. L., Walenga, J., Soloman, J., Statland, B. T., Ito, R., Perry, J. F., and Wehrly, J. A.,** A clinical evaluation of Dupont ACATH antithrombin III assay, *Clin. Chem.*, 27, 1108, 1981.
58. **Conard, J.,** Automation of antithrombin III methods on routinely available instruments, *Sem. Thromb. Hemostas.*, 9, 257, 1983.

59. **Fareed, J., Messmore, H. L., and Fenton, J. W.,** The application of various molecular forms of human thrombin in the quantitation of antithrombin III (heparin cofactor), in Progress in Clinical Enzymology, Goldberg, D. M. and Werner, M., Eds., Masson, New York, 1980, 257.
60. **Fareed, J., Walenga, J. M., Svendsen, L. G., and Bermes, E. W.,** Coagulant versus amydolytic properties of human and bovine thrombins: implications in standardization and diagnostic usage, *Sem. Thromb. Haemostas.*, 12, 310, 1986.
61. **Latallo, Z. S. and Jackson, C. M.,** Reaction of thrombins with human antithrombin III. II. Dependence of rate of inhibiton on molecular form and origin of thrombin, *Thromb. Res.*, 43, 523, 1986.
62. **Bounameaux, H., Duckert, F., Walter, M., and Bounameaux, Y.,** Comparison of six methods. Effect of oral contraceptive therapy, *Thromb. Haemostas.*, 39, 607, 1978.
63. **Bick, R. L. and McClain, B. J.,** A clinical comparison of chromogenic, fluorometric and natural (fibrinogen) substrate assays for the determination of antithrombin III., *Thromb. Haemostas.*, 46, 364, 1981.
64. **Philo, R. D. and Gaffney, P. J.,** Comparison of antithrombin III assays using biological and chromogenic substrates, *Br. J. Haematol.*, 50, 147, 1982.
65. **Fahey, J. L. and McKelvey, E. M.,** Quantitative determination of serum immunoglobulins in antibody-agar plates, *J. Immunol.*, 94, 84, 1965.
66. **Lundblad, R. L., Kingdon, H. S., and Mann, K. G.,** Thrombin, *Methods Enzymol.*, 45, 156, 1976.
67. **Abildgaard, U., Lie, M., and Ødegard, O. R.,** Antithrombin (heparin cofactor) assay with "new" chromogenic substrate, *Thromb. Res.*, 11, 549, 1977.
68. **Kirkwood, T. B. L., Barrowcliffe, T. W., and Thomas, D. P.,** An international collaborative study establishing a reference preparation for antithrombin III, *Thromb. Haemostas.*, 43, 10, 1980.
69. **Conard, J., Brosstad, F., Lie Larsen, M., Samama, M., and Abildgaard, U.,** Molar antithrombin concentration in normal human plasma, *Haemostasis*, 13, 363, 1983.
70. **Abildgaard, U.,** Inhibition of the thrombin-fibrinogen reaction by heparin and purified cofactor, *Scand. J. Haematol.*, 5, 440, 1968.
71. **Heimburger, N.,** On the proteinase inhibitors of human plasma with especial reference to antithrombin in 1st Int. Symp. Tissue Factors in the Haemostas. of the Coagulation-Fibrinolysis Syst., Florence, 1967.
72. **Murano, G., Williams, L., Miller-Andersson, M., Aronson, D. L., and King, C.,** Some properties of antithrombin III and its concentration in human plasma, *Thromb. Res.*, 18, 259, 1980.
73. **Collen, D., Schetz, J., de Cock, F., Holmer, E., and Verstraete, M.,** Metabolism of antithrombin III (heparin cofactor), in Man: Effects of Venous Thrombosis and of Heparin Administration, *Eur. J. Clin. Invest.*, 7, 27, 1977.
74. **Ødegard, O. R., Fagerhol, M. K., and Lie, M.,** Heparin cofactor activity and antithrombin III concentration in palsma related to age and sex, *Scand. J. Haematol.*, 17, 258, 1976.
75. **Panicucci, F., Sagripanti, A., Conte, B., Pinori, E., Vispi, M., and Lecchini, L.,** Antithrombin III, heparin cofactor and antifactor Xa in relation to age, sex and pathological condition, *Haemostasis*, 9, 297, 1980.
76. **Egeberg, O.,** Inherited antithrombin III deficiency causing thrombophilia, *Thromb. Diath. Haemorrh.*, 13, 516, 1965.
77. **van der Meer, J., Stoepman-van Dalen, E. A., and Jansen, J. M. S.,** Antithrombin III deficiency in a Dutch family, *Am. J. Clin. Pathol.*, 26, 532, 1973.
78. **Marciniak, E., Farley, C. H., and DeSimone, P. A.,** Familial thrombosis due to antithrombin III deficiency, *Blood*, 43, 219, 1974.
79. **Sas, G., Blaskó, G., Bánhegyi, D., Jákó, J., and Pálos, L. Á.,** Abnormal antithrombin III (antithrombin III "Budapest") as a cause of a familial thrombophilia, *Thromb. Diath. Haemorrh.*, 32, 105, 1974.
80. **Nagy, I., Losonczy, H., Szaksz, I., Temesi, C., and Hergert, K.,** An analysis of clinical and laboratory data in patients with congenital antithrombin III (AT-III) deficiency, *Acta Med. Acad. Sci. Hung.*, 36, 53, 1979.
81. **Wolf, M., Boyer, C., Lavergne, J. M., and Larrieu, M. J.,** A new variant of antithrombin III. Study of three related cases, *Thromb. Haemostas.*, 42, 186, 1979.
82. **Sas, G., Pető, I., Bánhegyi, D., Blaskó, G., and Domján, G.,** Heterogeneity of the "classical" antithrombin III deficiency, *Thromb. Haemostas.*, 43, 133, 1980.
83. **Sas, G.,** Hereditary antithrombin III deficiency: biochemical aspects, *Haematologia*, 17, 81, 1984.
84. **Schmidt, B., Wais, U., Pringsheim, W., Witt, I., and Künzer, W.,** Decreased production or increased turnover of antithrombin III in severe acquired coagulopathy? *Klin. Wochenschr.*, 59, 1349, 1981.
85. **Anker, E., Abildgaard, U., Andersen, R., Fagerhol, M., and Bjune, G.,** Low antithrombin in severe disease: consumption or decreased synthesis? *Scand. J. Haematol.*, 30, 59, 1983.
86. **Knot, E., ten Cate, J. W., Drijfhout, H. R., Kahlé, L. H., and Tytgat, G. N.,** Antithrombin III metabolism in patients with liver disease, *J. Clin. Pathol.*, 37, 523, 1984.
87. **Nagy, I., Losonczy, H., and Szilágyi, C.,** Durch hereditäre Antithrombin-III-Verminderung verursachte rezidivierende Thromboembolien bei Jugendlichen, *Folia. Haematol.*, 102, 233, 1975.

88. **Juillet, Y., Vayssairat, M., Fiessinger, J. N., Aiach, M., and Housset, E.,** Thrombose des veines porte et mésenterique supérieure au cours d'un déficit congénital et familial en antithrombine III, *Ann. Med. Interne,* 130, 53, 1979.
89. **Lechner, K., Thaler, E., Niessner, H., Nowotny, Ch., and Partsch, H.,** Antithrombin-III-Mangel und Thromboseneigung, *Wien. Klin. Wochenschr.,* 89, 215, 1977.
90. **Manotti, C., Quintavalla, R., Megha, A., Ponari, O., and Dettori, A. G.,** Inherited deficiency of antithrombin III in two Italian families: different response to oral anticoagulant treatment, *Haemostasis,* 12, 300, 1982.
91. **Scully, M. F., De Haas, H., Chan, P., and Kakkar, V. V.,** Hereditary antithrombin III deficiency in an English family, *Br. J. Haematol.,* 47, 235, 1981.
92. **Conard, J., Cazenave, B., Horellou, M. H., and Samama, M.,** Déficits congénitaux en antithrombine III, *Med. Hyg.,* 39, 4259, 1981.
93. **Stathakis, N. E., Papayannis, A. G., Antonopoulos, M., and Gardikas, C.,** Familial thrombosis due to antithrombin III deficiency in a Greek family, *Acta Haematol.,* 57, 47, 1977.
94. **Mackie, M., Bennett, B., Ogston, D., and Douglas, A. S.,** Familial thrombosis: inherited deficiency of antithrombin III, *Br. Med. J.,* 1, 136, 1978.
95. **Johansson, L., Hedner, U., and Nilsson, I. M.,** Familial antithrombin III deficiency as pathogenesis of deep venous thrombosis, *Acta Med. Scand.,* 204, 491, 1978.
96. **Fontcuberta, J., Felez, J., Borrell, M., and Ruttlant, M. L.,** Deficit congenito de AT III, *Biol. Clin. Hematol.,* 1, 229, 1979.
97. **von Kaulla, E. and von Kaulla, K. N.,** Deficiency of antithrombin III activity with hereditary thrombosis tendency, *J. Med.,* 3, 349, 1972.
98. **Gruenberg, J. C., Smallridge, R. C., and Rosenberg, R. D.,** Inherited antithrombin III deficiency causing mesenteric venous infarction: a new clinical entity, *Ann. Surg.,* 181, 791, 1975.
99. **Filip, D. J., Eckstein, J. D., and Veltkamp, J. J.,** Hereditary antithrombin III deficiency and thromboembolic disease, *Am. J. Haematol.,* 2, 343, 1976.
100. **Carvalho, A. and Ellman, L.,** Hereditary antithrombin III deficiency, *Am. J. Med.,* 61, 179, 1976.
101. **Arko, F. R., Jewell, C. T., Dainer, P., and MacLeod, W. A. J.,** Primary mesenteric vein thrombosis associated with antithrombin III deficiency, *J. Am. Med. Assoc.,* 242, 2324, 1979.
102. **Ambruso, D. R., Linda, M. D., Jacobson, L. J., and Hathaway, W. E.,** Inherited antithrombin III deficiency and cerebral thrombosis in a child, *Pediatrics,* 65, 125, 1980.
103. **Halal, F., Quenneville, G., Laurin, S., and Loulou, G.,** Clinical and genetic aspects of antithrombin III deficiency, *Am. J. Med. Genet.,* 14, 737, 1983.
104. **Zucker, M. L., Gomperts, E. D., and Marcus, R. G.,** Prophylactic and therapeutic use of anticoagulants in inherited antithrombin III deficiency, *S. Afr. Med. J.,* 50, 1743, 1975.
105. **Gomperts, E. D., Feesey, M., and van der Walt, L.,** Two dimensional immonoelectrophoretic studies in antithrombin III deficiency, *Thromb. Res.,* 8, 713, 1976.
106. **Matsuo, T., Ohki, Y., Kondo, S., and Matsuo, O.,** Familial antithrombin III deficiency in a Japanese family, *Thromb. Kes.,* 16, 815, 1979.
107. **Concannon, A. J. and Low, J.,** Antithrombin III deficiency in a Chinese family, *Med. J. Aust.,* 1, 521, 1981.
108. **Pitney, W. R., Manoharan, A., and Dean, S.,** Antithrombin III deficiency in an Australian family, *Br. J. Haematol.,* 46, 147, 1980.
109. **Ødegard, O. R. and Abildgaard, U.,** Antithrombin III: critical review of assay methods, *Haemostasis,* 7, 127, 1978.
110. **Rosenberg, R. D.,** Action and interacton of antithrombin and heparin, *N. Engl. J. Med.,* 292, 146, 1975.
111. **Winter, J. H.,** Prevalence of antithrombin deficiency, in Antithrombin Deficiency, Böttiger, L. E., Ed., KabiVitrum AB., Stockholm, 1987, 25.
112. **Juillet, Y., Aiach, M., Fiessinger, J. N., Leclerc, M., and Housset, E.,** Antithrombine III et thromboses veineuses, *Sem. Hop.,* 54, 1126, 1978.
113. **Ambruso, D. R., Leonard, B. D., Bies, R. D., Jacobson, L., Hathaway, W. E., and Reeve, E. B.,** Antithrombin III deficiency: decreased synthesis of a biochemically normal molecule, *Blood,* 60, 78, 1982.
114. **Knot, E. A. R., de Jong, E., ten Cate, J. W., Ilburg, A. H. C., Henny, Ch. P., Bruin, T., and Stibbe, J.,** Purified radiolabeled antithrombin III metabolism in three families with hereditary AT III deficiency: application of a three-compartment model, *Blood,* 67, 93, 1986.
115. **Cosgriff, T. M., Bishop, D. T., Hershgold, E. J., Skolnick, M. H., Martin, B. A., Baty, B. J., and Carlson, K. S.,** Familial antithrombin III deficiency: its natural history, genetics, diagnosis and treatment, *Medicine,* 62, 209, 1983.
116. **Williams, L. and Murano, G.,** Human antithrombin III heterogeneity, *Blood,* 57, 229, 1981.
117. **Leone, G., Cotumaccio, R., De Stefano, V., and Zanetti, L.,** Antithrombin III Roma: a familial quantitative-qualitative AT-III deficiency identifiable by crossed immunoelectrofocusing and by crossed immunoelectrophoresis, *Haematologica,* 68, 765, 1983.

118. **Abildgaard, U.,** Antithrombin and related inhibitors of coagulation, in Recent Advances in Blood Coagulation, Vol. 3, Poller, L., Ed., Churchill Livingstone, Edinburgh, 1981, 151.
119. **Prochownik, E. V., Antonarakis, S., Bauer, K. A., Rosenberg, R., Fearon, E. R., and Orkin, S. H.,** Molecular heterogeneity of inherited antithrombin III deficiency, *Engl. J. Med.*, 308, 1549, 1983.
120. **Sas, G., Köves, Á., Petõ, I., and Domján, G.,** On the inheritance of the abnormal antithrombin III ("AT-III Budapest"), *Thromb. Haemostas.*, 39, 530, 1978.
121. **Sørensen, P. J., Sas, G., Petõ, I., Blaskó, G., Kremmer, T., and Samu, A.,** Distinciton of two pathologic antithrombin III molecules: antithrombin III "Aalborg" and Antithrombin III "Budapest", *Thromb. Res.*, 26, 211, 1982.
122. **Tengborn, L., Frohm, B., Nisson, L.-E., and Nilsson, I. M.,** A Swedish family with abnormal antithrombin III, *Scand. J. Haematol.*, 34, 412, 1985.
123. **Murayama, H. and Matsuda, M.,** Abnormal antithrombin III with defective biological and immunological functions found in a thrombophilic patient — antithrombin III "Tokyo", *Thromb. Haemostas.*, 50, 358, 1983.
124. **Murayama, H. and Matsuda, M.,** Abnormal properties and behaviours of antithrombin III found in a thrombophilic patient: defective biological functions and dissimilar antigenic determinants, *Thromb. Haemostas.*, 56, 165, 1986.
125. **Bauer, K. A., Ashenhurst, J. B., Chediak, J., and Rosenberg, R. D.,** Antithrombin III "Chicago": a functionally abnormal molecule with increased heparin affinity causing familial thrombophilia, *Blood*, 62, 1242, 1983.
126. **Girolami, A., Marafioti, F., Rubertelli, M., Vicariato, M. A., Cappellato, G., and Mazzuccato, M.,** Antithrombin III Trento. A "new" congenital AT III abnormality with a peculiar crossed-immunoelectrophoretic pattern in the absence of heparin, *Acta Haematol.*, 72, 73, 1984.
127. **Girolami, A., Cappellato, M. G., Vicariato, M. A., Casonato, S., and Marafioti, F.,** Associated von Willebrand disease as a possible cause of lack of thrombosis in AT-III abnormality (AT III Trento), *Blut*, 52, 29, 1986.
128. **Brozovic, M., Stirling, Y., and Hamlyn, A. N.,** Thrombotic tendency and probable antithrombin III deficiency, *Thromb. Haemostas.*, 39, 778, 1978.
129. **Howarth, D. J., Samson, D., Stirling, Y., and Seghatchian, M. J.,** Antithrombin III "Northwick Park": a variant antithrombin with normal affinity for heparin but reduced heparin cofactor activity, *Thromb. Haemostas.*, 53, 314, 1985.
130. **Lane, D. A., Flynn, A., Ireland, H., Erdjument, H., Samson, D., Howarth, D., and Thompson, E.,** Antithrombin III Northwick Park: demonstration of an inactive high MW complex with increased affinity for heparin, *Br. J. Haematol.*, 65, 451, 1987.
131. **Wolf, M., Boyer, C., Tripodi, A., Meyer, D., Larrieu, M. J., and Mannucci, P. M.,** Antithrombin Milano: a new variant with monomeric and dimeric inactive antithrombin III, *Blood*, 65, 496, 1985.
132. **Sørensen, P. J., Dyerberg, J., Stoffersen, E., and Krogh Jensen, M.,** Familial functional antithrombin III deficiency, *Scand. J. Haematol.*, 24, 105, 1980.
133. **Barbui, T. and Rodeghiero, F.,** Hereditary dysfunctional antithrombin III (AT-III Vicenza), *Thromb. Haemostas.*, 45, 97, 1981.
134. **Barbui, T., Finazzi, G., Rodeghiero, F., and Dini, E.,** Immunoelectrophoretic evidence of a thrombin-induced abnormality in a new variant of hereditary dysfunctional antithrombin III (AT III "Vicenza"), *Br. J. Haematol.*, 54, 561, 1983.
135. **Finazzi, G., Tran, T. H., Babui, T., and Duckert, F.,** Purification of antithrombin "Vicenza" a molecule with normal heparin affinity and impaired reactivity to thrombin, *Br. J. Haematol.*, 59, 259, 1985.
136. **Jørgensen, M., Petersen, L. C., and Thorsen, S.,** Purification and characterization of hereditary abnormal antithrombin III with impaired thrombin binding, *J. Lab. Clin. Med.*, 104, 245, 1984.
137. **Sambrano, J. E., Jacobson, L. J., Reeve, E. B., Manco-Johnson, M. J., and Hathaway, W. E.,** Abnormal antithrombin III with defective serine protease binding (Antithrombin III "Denver"), *J. Clin. Invest.*, 77, 887, 1986.
138. **Stephens, A. W., Thalley, B. S., and Hirs, C. H. W.,** Antithrombin III Denver, a ser to leu^{394} variant without protease inhibitory activity, *Thromb. Haemostas.*, 54, 49, 1985.
139. **Aiach, M., Nora, M., Fiessinger, J. N., Roncato, M., Francois, D., and Gelas, M. A.,** A functional abnormal antithrombin III (AT III) deficiency: AT III Charleville, *Thromb. Res.*, 39, 559, 1985.
140. **Tripodi, A., Krachmalnicoff, A., and Mannucci, P. M.,** Characterization of an abnormal antithrombin (Milano 2) with defective thrombin binding, *Thromb. Haemostas.*, 56, 349, 1986.
141. **Leone, G., De Stefano, V., Di Donfrancesco, A., Ferrelli, R., Traisci, G., and Bizzi, B.,** Antithrombin III Perscara: a defective AT III variant with no alterations of plasma crossed immunoelectrophoresis, but with an abnormal crossed immunoelectrofocusing pattern. *Br. J. Haematol.*, 65, 187, 1987.
142. **Penner, J. A., Hassouna, H., Hunter, M. J., and Chockley, M. A.,** A clinically silent antithrombin III defect in an Ann Arbor family, *Thromb. Haemostas.*, 42, 186, 1979.

143. **Tran, T. H., Bounameaux, H., Bondeli, C., Honkanen, H., Marbet, G. A., and Duckert, F.,** Purification and partial characterization of a hereditary abnormal antithrombin III fraction of a patient with recurrent thrombophlebitis, *Thromb. Haemostas.*, 44, 87, 1980.
144. **Tran, T. H., Bondeli, C., Marbet, G. A., and Duckert, F.,** Reactivity of a hereditary abnormal antithrombin III fraction in the inhibition of thrombin and Factor Xa, *Thromb. Haemostas.*, 44, 92, 1980.
145. **Chang, J.-Y. and Tran, T. H.,** Antithrombin III Basel. Identification of a Pro-Leu substitution in a hereditary abnormal antithrombin with impaired heparin cofactor activity, *J. Biol. Chem.*, 261, 1174, 1986.
146. **Wolf, M., Boyer, C., Lavergne, J. M., and Larrieu, M. J.,** A new familial variant of antithrombin III: "Antithrombin III Paris," *Br. J. Haematol.*, 51, 285, 1982.
147. **Girolami, A., Pengo, V., Cappellato, G., Vianello, C., Procidano, M., and Cartei, C.,** Antithrombin III Padua: a "new" congenital antithrombin III abnormality with normal or near normal activity, normal antigen, abnormal migration and no thrombotic disease, *Folia Haematol. Leipzig*, 110, 98, 1983.
148. **Girolami, A., Fabris, F., Cappellato, G., Sainati, L., and Boeri, G.,** Antithrombin III (AT III) Padua$_2$: a "new" congenital abnormality with defective heparin co-factor activities but no thrombotic disease, *Blut*, 47, 93, 1983.
149. **Sakuragawa, N., Takahashi, K., Kondo, S., and Koide, T.,** Antithrombin III Toyama: a hereditary abnormal antithrombin III of a patient with recurrent thrombophlebitis. *Thromb. Res.*, 31, 305, 1983.
150. **Koide, T., Takahashi, K., Odani, S., Ono, T., and Sakuragawa, N.,** Isolation and characterization of a hereditary abnormal antithrombin III "Antithrombin III Toyama," *Thromb. Res.*, 31, 319, 1983.
151. **Koide, T., Odani, S., Takahashi, K., Ono, T., and Sakuragawa, N.,** Antithrombin III Toyama: replacement of arginine-47 by cysteine in hereditary abnormal antithrombin III that lacks heparin-binding ability, *Proc. Natl. Acad. Sci. U.S.A.*, 81, 289, 1984.
152. **Fischer, A. M., Gazengel, C., Dautzenberg, M. D., Benhamno, J., Béguin, S., and Vergoz, D.,** A new case of abnormal antithrombin III: biological characteristics and thromboembolic accidents mangement, *Thromb. Haemostas.*, 50, 358, 1983.
153. **Chasse, J. F., Esnard, F., Guitton, J. D., Mouray, H., Perigois, F., Fauconneau, G., and Gauthier, F.,** An abnormal plasma antithrombin with no apprent affinity for heparin, *Thromb. Res.*, 34, 297, 1984.
154. **Duchange, N., Chasse, J. F., Cohen, G. N., and Zakin, M. M.,** Molecular characterization of the antithrombin III Tours deficiency, *Thromb. Res.*, 45, 115, 1987.
155. **Fischer, A. M., Cornu, P., Sternberg, C., Mériane, F., Dautzenberg, M. D., Chafa, O., Béguin, S., and Desnos, M.,** Antithrombin III Alger: a new homozygous AT III variant, *Thromb. Haemostas.*, 55, 218, 1986.
156. **Boyer, C. Wolf, M., Vedrenne, J., Meyer, D., and Larrieu, M. J.,** Homozygous variant of antithrombin III: AT III Fontainebleau, *Thromb. Haemostas.*, 56, 18, 1986.
157. **de Moerloose, P. A., Reber, G., Vernet, Ph., Minazio, Ph., and Bouvier, C. A.,** Antithrombin III Geneve: a hereditary abnormal AT III with defective heparin cofactor activity, *Thromb. Haemostas.* 57, 154, 1987.
158. **Tullis, J. L. and Wantanabe, K.,** Platelet antithrombin deficiency. A new clinical entity, *Am. J. Med.*, 65, 472, 1978.
159. **Carvalho, A. and Ellman, L.,** Hereditary antithrombin III deficiency. Effect of antithrombin III deficiency on platelet function, *Am. J. Med.*, 61, 179, 1976.
160. **Petõ, I., Blaskó, G., and Sas, G.,** Platelet functions in different types of congenital antithrombin-III deficiencies, *Thromb. Res.*, 23, 471, 1981.
161. **Thaler, E. and Lechner, K.,** Antithrombin III deficiency and thromboembolism, *Clin. Haematol.*, 10, 369, 1981.
162. **Michiels, J. J. and Van Vliet, H. H. D. M.,** Hereditary antithrombin III deficiency and venous thrombosis, *Neth. J. Med.*, 27, 226, 1984.
163. Anon., Familial antithrombin III deficiency, *Lancet*, 1, 1021, 1983.
164. **Bjarke, B., Herin, P., and Blombäck, M.,** Neonatal aortic thrombosis, *Acta Paediatr. Scand.*, 63, 297, 1974.
165. **Haas, H. A., Scully, M. F., Clark, S. E., and Kakkar, V. V.,** A case of familial AT III deficiency in an English family, *Thromb. Haemostas.*, 42, 185, 1979.
166. **Leone, G., Valori, V. M., Storti, S., and Myers, T. J.,** Inferior vena cava thrombosis in a child with familial antithrombin III deficiency, *Thromb. Haemostas.*, 43, 74, 1980.
167. **Ødegard, O. R. and Abildgaard, U.,** Antifactor Xa activity in thrombophilia. Studies in a family with AT-III deficiency, *Scand. J. Haematol.*, 18, 86, 1977.
168. **Karl, R., Garlick, I., Zarins, C., Cheng, E., and Chediak, J.,** Surgical implications of antithrombin III deficiency, *Surgery*, 89, 429, 1981.
169. **Sas, G.,** Defects in serine protease inhibitors, *Thromb. Haemostas.*, 58, 248, 1987.
170. **Boyer, C., Wolf, M., Lavergne, J. M., and Larrieu, M. J.,** Thrombin generation and formation of thrombin-antithrombin III complexes in congenital antithrombin III deficiency, *Thromb. Res.*, 20, 207, 1980.

171. **Pálos, L. A., Sas, G., and Csurgay, Á.,** Reaction kinetics of thrombin activity in decalcified plasma and blood, *Thromb. Diathes. Haemorrh.*, 21, 580, 1969.
172. **Borg, J. Y., Soria, C., Soria, J., Mirshahi, M., Monconduit, M., and Caen, J.,** Evaluation of the thromboembolic risk in hereditary quantitative and qualitative antithrombin III (AT-III) deficiency by measurement of plasmatic fibrin degradation products (FDP) using a monoclonal anit-D-neo antibody, *Thromb. Res. Suppl.*, 6, 53, 1986.
173. **Marcum, J. A., McKenney, J. B., and Rosenberg, R. D.,** Acceleraton of thrombin-antithrombin complex formation in rat hindquarters via heparin-like molecules bound to endothelium, *J. Clin. Invest.*, 74, 341, 1984.
174. **Marcum, J. A. and Rosenberg, R. D.,** Heparin-like molecules with anticoagulant activity are synthesized by cultured endothelial cells, *Biochem. Biophys. Res. Commun.*, 126, 365, 1985.
175. **Nagy, I. and Losonczy, H.,** The significance of the chronic anticoagulant treatment in recurrent thromboembolism caused by hereditary antithrombin III deficiency, in Abstr. 5th Congr. Int. Soc. on Thromb. and Haemostas., Paris, 170, 1975.
176. **McDonald, M. M., Hathaway, W. E., Reeve, E. B., and Leonard, B. D.,** Biochemical and functional study of antithrombin III in newborn infants, *Thromb. Haemostas.*, 47, 56, 1982.
177. **Carter, C. J., Johnson, M., Brain, M. C., and Glynn, M. F. X.,** A new antithrombin III variant presenting as familial thrombophilia, *Blood,* 58, 231a, 1981.
178. **Mannucci, P. M. and Tripodi, A.,** Laboratory screening of inherited thrombotic syndromes, *Thromb. Haemostas.*, 57, 247, 1987.
179. **Sas, G. and Petõ, I.,** Late results of streptokinase heparin treatment in deep venous thrombosis (DVT), *Thromb. Haemostas.*, 54, 174, 1985.
180. **Hellgren, M., Tengborn, L., and Abildgaard, U.,** Pregnancy in women with congenital antithrombin III deficiency: experience of treatment with heparin and antithrombin, *Gynecol. Obstet. Invest.*, 14, 127, 1982.
181. **Bolwerk, C. J. M., Henny, C. P., Büller, H. R., and ten Cate, J. W.,** Hereditary AT III deficiency and heparin, *Thromb. Res.*, 28, 689, 1982.
182. **Mannucci, P. M., Boyer, C., Wolf, M., Tripodi, A., and Larrieu, M. J.,** Treatment of congenital antithrombin III deficiency with concentrate, *Br. J. Haematol.*, 50, 531, 1982.
183. **Marciniak, E. and Gockerman, J. P.,** Heparin induced clearance in circulating antithrombin III, *Lancet,* 2, 581, 1977.
184. **Lane, D. A., Lowe, G. D. D., Flynn, A., Ireland, H., Thompson, E., and Erdjument, H.,** Antithrombin III Glasgow: a variant with increased heparin affinity and reduced ability to inactivate thrombin, associated with familial thrombosis, *Thromb. Haemostas.*, 58, 427, 1987.
185. **Owen, M. C., Borg, V. Y., Soria, C., Soria, J., Caen, J., and Carrel, R. W.,** Heparin binding reduction in a new antithrombin III variant: Rouen, 47 Arg to His, *Blood,* 69, 1275, 1987.
186. **Borg, J. Y., Owen, M. C., Soria, C., Soria, J., Caen, J., and Carrell, R. W.,** Antithrombin Rouen-I (47 Arg-His) and Rouen-III (47 Ser); two new variants with decreased heparin affinity, *Thromb. Haemostas.*, 58, 238, 1987.
187. **Roussel, B., Dieval, J., Gross, S., Claisse, J. F., and Delobel, J.,** A new asymptomatic type III variant of antithrombin III with decreased heparin cofactor activity: AT III Amiens, *Thromb. Haemostas.*, 58, 427, 1987.
188. **Aiach, M., Roncato, M., Sorin, G., Dezullus, P. and Fiessinger, J. N.,** A new AT III variant with defective protease binding site, *Thromb. Haemostas.*, 58, 38, 1987.
189. **Hedner, U. and Nilsson, I. M.,** Antithrombin III in a clinical material, *Thromb. Res.*, 3, 631, 1973.
190. **Mannucci, L., Dioguardi, N., Del Ninno, E., and Mannucci, P. M.,** Value of Normotest and antithrombin III in the assessment of liver function, *Scand. J. Gastroenterol. Suppl.*, 8, 19, 103, 1973.
191. **Chan, V. and Chan, T. K.,** Antithrombin III in fresh and cultured human endothelial cells: a natural anticoagulant from the vascular endothelium, *Thromb. Res.*, 15, 209, 1979.
192. **Fair, D. S. and Bahnak, B. R.,** Human hepatoma cells secrete single chain factor X, prothrombin and antithrombin III, *Blood,* 64, 194, 1984.
193. **Nagy, I., Losonczy, H., and Pár, A.,** Heparin induced change of antithrombin III (AT III) activity in chronic active hepatitis and liver cirrhosis, in Current Views in Gastroenterology, Vol. 2, Varró, V. and Bálint, G. A., Eds., Hungarian Society of Gastroenterology, Budapest, 1978, 331.
194. **Rák, K.,** Attempt to better assess the haemostatic functions in patients with chronic liver diseases (CLD), *Thromb. Haemostas.*, 50, 273, 1983.
195. **Mannucci, P. M.,** Estimation of prothrombin in liver disease, *Am. J. Pathol.*, 23, 291, 1970.
196. **Damus, P. S. and Wallace, G. A.,** Immunologic measurement of antithrombin III-heparin cofactor and α_2-macroglobulin in disseminated intravascular coagulation and hepatic failure coagulopathy, *Thromb. Res.*, 6, 27, 1975.
197. **Boneu, B., Sie, P., Caranobe, C., Cassigenul, J., and Pascal, J.,** Progressive antithrombin activity and the concentration of three thrombin inhibitors in liver cirrhosis, *Thromb. Haemostas.*, 47, 78, 1982.

198. **Büller, H. R. and ten Cate, J. W.,** Antithrombin III infusion in patients undergoing peritoneovenous shunt operation: failure in the prevention of disseminated intravascular coagulation, *Thromb. Haemostas.*, 49, 128, 1983.
199. **Korninger, C., Klepetko, W., Miholic, J., Schwarz, Ch., and Lechner, K.,** Randomized trial of antithrombin III versus placebo in patients undergoing peritoneo-venous shunt operation. *Thromb. Haemostas.*, 58, 426, 1987.
200. **Kauffmann, R. H., Keltkamp, J. J., Tilburg, N. H., and van Es, L. A.,** Acquired Antithrombin III deficiency and thrombosis in the nephrotic syndrome, *Am. J. Med.*, 65, 607, 1978.
201. **Kuhlmann, U., Blatter, W., Pouliadis, G., and Siegenthaler, W.,** Komplikationen des nephrotischen Syndroms unter besonderer Berücksichtingung thrombotischer Zwischenfälle, *Schweiz. Med. Wochenschr.*, 109, 200, 1979.
202. **Schrader, J., Köstering, H., and Scheler, F.,** Antithrombin III bei Patienten mit Nieren-und Hochdruckheiten, in Antithrombin III, Köstering, H., Ed., Schattauer, Stuttgart, 1984, 104.
203. **Thaler, E., Balzar, E., Kopsie, H., and Pinggera, W. F.,** Acquired antithrombin III deficiency in patients with glomerular proteinuria, *Haemostasis,* 7, 257, 1978.
204. **Kobayashi, N. and Takeda, Y.,** Studies of the effects of estradiol, progesterone, cortisol, thrombophlebitis and typhoid vaccine on synthesis and catabolism of antithrombin in the dog, *Thromb. Haemostas.*, 37, 111, 1977.
205. **Jørgensen, K. A. and Stoffersen, E.,** Antithrombin III and the nephrotic syndrome, *Scand. J. Haematol.*, 22, 442, 1978.
206. **Bouissou, F., Barthe, Ph., and Boneu, B.,** Déficits acquis en facteur XII et antithrombine III (AT III) dans les néphroses de l'enfant, *Nouv. Presse. Med.*, 9, 1778, 1980.
207. **Brandt, P. and Jespersen, J.,** Renal diseases, disseminated intravascular coagulation and antithrombin III, *Nephron,* 34, 203, 1983.
208. **Hoie, J.,** Renal vascular resistance changes following thrombin-induced intravascular coagulation: role of platelets and fibrin emboli, *Acta Chir. Scand.*, 141, 167, 1975.
209. **Köstering, H.,** Antithrombin III — Grundlagen, Diagnostik, Klinische Bedeutung und Therapie, Schattauer, Stuttgart, 1984.
210. **Schuster, H. P., Konz, M. W., Blair, J., Seddnsky, J. A., and Mammen, E.,** The influence of disseminated intravascular coagulation or renal function after experimental hemorrhagic shock, *Resuscitation,* 8, 3, 1980.
211. **Schrader, J.,** Antithrombin III in renal disease: importance and treatment, in Antithrombin Deficiency, Böttiger, L. E., Ed., KabiVitrum, Stockholm, 1986, 43.
212. **Schipper, H. G. and ten Cate, J. W.,** Antithrombin-III transfusion in patients with liver cirrhosis, in Antithrombin III and Human Antithrombin III Concentrates. Clinical and Experimental Studies, Schipper, H. G., Ed., Rodopi, Amsterdam, 1980, 65.
213. **Thompson, A. R.,** Factor XII and other hemostatic protein abnormalities in nephrotic syndrome patients., *Thromb. Haemostas.*, 48, 27, 1982.
214. **Stathakis, N., Papayannis, A. G., and Gardikas, C. D.,** Postoperative antithrombin III concentration, *Lancet,* 1, 430, 1973.
215. **Aberg, M., Nilsson, I. M., and Hedner, U.,** Antithrombin III after operation, *Lancet,* 2, 1337, 1973.
216. **Jørgensen, K. A., Stofferesen, E., Sørensen, P. J., Ingeberg, S., Hüttel, M., and Ahlbom, G.,** Alterations in plasma antithrombin III following total hip replacement and elective cholecystectomy, *Scand. J. Haematol.*, 24, 101, 1980.
217. **Sagar, S., Thomas, D. P., Stamatakis, J. D., and Kakkar, V. V.,** Oral contraceptives, antithrombin III activity and postoperative deep-vein thrombosis, *Lancet,* 1, 509, 1976.
218. **Gitel, S. N., Salvati, E. A., Wessler, S., Robinson, H. J., and Worth, M. H.,** The effect of total hip replacement and general surgery on antithrombin III in relation to venous thrombosis, *J. Bone J. Surg.*, 61, 653, 1979.
219. **Chandra, S., Bang, N. U., and Marks, C.,** Radio labeled AT-III as a probe for the detection of activation of blood coagulation *in vivo, Thromb. Res.*, 9, 9, 1976.
220. **Bick, R. L., Dukes, M. L., Wilson, W. L., and Fekete, L. F.,** Antithrombin III (AT-III) as a diagnostic aid in disseminated intravascular coagulation, *Thromb. Res.*, 10, 721, 1977.
221. **Bick, R. L., Bick, M. D., and Fekete, L. F.,** Antithrombin III patterns in disseminated intravascular coagulation., *Am. J. Clin. Pathol.*, 73, 577, 1980.
222. **Büller, H. R., Bolwerk, C., ten Cate, J., Roos, J., Kahlé, L. H., and ten Cate, J. W.,** Post-operative haemostatic profile in relation to gram negative septicaemia, *Crit. Care Med.*, 10, 311, 1982.
223. **Smit-Erichsen, N.,** Antithrombin III in septicaemia, in Antithrombin Deficiency, Böttiger, L. E., Ed., KabiVitrum Stockholm, 1986, 61.
224. **Laursen, B., Faber, V., Brock, A., Gormsen, J., and Sørensen, H.,** Disseminated intravascular coagulation, antithrombin III, and complement in meningococcal infections, *Acta Med. Scand.*, 209, 221, 1981.

225. **Rubli, E., Büssard, S., Frei, E., Lundsgaard-Hansen, P., and Pappova, E.,** Plasma fibronectin and associated variables in surgical intensive care patients, *Ann. Surg.*, 197, 310, 1983.
226. **Henny, Ch. P., Knot, E. A. R., ten Cate, J. W. Peters, M., ten Veen, J. H., and Roos, J.,** An acquired antithrombin III deficiency in the course of toxic shock syndrome after elective orthopaedic surgery, *Neth. J. Med.*, 26, 133, 1983.
227. **Schipper, H. G., Kahlé, L. H., Jenkins, C. S. P., and ten Cate, J. V.,** Antithrombin III transfusion in disseminated intravascular coagulation, *Lancet,* 2, 854, 1978.
228. **Thaler, E. and Kleinberger, G.,** Sepsis und Blutgerinnung, *Intensivmedizin,* 16, 54, 1979.
229. **Braunstein, K. M., Dodds, K. A., Stewart, G., Shull, K. C., and Eurenius, K.,** Heparin cofactor activity following thermal injury., *Am. J. Clin. Pathol.*, 70, 632, 1978.
230. **Losito, R., Beaudry, P., Valderrama, J. C., Cousineau, L., and Longpre, B.,** Antithrombin III and factor VIII in patients with neoplasms, *Am. J. Clin. Pathol.*, 68, 258, 1977.
231. **Rubin, R. B., Kies, M. S., and Posch, J. J., Jr.,** Measurement of antithrombin III in solid tumor patients with and without hepatic metastases, *Thromb. Res.*, 18, 353, 1980.
232. **Brennan, S. O., George, P. M., Carrell, R. W., and Jordan, R.,** The physiological antithrombin (beta) variant with increased heparin affinity lacks carbohydrate as Asn 135, *Thromb. Haemostas.*, 58, 238, 1987.
233. **Bock, S. C., Harris, J. F., Schwartz, C. E., Ward, J. H., Hershgold, E. J., and Skolnick, M. H.,** Hereditary thrombosis in a Utah kindred is caused by a dysfunctional antithrombin III gene, *Am. J. Hum. Genet.*, 37, 32, 1985.
234. **Nalli, G., Majolino, I., Panizza, P., and Ascari, E.,** Antithrombin III immunoelectrophoretic pattern in DIC, *Thromb. Res.*, 13, 303, 1978.
235. **Kwaan, H. C., Andersson, M. C., and Gramatica, L. E.,** A study of pancreatic enzymes as a factor in the pathogenesis of disseminated intravascular coagulation during acute pancreatitis, *Surgery,* 69, 663, 1971.
236. **Aasen, A. O., Kierulf, P., Ruud, T. E., Godal, H. C., and Aune, S.,** Studies on pathological plasma proteolysis in patients with acute pancreatitis. A preliminary report, *Acta Chir. Scand. Suppl.*, 509, 83, 1982.
237. **Aasen, A. O.,** Antithrombin III in pancreatitis, in Antithrombin Deficiency, Böttiger, L. A., Ed., KabiVitrum, Stockholm, 1986, 57.
238. **Lake, A. M., Stauffer, J. Q., and Stuart, M. J.,** Hemostatic alterations in inflammatory bowel disease: response to therapy, *Am. J. Dig. Dis.*, 23, 897, 1978.
239. **Muntean, W. and Rossipal, E.,** Verlust von Inhibitoren des Gerinnungssystem bei der exsudativen Enteropathie, *Klin. Paediatr.*, 191, 20, 1979.
240. **Schmitz-Huebner, U., Briest, R., and Schönleben, K.,** Antithrombin-III-Verminderung nach operativer Dünndarmausschaltung, in Fibrinolyse, Thrombose, Hämostase, Deutsch, E. and Lechner, K., Eds., Schattauer, Stuttgart, 1980, 503.
241. **Fuller, J. H., Keen, H., Jarrett, R. J., Omer, T., Meade, T. W., Chakrabarti, R. North, W. R. S., and Stirling, V.,** Haemostatic variables associated with diabetes and its complications, *Br. Med. J.*, 2, 964, 1979.
242. **Hughes, A., McVerry, B. A., Wilkinson, L., Goldstone, A. H., Lewis, D., and Bloom, A.,** Diabetes, a hypercoagulable state? Haemostatic variables in newly diagnosed type 2 diabetic patients, *Acta Haematol.*, 69, 254, 1983.
243. **Bannerjee, R. N., Sahni, A. L., Kumere, V., and Arza, N.,** Antithrombin III deficiency in maturity onset diabetes and atherosclerosis, *Thromb. Diath. Haemorrh.*, 31, 339, 1974.
244. **Monnier, L., Follea, G., and Mirouze, J.,** Antithrombin III deficiency in diabetes mellitus: influence on vascular degenerative complications, *Horm. Metab. Res.*, 10, 470, 1978.
245. **Corbella, E., Miragliotta, G., Masperi, R., Villa, S., Bini, A., de Geatano, G., and Chiumello, G.,** Platelet aggregation and antithrombin III levels in diabetic children, *Haemostasis,* 8, 30, 1979.
246. **Elder, G. E., Mayne, E. E., Daly, J. G., Kennedy, A. L., Hadden, D. R., Montgomery, D. A. D., and Weaver, J. A.,** Aniththrombin III activity and other coagulation changes in proliferative diabetic retinopathy, *Haemosatsis,* 9, 288, 1980.
247. **Perez-Requejo, J. L., Di Pasquale, S., Arocha-Pinango, C. L., and Rodriquez, S.,** Differences between immunological and amidolytic activities of antithrombin III in diabetic patients, *Thromb. Haemostas.*, 50, 1243, 1983.
248. **Small, M., Douglas, J. T., Lowe, G. D. O., MacCuish, A. C., and Forbes, C. D.,** Effect of insulin therapy on coagulation and platelet function in type III (Non-insulin-dependent) diabetes mellitus, *Haemostasis,* 16, 417, 1986.
249. **Ceriello, A., Dello Russo, P., Zuccotti, C., Florio, A., Nazzaro, S., Pietrantuono, C., and Rosato, G. B.,** Decreased antithrombin III activity in diabetes may be due to nonenzymatic glycosylation — a preliminary report, *Thromb. Haemostas.*, 50, 633, 1983.
250. **Brownlee, M., Vlassara, H., and Cerami, A.,** Inhibition of heparin-catalysed human antithrombin III activity by nonenzymatic glycosylation. Possible role in fibrin deposition in diabetes, *Diabetes,* 33, 532, 1984.

251. **Ceriello, A., Giugliano, D., Quatraro, A., Stante, A., Consoli, G., Dello Russo, P., and D'Onofrio, F.**, Heparin preserves antithrombin III biological activity from hyperglycemia-induced alterations in insulin-dependent diabetics, *Haemostasis,* 16, 458 1986.
252. **Hansen, M. S. and Jørgensen, B. M.**, Functional changes in antithrombin III in insulin-dependent diabetes mellitus, *Thromb. Haemostas.*, 58, 88, 1987.
253. **Aiach, M., Francois, D., Priollet, P., Capron, L., Roncato, M., Alhenc-Gelas, M., and Fiessinger, J.-N.**, An abnormal antithrombin III (AT III) with low heparin affinity: AT III Clichy, *Br. J. Haematol.*, 66, 515, 1987.
254. **Lane, D. A., Lowe, G. D. O., Flynn, A., Thompson, E., Ireland, H., and Erdjument, H.**, Antithrombin III Glasgow: a variant with increased heparin affinity and reduced ability to inactivate thrombin associated with familial thrombosis, *Br. J. Haematol.*, 66, 523, 1987.
255. **Hedner, U. and Nilsson, I. M.**, Antithrombin III in a clinical material, *Thromb. Res.*, 3, 631, 1973.
256. **Yue, R. H., Gertler, M. M., Starr, T., and Koutrouby, R.**, Alteration of plasma antithrombin III levels in ischaemic heart disease, *Thromb. Haemostas.*, 35, 598, 1976.
257. **O'Brien, J. R., Etherington, M. D., Hamieson, S., Lawford, P., Lincoln, S. V., and Alkjaersig, N.**, Blood changes in atherosclerosis and lung after myocardial infarction and venous thrombosis, *Thromb. Diath. Haemorrh.*, 34, 483, 1975.
258. **Gonzalez, R., Vicente, V., Alegre, A., Pabon, P., and Alberca, I.**, Protein C and antithrombin III in acute myocardial infarction, *Thromb. Res.*, 43, 681, 1986.
259. **Innerfield, I., Goldfischer, J., Reicherreiss, H., and Greenberg, J.**, Serum antithrombin in coronary-artery disease, *Am. J. Clin. Pathol.*, 65, 64, 1976.
260. **Marciniak, E. and Gockerman, J. P.**, Heparin induced decrease in circulating antithrombin III, *Lancet,* 2, 581, 1977.
261. **Rao, A. K., Niewiarowski, S., Guzzo, J., and Day, H. J.**, Antithrombin III levels during heparin therapy, *Thromb. Res.*, 24, 181, 1981.
262. **Levesque, G., Samama, M., Kher, A., Barbier, P., Horellou, M. H., and Conard, J.**, Low-dose heparin in gynecologic surgery: effect on blood coagulation tests, *Haemostasis,* 10, 97, 1981.
263. **Kakkar, V. V., Bentley, P. G., Scully, M. F., MacGregor, I. R., Jones, N. A. G., and Webb, P. J.**, Antithrombin III and heparin, *Lancet,* 2, 103, 1980.
264. **Bolwerk, C. J. M., Henny, Ch. P., and Büller, H. R.**, Hereditary AT III deficiency and heparin, *Thromb. Res.*, 28, 689, 1982.
265. **Tilsner, V., Müller, U., Reuter, H., and Raedler, A.**, Results of low-dose heparin prophylaxis of venous thrombosis considering plasma heparin and antithrombin III concentration, *Thromb. Res.*, 17, 519, 1980.
266. **Refvem, O., Fagerhol, M. K., and Abildgaard, U.**, Changes in antithrombin III levels following cessation of anticoagulant therapy, *Acta Med. Scand.*, 193, 307, 1973.
267. **O'Brien, J. R. and Etherington, M. D.**, Effect of heparin and warfarin on antithrombin III, *Lancet,* 2, 1232, 1977.
268. **Bull, H., Mackie, I., Brozovic, M., and Woodings, D.**, Antithrombin III in patients on long-term oral anticoagulants, *J. Clin. Pathol.*, 33, 1202, 1980.
269. **Andersson, G., Fagrell, B., Holmgren, K., Johnson, H., Ljunberg, B., and Wilhelmsson, S.**, Antithrombin III in patients with acute deep vein thrombosis during heparin treatment with oral coumarins, *Thromb. Res.*, 34, 333, 1984.
270. **Ødegard, O. R. and Teien, A. N.**, Antithrombin III, heparin cofactor and antifactor Xa in a clinical material, *Thromb. Res.*, 8, 173, 1976.
271. **Frost, T. and Loveday, D.**, Oral anticoagulants and antithrombin III, *Med. J. Aust.*, 2, 220, 1980.
272. **De Stefano, V., Leone, G., De Martini, D., Di Donfrancesco, A., Accorrá, F., and Bizzi, B.**, Effect of oral anticoagulant treatment on plasma and serum antithrombin III: a study on 172 patients at different levels of anticoagulation, *Haemostasis,* 17, 195, 1987.
273. **Hultin, M. B.**, Studies of factor IX concentrate therapy in haemophilia, *Blood,* 62, 677, 1983.
274. **Hoffman, C. and Hultin, M. B.**, Factor IX concentrate therapy and thrombosis: relation to changes in plasma antithrombin III, *Thromb. Res.*, 43, 143, 1986.
275. **Hultin, M. B. and Abildgaard, U.**, Antithrombin antigen of high molecular weight associated with neoantigen in hemophilic plasma after factor IX concentrate therapy, *Thromb. Res.*, 45, 175, 1987.
276. **Conard, J., Samama, M., Bilski-Posquier, G., and Bousser, J.**, Toxicité *in vivo* de la L-asparaginase sur les facteurs de coagulation ez en particular sur l'anti-thrombine III: a propos de 25 observations, *Coagulation,* 4, 195, 1971.
277. **Wada, J. K., Patch, M. J., and McGehee, W. G.**, Low levels of antithrombin III (AT III) due to L-asparaginase (ASP), *Blood,* 54, (Suppl. 1), 308, 1979.
278. **Buchanan, G. R. and Holtkamp, C. A.**, Reduced antithrombin III levels during L-asparaginase therapy, *Med. Pediatr. Oncol.*, 8, 7, 1980.
279. **Pitney, W. R., Phadke, K. P., and Dean, S.**, Antithrombin III deficiency during asparaginase therapy, *Lancet,* 1, 493, 1980.

280. **Conard, J., Cazenave, B., Maury, J., Horellou, M. H., and Samama, M.,** L-asparaginase, antithrombin III and thrombosis, *Lancet,* 1, 1091, 1980.
281. **Bauer, K. A., Teitel, J. M., and Rosenberg, R. D.,** L-asparaginase induced antithrombin III deficiency: evidence against the production of a hypercoagulable state, *Thromb. Res.,* 29, 437, 1983.
282. **Gralnick, H. R. and Henderson, E.,** Hypofibrinogenemia and coagulation factor deficiencies with L-asparaginase therapy, *N. Engl. J. Med.,* 301, 252, 1979.
283. **Ramsay, N. K. C., Coccia, P. F., Krivit, W., Nesbit, M. E., and Edson, J. R.,** The effect of L-asparaginase on plasma coagulation factors in acute lymphoblastic leukemia, *Cancer,* 40, 1398, 1977.
284. **Vellenga, E., Mulder, N. H., and Nieweg, H. O.,** Antithrombin III deficiency during asparaginase therapy, *Lancet,* 1, 649, 1980.
285. **Nagasawa, H., Kim, B. K., Steiner, M., and Baldini, M. G.,** Inhibition of thrombin-neutralizing activity of antithrombin III by steroid hormones, *Thromb. Haemostas.,* 47, 157, 1982.
286. **Henny, C. P., ten Cate, H., Dabhoiwala, N. F., Büller, H. R., and ten Cate, J. W.,** Effect of hormonal manipulation on antithrombin activity in patients with prostatic carcinoma, *Eur. Urol.,* 10, 202, 1984.
287. **Büller, H. R., Boon, T. A., Henny, C. P., Dabhoiwala, N. F., and ten Cate, J. W.,** Estrogen-induced deficiency and decrease in antithrombin III activity in patients with prostatic cancer, *J. Urol.,* 128, 72, 1982.
288. **Drijfhout, H. H., Knot, E. A. R., and ten Cate, J. W.,** Antithrombin III metabolism in two patients with a nephrotic syndrome caused by minimal change nephritis and primary amyloidosis, *Haemostasis,* 17, 286, 1987.
289. **Collen, D. and De Cock, F.,** Emergence in plasma during activation of the coagulation or fibrinolytic systems of neoantigens, associated with the complexes of thrombin or plasmin with their inhibitors, *Thromb. Res.,* 5, 777, 1974.
290. **Collen, D. and De Cock, F.,** Neoantigenic expression in enzyme-inhibitor complexes: a means to demonstrate activation of enzyme systems, *Biochem. Biophys. Acta,* 525, 287, 1978.
291. **Collen, D., De Cock, F., and Verstraete, M.,** Quantitation of thrombin-antithrombin III complexes in human blood, *Eur. J. Clin. Invest.,* 7, 407, 1977.
292. **Collen, D. and Verstraete, M.,** Quantitation of thrombin-antithrombin III complex during coagulation of blood, in Physiological Inhibitors of Coagulation and Fibrinolysis, Collen, D., Wiman, B., and Verstraete, M., Eds., Elsevier, Amsterdam, 1979.
293. **Lau, H. K. and Rosenberg, R. D.,** The isolation and characterization of a specific antibody population directed against the thrombin-antithrombin complex, *J. Biol. Chem.,* 255, 5885, 1980.
294. **Teitel, J. M., Bauer, K. A., Lau, H. K., and Rosenberg, R., D.,** Studies of the prothrombin activation pathway utilizing radioimmunoassays for the F_2/F_{1+2} fragment and thrombin-antithrombin complex, *Blood,* 59, 1086, 1982.
295. **Bauer, K. A. and Rosenberg, R. D.,** Thrombin generation in acute promyelocytic leukemia, *Blood,* 64, 791, 1984.
296. **Pelzer, H., Schwartz, A., and Heimburger, N.,** Enzyme immunoassay for determination of thrombin/antithrombin III complex, *Thromb. Res. Suppl.,* 6, 51, 1986.
297. **Wolf, M., Boyer-Neumann, C., Meyer, D., Tripodi, A., Mannucci, P. M., and Larrieu, M. J.,** Purification and further characterization of antithrombin III Milano: lack of reactivity with thrombin, *Thromb. Haemostas.,* 58, 888, 1987.
298. **Milner, A. E., Burnett, D., Rutter, J., and Bradwell, A. R.,** Detection of antithrombin III microheterogeneity, *Thromb. Res.,* 37, 127, 1985.
299. **Daly, M., O'Meara, A., and Hallinan, F. M.,** Identification and characterization of a new antithrombin III familial variant (AT Dublin) with possible increased frequency in children with cancer, *Br. J. Haematol.,* 65, 457, 1987.
300. **Kamboh, M. I.,** Biochemical and genetic aspects of human serum α_1-proteinase inhibitor protein, *Dis. Markers,* 3, 135, 1985.

Chapter 3

ANTITHROMBIN III IN OBSTETRICS, GYNECOLOGY, AND NEONATOLOGY

I. Rákóczi

TABLE OF CONTENTS

I. INTRODUCTION

Antithrombin III (AT-III) is the major physiological inhibitor of blood coagulation. Deficiency of this protein is associated with an increased risk of thromboembolic disease (see Chapter 2). This review summarizes the present knowledge of hereditary or acquired AT-III deficiency in connection with pregnancy and with oral contraception usage, as well as with the newborn period.

II. AT-III IN PREGNANCY

A. ACQUIRED AT-III DEFICIENCY IN PREGNANCY

1. AT-III in a Normal Pregnancy

In a number of articles, it is stated that AT-III levels decrease during pregnancy.[1,2] Both inherited and acquired AT-III deficiencies are associated with a high risk of thromboembolism, especially during pregnancy.[3] However, AT-III plasma levels are not or only very slightly depressed in a normal pregnancy.[4-6] Some authors have suggested that the decrease in AT-III levels to around 70% of normal may occur during pregnancy and puerperium.[7-9] This is thought to be one of the causes of the increased tendency of thrombosis during and immediately after pregnancy. However, Weenink et al.,[10] who studied 94 women during and after normal pregnancies, failed to show any reduction in AT-III levels as compared with tests performed 6 to 8 weeks after delivery. Recently, the same group has found slightly but significantly lower AT-III levels in 61 normal pregnant women at 37 to 42 weeks of gestation compared with their own mean control values at 6 to 8 weeks postpartum.[11] However, it should be stressed that this small decrease has no clinical significance because the mean value is still above that of the reference pool plasma. Discrepancies between the different results may in part be explained by differences in laboratory techniques. The selection of the patient material may also be a factor. In addition, the selection criteria have not always been reported. In early puerperium, AT-III levels increase rapidly after a vaginal delivery. This phenomenon is compatible with increased AT-III synthesis, which continues in the early postpartum days after increased consumption has stopped. In contrast, AT-III levels decrease after a Caesarean section.[10,11]These changes in AT-III levels may enhance the risk of thromboembolism. Since AT-III levels are not depressed during a normal pregnancy, in spite of the increase in plasma volume, an increased AT-III sythesis may be postulated rather than an oestrogen-induced decreased synthesis.[10] It is concluded that an AT-III deficiency can be established during pregnancy as plasma AT-III levels do not change significantly during a normal, uncomplicated pregnancy.

2. AT-III in Preeclampsia

The aetiology of preeclampsia in unknown. However, considerable evidence has been accumulated that intravascular coagulation is a feature of preeclampsia.[12,13]It has been reported that pregnancy is normally associated with the increase in clotting and fibrinolytic activities, and that in preeclampsia, there appears to be an aggravation of this pattern.[13] Recent advances in haemostatic research suggested that vascular endothelial injuries played a central role in the haemostatic changes associated with preeclampsia. A vascular injury in preeclampsia could be caused by vasospasm or immune complexes.[14] This vascular damage may cause the activation of both clotting and fibrinolysis, and decreased prostacyclin production resulting in the generation of thrombin. The thrombin consumes AT-III and causes intravascular fibrin depositions.[15] If the haemostatic system is activated in preeclampsia, an increased comsumption of AT-III may be postulated. In the beginning of this process, increased synthesis may compensate for this depletion of AT-III levels, but if consumption exceeds increased synthesis, AT-III levels may decline. It has been found that a significant decrease in AT-III levels occur in preeclampsia.[16-19] Hellgren et al.[7] have found that low third trimester AT-III levels occur primarily in patients with preeclampsia. In contrast, there was no significant AT-III depression in pregnant women with chronic hypertension even when persistent proteinuria due to chronic renal disease was present.[18,19] Studies from two groups have shown that low AT-III levels correlate with the degree of maternal morbidity as determined by other parameters (blood pressure, proteinuria, disturbance of renal and liver function, thrombocytopenia).[17,18] In addition, they have also found that low AT-III levels correlated with placental infarction and poor fetal outcome.[17,18] Clinical evidence strongly suggests that AT-III depletion in preeclampsia is caused by increased consumption rather than decreased synthesis or urinary loss.[19] AT-III levels in preeclampsia correlate with hepato-renal damage. In preeclampsia, fibrin is deposited in the periportal areas and in renal glomeruli.[20] It has been, therefore, suggested that AT-III is consumed in the fibrin deposition process. An inverse correlation of hepatic enzymes (SGOT, SGPT, LDH) with plasma AT-III levels can be found.[19] In preeclampsia after vaginal delivery, AT-III levels returned to normal values within a few days. The decrease in AT-III levels after a Caesarean section is more pronounced than after a vaginal delivery.[11] Patients who underwent Caesarean sections can receive heparin prophylaxis. The further AT-III decrease in the postoperative phase after a caesarean section is a strong argument in favor of subcutaneous heparin prophylaxis. The increased risk of bleeding in preeclampsia must also be kept in mind. In addition, occasionally AT-III levels in preeclampsia may become extremely low and heparin may then not be effective since it needs AT-III for its action. In these cases, treatment with an AT-III concentrate prior to a Caesarean section may be indicated.[11,19] Unfortunately, routine coagulation tests such as the PT, the APTT, the ethanol gelation test, and levels of individual clotting factors are seldom abnormal in preeclampsia. Therefore, these tests are of no use for the routine monitoring of preeclamptic patients. The main clinical relevance of AT-III determinations in preeclampsia is the monitoring of individual patients. Exacerbations and remissions of the preeclamptic process are reflected by decreases and increases of AT-III levels. Weenink et al.[19] use AT-III determinations in their hospital as a routine test in monitoring preeclamptic patients. If AT-III levels fall below 0.80 U/ml and/or platelet counts fall below $100 \times 10^9/1$, they indicate more elaborated coagulation studies, especially if surgery is imminent. Weiner et al.[16] have recently also reported on the usefulness of the determination of plasma AT-III levels in establishing or refusing the diagnosis of preeclampsia in doubtful cases and in differentiating between true preeclampsia and chronic hypertension.

3. AT-III in DIC

Obstetric conditions classically associated with disseminated intravascular coagulation (DIC) include abruptio placentae, amniotic fluid embolism, septic abortion and intrauterin infection, retained dead fetus, hydatidiform mole, placenta accreta, preeclampsia and eclampsia, and prolonged shock from any cause.[20] The coagulation can be activated both endogenously and exogenously, giving rise to serine proteases which are neutralized by inhibitors and eliminated from the blood by the reticuloendothelial system. If the need for the activation of coagulation system persists, AT-III is consumed by complex formation with serine proteases, accompanied with impairment of synthesis in the liver. As a result, in DIC, the presence of finely dispersed fibrin is associated with organ failure (e.g. kidney, lung) and haemorrhage. The activation of the coagulation system is followed by reactive hyperfibrinolysis. A decreased inhibition of coagulation and/or a decreased fibrinolysis have been shown in experimental and clinical studies to be central in the pathogenesis of DIC following thrombogenic exposure.[20] Clinical observations have shown that episodes of thrombosis following such exposure occur more often in patients with a congenital or acquired deficiency of AT-III than in normal individuals. These observations have found support in results from animal studies. Mann et al.[21] have showed that intravenously injected AT-III prevented the formation of thrombin in chicken embryos in which solutions of tissue thromboplastin had been injected. Later, a corresponding effect has been demonstrated in rats.[22] Heparin administration to dogs has been shown to prevent the occurance of DIC following circulatory arrest and its subsequent consequences.[23] In patients with familial asymptomatic AT-III deficiencies, the administration of AT-III as plasma or in the form of a concentrate supplemented with heparin has a protective effect.[24-26] The treatment of patients with DIC is extremely time-consuming, complex, and often unrewarding. Although no single prognostic factor has proved to be conclusively dependable, several reports have indicated that consecutive measurements of AT-III alone or with other inhibitors may provide data useful in the prediction of the development of complications or a fetal outcome.[27-29] Heparin has long been used in the treatment of DIC.[30] Heparin combined with AT-III in the blood greatly enhances the reactivity of AT-III with serine proteases.[31] However, the treatment of DIC with heparin is often unsuccessful due to the marked consumption and reduction of AT-III.[32,33] Clinical studies have showed that heparin may even worsen bleeding in patients with DIC or aggravate DIC depending upon the administration or dosage of heparin.[34,35] Recently, an increasing number of reports have described the successful application of intravenous AT-III concentrate in acute DIC.[26,36-39] The results are of particular interest in cases of gram-negative sepsis because of its extremely high mortality.[40] Maki et al.[41] have investigated the clinical efficacy of therapy with AT-III in a well-controlled comparative study vs. the injectable synthetic protease inhibitor (FOY). The result of the trial showed that the AT-III group (92%; $n = 24$) was significantly superior in clinical efficacy to the other group (60%; $n = 15$). It could be concluded that a single therapy with an AT-III concentrate can sufficiently control symptoms of DIC in obstetrics without the risk of increased bleeding. It is impossible to calculate the amount of AT-III concentrate required to normalize AT-III, i.e., to 100% of a pool of normal plasma. Usually, treatment has been started between 500 and 1000 units as a bolus followed 1 to 2 hours later by the determination of the level of AT-III. This renders it possible to estimate the increment of AT-III level following additional doses of AT-III concentrate.

B. HEREDITARY AT-III DEFICIENCY IN PREGNANCY

The incidence of thromboembolism during pregnancy seems to have remained unchanged during the last 30 years, but the incidence in puerperium may have decreased.[20,42,43] This may be explained by early mobilization and less infections and traumatic complications during and after delivery. In contrast, women with congenital AT-III deficiencies have a markedly increased risk of suffering thromboembolic complications in connection with pregnancy.[44] The prevalence of thromboembolism in pregnancy in patients with congenital AT-III deficiencies, who receive no prophylactic therapy, is between 70% and 94% compared to a general prevalence of thromboembolism during pregnancy of about 0.1%.[3,43-46] Thromboembolic complications occur both during early and late pregnancy, and during puerperium. However, most of the events occur in antepartum periods compared to those patients who do not have AT-III deficiencies where the majority of complications occur after delivery.[3] The condition is often present for the first time before abortion and delivery, or when the patients take combined oral contraceptives.[47] The venous system is mainly affected and there does not appear to be any increased risk of arterial thromboembolism. The most common sites are the deep veins of the leg and the pulmonary circulation, but some of the patients had mesenteric vein thrombosis.[25,43,48,49] It has been reported that the AT-III level decreases further during delivery and during some obstetric comlications and, therefore, a sufficient inhibition against thrombosis is even more important than during pregnancy.[50,51]The prepregnancy counseling should be included in the routine management of women with AT-III deficiencies. Patients should be counseled about the genetic risk. In addition, they should be counseled that their treatment should be changed from warfarin to heparin before con-

TABLE 1
Management of AT-III Deficiency in Pregnancy

1. Substitute 12-hourly subcutaneous heparin for warfarin before conception, aiming for a 10-second prolongation of the partial thromboplastin time 10 hours post-injection (start dose of heparin = 10,000 units twice a day).
2. Check partial thromboplastin time at least every 2 weeks, increasing heparin as necessary.
3. When delivery is imminent, decrease heparin to 5000 units twice a day and start alternate day infusions of AT-III to achieve a level of biologically active AT-III greater than 80%. Start with AT-III 50 units/kg; check AT-III preinfusion immediately and adjust AT-III dose appropriately.
4. Induce delivery when AT-III levels are predictably greater than 80% and the partial thromboplastin time is normal.
5. Continue AT-III infusion and subcutaneous heparin 5000 units twice daily until 7 days postdelivery.
6. Restart warfarin.
7. Check cord blood AT-III. Infant will need therapy if affected (i.e., cord blood AT-III = 20 to 30%). See text.
8. Treat abortion as labor with AT-III infusion and decrease the heparin dose.
9. Treat established thromboembolism with intravenous heparin, 40 to 80,000 units, to double partial thromboplastin time. May need additional AT-III (Hellgren et al.[71]).

ception. Women should also be advised not to take combined oral contraceptives containing oestrogen or oestrogen preparations for post-menopausal hormonal replacement therapy because of the increased risk of thromboembolism in AT-III deficiencies.[52] The pill containing only progesterone does not affect AT-III levels.[47] The risk of thromboembolic events in women with congenital AT-III deficiencies is further increased during pregnancy.[3,53,54] Heparin prophylaxis can reduce the thromboembolic complications in pregnant women with normal AT-III levels.[45,48,51] Prophylaxis of thromboembolism with heparin has also been reported in women with congenital or acquired AT-III deficiencies.[3,54] Self-administration of long-term subcutaneous heparin injections during pregnancy are well-tolerated and complications are minimal.[45,48] Oral anticoagulans should not be given in early pregnancy because of teratogenic effects (e.g., chondrodysplasia punctata).[48] In addition, oral anticoagulants can pass the placenta and increase the risk of haemorrhagic complications in the fetus and in the neonate, as well as in the mother.[48,55]Although warfarin prophylaxis has been used succesfully in midpregnancy in isolated cases, for the reasons given above, oral anticoagulants should altogether be avoided during pregnancy if possible and a regimen of subcutaneous heparin be used.[56,57] The heparin effect varies during pregnancy. Only during the first trimester, 5000 units of heparin sustains a prophylactic level because of increased plasma volume, renal clearance, and the presence of a placental heparinase, or during labor, an increase in low-density lipids.[58] It is well known that heparin does decrease plasma AT-III levels in a dose-dependent manner.[45,59]A decrease has also been noted in AT-III levels from about 50% to about 25 to 30% of normal during the heparin treatment of women with congenital AT-III deficiencies. Complications of low-dose heparin can occur including thrombocytopenia, osteoporosis, thrombosis, and fat necrosis.[60] Both osteoporosis and fat necrosis have only been reported in patients receiving greater than 15,000 units/d for more than 3 months.[61] Vertebral fracture and osteoporosis in connection with heparin treatment has been reported during pregnancy.[45,62,63] The mechanism of heparin-induced osteoporosis is not fully understood, but changes in Ca homeostasis and a decrease in bone-mineralization have been noted.[64,65] There is no evidence that long-term heparin prophylaxis results in an overall increase in preterm delivery, placental abruption, or blood loss at delivery.[66] However, conduction anesthesia has been avoided in these patients. The management of an AT-III deficiency in pregnancy, taken from studies of Hellgren et al., DeSwiet, and Samson et al., are summarized in Table 1.[44,66,67] It was shown that a marked fall in AT-III levels occur in very early pregnancy independently of heparin administration.[67] Therefore, patients should be switched from warfarin prophylaxis to subcutaneous heparin. Unfortunately, there is a dilemma regarding the heparin dose during treatment of pregnant women with congenital AT-III deficiencies. High doses of heparin results in more markedly decreased AT-III activities. In contrast, small doses can be insufficient and thromboembolic complications may occur. Further studies are needed to solve this problem. The required initial dosage of subcutaneous heparin is 10,000 to 12,000 units twice daily. The dose of heparin should be adjusted to achieve a 5- to 10-second prolongation of the partial thromboplastin time (PTT) 10 h post injection. PTT is preferred to the chromogenic heparin assay in patients with AT-III deficiencies because of the uncertain quantification of the anticoagulant effect of heparin. A platelet count (to detect thrombocytopenia) and PTT should be repeated every 2 weeks after the stabilization of the heparin effect. During late pregnancy, control of the heparin effect is recommended once a week because it is likely that the heparin requirements will increase as the pregnancy continues. At delivery and obstetric complications, the inhibitory capacity of AT-III is advised to be normalized with plasma or an AT-III concentrate.[44,45,50] It is very important to reduce the heparin dosage to 5000 units every 12 hours in connection with the AT-III concentrate. The reduction of the heparin dosage should achieve a normal PTT and this avoids bleeding complications. An AT-III concentrate is given in order to normalize the AT-III level the day before delivery or as soon as the obstetric complication is diagnosed. The half-life of the AT-III infusion is about 36 h and this reduces the risk of thromboembolism.[49,67] The initial dosage of the AT-III concentrate is 50 units/kg. One unit of the AT-III concentrate per kg body weight (b.w.) increases the AT-III activity by 1 to 1.5% of normal AT-III activity, i.e., 50 units per kg b.w. increase the AT-III activity by about 50 to 75% of normal.[44] The subsequent doses should be adjusted to achieve an AT-III level of 80%. Usually, daily repeated infusions of an AT-III concentrate are needed to maintain a normal AT-III activity twice daily. The treatment should be monitored by the determination of plasma AT-III activity twice daily. Labor should be induced or a Caesarean section should be performed if AT-III levels are satisfactory and the PTT is normal. However, a Cesarian section should be avoided if possible because of the additional risk of thromboembolism. In addition, epidural anaesthesia should not be used because of bleeding. An AT-III concentrate and subcutaneous heparin should be maintained for 1 week post partum because of the risk of thromboembolism in the puerperium. After that, the restart of warfarin can be recommended at least 8 weeks after delivery or for lifelong if earlier thromboembolism has occurred.[45] Treatment with warfarin can be given after an initial period of AT-III treatment, combined with heparin or dextran, until an appropriate anticoagulant effect is achieved.[44,67] During obstetrical complications, normal AT-III activity is maintained until heparin treatment can be given without danger. Dextran prophylaxis is advised in combination with an AT-III concentrate if the thrombosis prophylaxis with heparin is withdrawn as women with congenital AT-III deficiencies can have other defects in haemostasis predisposing thromboembolic complications as well.[44] The AT-III level of a neonate in cord blood should be checked immediately on delivery. AT-III is usually subnormal in the neonatal period compared to the values seen in adults (50% of normal).[67,68] Newborns with low AT-III activities for their gestational ages may have an increased risk of thromboembolism and DIC, as well as increased morbidity and mortality.[69,70] If the AT-III level of cord blood suggests an AT-III deficiency for a gestational age, treatment with an AT-III concentrate should be taken into consideration. Hellgren et al. reported three AT-III-deficient newborns, two of them died from thromboembolic and respiratory diseases.[71] AT-III levels are normally reduced in the neonatal period and do not reach normal levels for about the first 6 months. This makes it very difficult for the precise diagnosis of AT-III deficiency on delivery.[68] Follow-up studies at 6 and 12 months of age are advised in order to rule out or verify a congenital AT-III deficiency. Women with abortions should be treated with AT-III concentrates like patients during delivery to reach an AT-III level of 80% and treated with reduced heparin dosage. Fresh frozen plasma and normal plasma might be alternatives to an AT-III concentrate.[56] Unfortunately, it would be impossible to give adequate quantities of fresh frozen plasma to restore AT-III levels to the accepted level (80% of normal). A pregnant woman who has a thromboembolic episode during pregnancy should be treated with a heparin infusion (25,000 to 50,000 units/d). She may need an additional AT-III infusion to achieve the sufficient therapeutic effect, i.e., to double the PTT.[73]

III. AT-III IN GYNECOLOGY

A. AT-III DURING HORMONAL TREATMENT

In the last 2 decades, it has become clear that the most important concern about the effects of oral contraceptives on women's health is the increased risk of cardiovascular disease, especially venous thromboembolic disease, myocardial infarction, and stroke.[74,75] A positive correlation between the dose of estrogen in oral contraceptives and the risk of thromboembolism has been reported.[76] Estrogen therapy to suppress lactation also increases the risk of thromboembolism and it should no longer be used.[77] In uncontrolled studies, thrombophlebitis has been reported with estrogen replacement therapy, whereas this association has not been present in controlled experiments.[78] Estrogen exerts several effects on the haemostatic mechanism, which may contribute or be responsible for a generalized hypercoagulable state. Some of these effects are exerted through the action of estrogen on the hepatic function. Estrogen treatment is known to influence the clotting mechanism by increasing the levels of factors II, VII, VIII, IX, and X; fibrinogen; and soluble fibrin.[79,80] Estrogen replacement treatment can also lower levels of AT-III.[79] The potential importance of a reduction of AT-III during estrogen therapy is suggested by the recurrence of intravascular clotting in patients with hereditary AT-III deficiencies.[53] A reduction of 20% or more in AT-III levels has been found to be highly predictive of the occurence of subclinical venous thromboembolism that is extensive enough to be detected by the ^{125}I-fibrinogen technique.[81] The effects of estrogen-containing oral contraceptives on haemostasis have been recently reviewed.[82,83] The factors that result in venous thrombosis may indeed be related to the estrogen component of the oral contraceptive pill because studies have shown a definitive decrease in the incidence of venous thromboembolic events as the dosage of estrogen in the pill is lowered. This does not apply for arterial thrombosis.[84] The pathogenesis of venous thromboembolism in women taking contraceptive pills may relate to changes in the levels of coagulation factors and inhibitors, and altered fibrinolytic and platelet activity.[83] In addition, there is evidence which suggests that endogenous and exogenous estrogen may also cause endothel proliferation and changes in the rate of venous flow.[85,86] The pathogenesis of arterial vascular complications in pill users appears to be much more complex than that responsible for venous thromboembolic complications.[87] The progesteron component of the pill is now considered to be an important factor in connection with arterial vascular complications.[47] It is well known that a deficiency of AT-III is associated with an increased liability of thrombosis (see Chapter 2). The von Kaulla's were the first to describe decreased AT-III serum levels in women who used estrogen-containing contraceptives and to suggest this as a possible cause of thrombosis.[88] Since then, a number of studies have shown a statistically significant decrease in AT-III antigens and activities in women taking combined oral contraceptives.[89,92] Early studies on decreased AT-III activities in women on the pill were based on a serum determination which is mainly reflected *in vitro* clotting.[88,89] At present, it is generally accepted that an AT-III assay should be done in plasma and not in serum. The decrease of plasma AT-III seems to be dose-related because lower-dose pills (those containing 30 to 35 μg of ethinyl estradiol) are associated either with no significant change or a much reduced effect when compared to higher-dose oral contraceptives (50 μg of ethinyl estradiol or more).[93-97] Recently, Bonnar reported a study which shows clearly that AT-III levels decreased significantly in women who received 50 μg estrogen-containing oral contraceptives and, to a lesser extent, in those receiving pills with 30 μg estrogen combined with norethindrone acetate.[87] In patients who received pills with 30 μg estrogen but contained levonorgestrel, AT-III levels did not significantly decrease during the observed period.[87] When interpreting the clinical significance of depressed AT-III levels, one point needs to be considered: the level of its activity. In a recent study, Weenink et al.[98] have found that the mean AT-III level decreased by 9% of the pretreatment value. A decrease of the same magnitude was observed by Howie, who determined progressive antithrombin activity before and during the usage of pills containing 50 μg ethinylestradiol.[99] The level at which the AT-III deficiency would cause thrombosis is not known, but it would probably have to be reduced to about 50% of its normal activity. Observations made by Weenink et al.[100] in "morning after pill" users show that AT-III levels do not decrease until the third or fourth day of treatment with this very high-dose estrogen. Conard et al.[101] have shown that only the progesteron preparation (containing norgestrienone) has no effect on AT-III activity. In addition, no decrease in AT-III levels was observed either with chlormadinone acetate or with ethynodiol diacetate and ethinyl-thio-retroprogesterone.[90,101,103] Reduced AT-III levels, caused by estrogens, have been attributed to increased consumption or depressed synthesis.[101,104] An alternative explanation would be the haemodilution caused by the retention of salt and water under the influence of estrogens.[98] Walters and Lin found that plasma volume increased by 11% while taking pills.[105] This corresponds well with the decrease in AT-III levels.[89,92] It has been suggested that it may be questioned whether or not the determination of AT-III levels has interest before or during oral contraceptive medication.[101] It is now clear that the low-dose oral contraceptives in current use produce a significantly less change in the haemostatic system than do preparations that contain 50 μg of estrogen. If new formulations of pills still produce a hypercoagulability mass screening for AT-III deficiencies in women, taking oral contraceptives will probably not identify those at risk of thromboembolism with the possible exception of the rare cases of congenital AT-III deficiencies.[98] In addition, accumulating evidence suggests that a depressed AT-III level is only one of many risk factors associated with venous thromboembolism and combined oral contraceptives. The decrease in AT-III levels in itself does not necessarily cause thromboembolism. If, however, the haemostatic system is further disturbed by prolonged stasis, endothel damage, postsurgical hypercoagulability, etc., intravascular clotting may well be precipitated. In such instances, the decreased AT-III level may become an important factor in the manifestation of thrombosis. Current research is aimed at finding low-dose formulations of the estrogen/progestagen ratio that will produce the least change in the haemostatic system.

IV. AT-III IN THE NEONATAL PERIOD

A. AT-III IN FULL-TERM AND PREMATURE INFANTS

In healthy full-term newborns, AT-III levels are about 50% as compared to the adult values, which are reached by 6 months of age.[106,109] The data on AT-III biological activity vs. its antigenic level in a newborn is controversial. Peters et al.[108] have studied the functional and immunochemical characteristics of neonatal AT-III.[106,110-111] In contrast to healthy adult controls, a reduced activity/antigen ratio (consistently higher antigen level) was observed, irrespective of the state of health of the newborn. Experiments with crossed-immunoelectrophoresis have excluded the possibility of AT-III-thrombin complexes being the cause of this decreased ratio. In addition, their results indicate that an AT-III molecule with a decreased or absent affinity for either heparin and/or thrombin may circulate in plasma during the newborn period.[108] McDonald et al.[112] have isolated AT-III by heparin affinity chromatography from adult venous blood and from umbilical cord blood of term and preterm neonates. This structural evaluations revealed a fetal AT-III of molecular weight, charge, and electrophoretic migration indistinquishable from adult AT-III. Functional studies showed that on an equimolar basis, the rates of thrombin and X_a interactions with fetal AT-III were as rapid as those with adult AT-III. In addition, the catalytic rates of various concentrations of heparin were also equal. Therefore, they have finally concluded that the newborn infant displays a quantitative but not qualitative deficiency of AT-III. De Stefano et al.[113] have investigated AT-III in healthy normal term and preterm infants and have reported the results obtained from four neonates born to mothers affected from AT-III hereditary deficiencies. Crossed immunoelectrophoresis on heparin agarose (H-CIE) was carried out on a sample and the distribution of isoantithrombins was investigated on plasma by the technique of crossed immunoelectro focusing (CIEF). In all infants, AT-III H-CIE runs displayed a single, fast moving anodal peak, so that a normal binding to heparin was demonstrated. In addition, the CIEF AT-III plasma pattern of the adults, as well as of all newborn infants, displayed three major peaks. It was concluded that the distribution of the isoantithrombins of plasma in neonatal age is identical to that of adults. If healthy full-term neonates have about 20 to 30% AT-III plasma levels, this strongly suggests a hereditary congenital deficiency since a lower normal limit, around 40%, has been recognized in term newborns in previous reports.[107,108] In preterm infants or with pathological conditions where AT-III levels can be markedly reduced, a precise diagnosis of an AT-III hereditary deficiency can not be established. In an AT-III qualitative hereditary defect, a precocious diagnosis can be firmly established by immunoelectrophoretic techniques (particulary by CIEF) which have been demonstrated to distinguish different AT-III molecular defective variants.[113,114] It has been shown that AT-III is further reduced in premature infants.[107,108,115] Peters et al.[108] have determined daily plasma AT-III levels during the first week of life in healthy preterm infants. The mean plasma levels of AT-III in the preterm group were significantly lower as compared to the corresponding values in the group of term infants. A gestational age dependency was found for AT-III levels. The mean plasma levels of AT-III in the premature newborn infants increased significantly and reached term values within the first week of life, independent of immaturity of the infant.[116] In contrast, Hathaway et al.[107] found a more gradual increase of plasma AT-III levels in premature infants, and so the term values were reached by 3 to 4 weeks of age.

B. AT-III IN PATHOLOGICAL CONDITIONS

1. AT-III in Neonates with Idiopathic Respiratory Distress Syndrome (IRDS)

Numerous studies have suggested that a reduced AT-III level occurs in the cord blood samples of premature infants who developed IRDS.[117-119] Karmazsin et al.[119] measured plasma AT-III activity and AT-III concentration. They found that both AT-III activity and concentration showed a linear correlation with the degree of maturity. The lowest values were found in premature babies affected by IRDS who later developed pulmonary haemorrhage. Peters et al.[120] in a comprehensive study found severe coagulation abnormalities in premature infants suffering from IRDS. Among them, markedly reduced AT-III levels were observed and associated with haemorrhage and fibrin depositions in various organs at autopsy. It was particularly interesting that they found very low AT-III levels in those infants who died as compared with survivors. In addition, AT-III was the only parameter which distinguished between survivors and non survivors in the IRDS patients. This severe AT-III deficiency may be a result of both increased turnover because of DIC and/or decreased synthesis due to liver damage. Their findings indicate that very low levels of AT-III are associated with DIC in neonates with IRDS and suggest that a deficiency of AT-III is predictive of a poor outcome. Several therapeutic regimens (heparin, plasma substitution, plasminogen) have been tried in an attempt to decrease mortality in IRDS neonates without any significant success.[121-123] As AT-III deficiencies are quite pronounced in premature infants with DIC or IRDS, it is anticipated that human AT-III concentrates may be effective in the prevention or treatment of these complications.[116]

2. AT-III in Neonates Small for Gestational Age

Small for gestational age (SGA) infants frequently have polycythemia, which is a primary cause of hyperviscosity syndrome.[124,125] The results of haemostatic studies in SGA neonates suggest that intravascular coagulation does occur in such infants.[126,127] It has been previously reported that premature infants with low AT-III levels were found to be associated with fibrin depositions in the vital organs. Peters et al.[128] have investigated several coagulation and fibrinolytic factors in neonates small for gestational age during the first 9 days of life. They found that the mean AT-III level in the SGA group was initially significantly lower than that in the control infants and remained on that level for the observed period. It is concluded that the persistent AT-III deficiency and the reduced blood flow associated with polycythemia may explain the increased risk of thromboembolic complications in SGA infants.[116]

3. AT-III in Neonatal Septicemia

In recent years, the postoperative behavior of AT-III has been claimed to be useful as an early warning sign of emerging septicemia.[127,129] These studies confirm that there is a marked reduction in functional AT-III activity in adult patients with surgical and medical septicemia. In medical septicemia, low AT-III activities indicate a poor prognosis. The data suggested that the serial determination of AT-III activity during surgical septicemia can be a useful tool in the monitoring of therapy.[129] Septicemia in neonates is difficult to diagnose and the mortality in these critically sick infants is high.[130] DIC is one of the possible causes which may play a role in the pathological process of septicemia.[131] Peters et al.[116] reported the results of a retrospective follow-up study on the behavior of the coagulation and fibrinolytic parameters in septic newborns. The results of this study showed that the only consistent abnormality was a significantly decreased plasma AT-III level. All neonates with Gram-negative septicemia (*E. coli*) displayed low AT-III levels, while a similar decrease in AT-III levels was found only in 4 out of 16 newborns with a gram-positive septicemia (B-hemolytic streptococcal infection). It is concluded that a very low AT-III level on the first day of life in newborns with clinical symptoms suggests septicemia.

REFERENCES

1. **Tatra, G. and Gruber, W.,** Quantitative immunological determination of antithrombin III concentration during normal pregnancy and post partum, *Arch. Gynecol.*, 217, 127, 1964.
2. **Billand, L. and Duckert, F.,** Coagulation factors of the newborn and his mother, *Thromb. Diath. Haemorrh.*, 29, 644, 1973.
3. **Brandt, P. and Stejnbgerg, S.,** Subcutaneous heparin for thrombosis in pregnant women with hereditary antithrombin deficiency, *Lancet,* 1, 100, 1979.
4. **Gjönnaess, H. and Fagerhol, M. K.,** Studies on coagulation and fibrinolysis in pregnancy, *Acta Obstet. Gynecol. Scand.*, 54, 363, 1975.
5. **Weiner, C. P. and Brand, J.,** Plasma antithrombin III activity in normal pregnancy, *Obstet. Gynecol.*, 56, 601, 1980.
6. **Hellgren, M. and Blombäck, M.,** Studies on blood coagulation and fibrinolysis in pregnancy during delivery and in the puerperium, *Gynecol. Obstet. Invest.*, 13, 141, 1981.
7. **Hellgren, M., Nygards, E. B., and Robbe, H.,** Antithrombin III in late pregnancy, *Acta. Obstet. Gynecol. Scand.*, 61, 187, 1982.
8. **Nelson, D. M., Stemple, L. E., and Brandt, J. T.,** Hereditary AT III deficiency and pregnancy: report of two cases and review of the literature, *Obstet. Gynecol.*, 65, 848, 1985.
9. **Leclerc, Y. R., Geerts, W., Panju, A., Nguyen, P., and Hirsh, P.,** Management of antithrombin III deficiency during pregnancy without administration of antithrombin III, *Thromb. Res.*, 41, 567, 1986.
10. **Weenink, G. H., Treffers, P. E., Kahlé, L. H., and Ten Cate, J. W.,** Antithrombin III in normal pregnancy, *Thromb. Res.*, 26, 281, 1982.

11. **Weenink, G. H., Borm, J. J. J., Ten Cate, J. W., and Treffers, P. E.,** Antithrombin III levels in normotensive and hypertensive pregnancy, *Gynecol. Obstet. Invest.*, 16, 230, 1983.
12. **Howie, P. W.,** The haemostatic mechanism in preeclampsia, *Clin. Obstet. Gynecol.*, 4, 595, 1977.
13. **McKay, D. G.,** Chronic intravascular coagulation in normal pregnancy and preeclampsia, *Contrib. Nephrol.*, 25, 108, 1982.
14. **Saleh, A. A., Bottoms, S. F., Welch, R. A., Ali, A. M., Mariona, F. G., and Mammen, E. F.,** Preeclampsia, delivery and hemostatic system, *Am. J. Obstet. Gynecol.*, 157, 381, 1987.
15. **Vassahli, P., Morris, R. H., and McCluskey, H. I.,** The pathogenic role of fibrin deposition in the glomerular lesions of toxemia of pregnancy, *J. Exp. Med.*, 118, 467, 1963.
16. **Weiner, C. P. and Brandt, J.,** Plasma antithrombin III activity, an aid in the diagnosis of preeclampsia-eclampsia, *Am. J. Obstet. Gynecol.*, 142, 275, 1982.
17. **Weenink, G. H., Treffers, P. E., Vijn, P., Smoren-Schoorl, M. E., and Ten Cate, J. W.,** Antithrombin III levels in preeclampsia correlate with maternal and fetal morbidity, *Am. J. Obstet. Gynecol.*, 148, 1092, 1984.
18. **Weiner, C. P., Kwaan, H. C., Xu, C., Paul, M., Burmeister, L., and Hauck, W.,** Antithrombin III activity in women with hypertension during pregnancy, *Obstet. Gynecol.*, 65, 301, 1985.
19. **Weenink, G., Ten Cate, J. W., and Treffers, E. P.,** Hypertensive disorders, *Clin. Obstet.*, 28, 37, 1985.
20. **Letsky, E. A.,** Coagulation Problems During Pregnancy, Churchill Livingstone, Edinburgh, 1985, 62.
21. **Mann, L. T., Jensenius, J. C., and Simonsen, M.,** Antithrombin III: protection against death after injection of thromboplastin, *Science*, 166, 517, 1966.
22. **Gierckskу, E. K., Björklid, E., and Prydz, H.,** The effect of intravenous injection of purified thromboplastin in rats, *Scand. J. Haematol.*, 16, 300, 1976.
23. **Takemoto, Y., Tananabe, J., Tanaha, S., Fukunda, A., Fujii, C., Kohama, A., and Shibata, S.,** The effect of prophylactic heparinization of DIC arising from transitory circulatory arrest in dogs, *Circ. Shock*, 15, 131, 1985.
24. **Brandt, P.,** Observation during the treatment of antithrombin III deficient women with heparin and antithrombin III concentrate during pregnancy, parturition and abortion, *Thromb. Res.*, 22, 15, 1981.
25. **Jespersen, J.,** Termination of pregnancy in a women with hereditary antithrombin deficiency under antithrombotic protection with subcutaneous heparin and infusion of plasma, *Gynecol. Obstet. Invest.*, 5, 267, 1985.
26. **Jespersen, J., Gram, J., Kluft, C., and Astrup, T.,** Protection against venous thrombosis in an antithrombin III deficient patient suffering from episodes of arterial thrombosis requiring major surgery, *Am. J. Clin. Pathol.*, 83, 768, 1985.
27. **Schipper, H. G., Roos, J. V. D., Meulen, F., and Ten Cate, J. W.,** Antithrombin deficiency in surgical intensive care patients, *Thromb. Res.*, 21, 73, 1981.
28. **Smith-Erichsen, N., Aasen, A. O., Gallimore, M. J., and Amudsen, E.,** Studies of components of the coagulation systems in normal individuals and septic shock patients, *Circ. Shock*, 9, 491, 1982.
29. **Hellgren, M., Egberg, N., and Eklund, J.,** Blood coagulation and fibrinolytic factors and their inhibitors in critically ill patients, *Intensive Care Med.*, 10, 23, 1984.
30. **Jespersen, J.,** A study of the antithrombotic potential in women on oral contraceptives low in oestrogen. Its relation to the present knowledge of the mechanism and pathophysiological aspects of the thrombo-haemorrhagic balance, in Clinical Aspects of Fibrinolysis and Thrombolysis, Jespersen, J., Keuft, C., and Korsgraad, O., Eds., South Jutland University Press, Esbjerg, Denmark, 1983, 399.
31. **Rosenberg, R. D.,** Heparin, antithrombin and abnormal clotting, *Ann. Rev. Med.*, 29, 367, 1978.
32. **Corrigan, J. J. and Jordan, C. M.,** Heparin therapy in septicaemia with disseminated intravascular coagulation, *N. Engl. J. Med.*, 283, 636, 1970.
33. **Lash, H. G. and Heene, D. H.,** Heparin therapy of diffuse intravascular coagulation (DIC), *Thromb. Diath. Haemorrh.*, 33, 105, 1974.
34. **Mant, M. J. and King, E. G.,** Severe, acute disseminated intravascular coagulation; a reappraisal of its pathophysiology, clinical significance and therapy based in 47 patients, *Am. J. Med.*, 67, 557, 1979.
35. **Klein, H. G. and William, R. G.,** Disseminated intravascular coagulation during heparin therapy, *Ann. Intern. Med.*, 80, 447, 1974.
36. **Astrup, T. and Jespersen, J.,** Disseminated intravascular coagulation and the balance between blood coagulation and fibrinolysis, *Folia Haematol.*, 111, 407, 1984.
37. **Astrup, T. and Jespersen, J.,** Thrombosis, disseminated intravascular coagulation and the dynamic haemostatic balance. Aspects of prophylaxis and treatment, *Intern. Anigo.*, 3, 331, 1984.
38. **Blauhut, B., Necek, S., Vinazzer, H., and Bergmann, H.,** Substitution therapy with antithrombin III concentrate in shock and DIC, *Thromb. Res.*, 27, 271, 1982.
39. **Hellgren, M., Javelin, L., Hägnevik, K., and Blombäck, M.,** Antithrombin III concentrate as adjuvant in DIC treatment. A pilot study in 9 severely ill patients, *Thromb. Res.*, 35, 459, 1984.
40. **Kaplan, R. L., Sahin, S. A., and Petty, T. L.,** Incidence and outcome of the respiratory distress syndrome in gram negative sepsis, *Arch. Intern. Med.*, 139, 867, 1979.

41. **Maki, M., Terao, T., Ikenone, T., Takemura, T., Sekiba, K., Shirakawa, K., and Soma, H.,** Clinical evaluation of antithrombin III concentrate (BI 6.013) for disseminated intravascular coagulation in obstetrics, *Gynecol. Obstet. Invest.*, 23, 230, 1987.
42. **Ullery, J. C.,** Thromboembolic disease complicating pregnancy and the puerperium, *Am. J. Obstet. Gynecol.*, 68, 1243, 1954.
43. **Henderson, S. R., Lund, C. J., and Creasman, W. T.,** Antepartum pulmonary embolism, *Am. J. Obstet. Gynecol.*, 1162, 476, 1971.
44. **Hellgren, M., Tengborn, L., and Abilgaard, U.,** Pregnancy in women with congenital antithrombin III deficiency: experience of treatment with heparin and antithrombin, *Gynecol. Obstet. Invest.*, 14, 127, 1982.
45. **Hellgren, M. and Nygards, E. B.,** Long-term therapy with subcutaneous heparin during pregnancy, *Gynecol. Obstet. Invest.*, 13, 76, 1982.
46. **Treffers, P E., Huidekoper, B. L., Weenink, G. H., and Klosterman, G. J.,** Epidemiological observations of thromboembolic disease during pregnancy and in the puerperium in 56,022 women, *Int. J. Gynecol. Obstet.*, 21, 327, 1983.
47. **Bergsjö, P., Fagerhol, M. K., and Abildgaard, V.,** Antithrombin III concentration in women using low-dose progesterone for contraception, *Am. J. Obstet. Gynecol.*, 112, 938, 1972.
48. **Bonnar, J.,** Venous thrombo-embolism and pregnancy, in Recent Advances in Obstetrics and Gynecology, Stallworthy, J. and Bourne, G., Eds., Churchill Livingstone, Edinburgh, 1979, 173.
49. The Lancet, Familial antithrombin III deficiency, *Lancet,* 1, 1021, 1983.
50. **Brandt, P., Jespersen, J., and Gregersen, G.,** Postpartum haemolyticuraemic syndrome successfully treated with antithrombin III, *Br. Med. J.*, 280, 449, 1980.
51. **Hellgren, M. and Blombäck, M.,** Studies on blood coagulation and fibrinolysis in pregnancy during delivery and in the puerperium, *Gynecol. Obstet. Invest.*, 12, 141, 1981.
52. **Winter, J. H., Fenech, A., and Ridley, W,** Familial antithrombin III deficiency, *Anat. J. Med.*, 304, 373, 1982.
53. **Egeberg, O.,** Inherited antithrombin deficiency causing thrombophilia, *Thromb. Diath. Haemorrh.*, 13, 516, 1965.
54. **Johansson, L., Hedner, U., and Nilsson, J. M.,** Familial antithrombin III deficiency and pathogenesis of deep venous thrombosis, *Acta Med. Scand.*, 201, 491, 1978.
55. **Hall, J., Pauli, R. M., and Wilson, K.,** Maternal and fetal sequelae of anticoagulation during pregnancy, *Am. J. Med.*, 68, 122, 1980.
56. **Zucker, M. L., Comperts, E. D., and Marcus, R. G.,** Prophylactic and therapeutic use of anticoagulants in inherited antithrombin III deficiency, *S. Afr. Med. J.*, 50, 1743, 1976.
57. **Vellenga, E., vanImhoff, G. W., and Aarnondse, J. G.,** Effective prophylaxis with oral anticoagulants and low dose heparin during pregnancy in an AT III deficient woman, *Lancet,* 2, 224, 1983.
58. **Weiner, C. P.,** Diagnosis and management of thromboembolic disease during pregnancy, *Clin. Obstet. Gynecol.*, 28, 107, 1985.
59. **Green, P. J.,** Antithrombin III and subcutaneous heparin, *Lancet,* 1, 103, 1980.
60. **Hrushesky, W. J.,** Subcutaneous heparin induced thrombocytopenia, *Arch. Int. Med.*, 138, 1489, 1978.
61. **Wise, P. H. and Hall, A. J.,** Heparin induced osteopenia in pregnancy, *Br. Med. J.*, 47, 110, 1980.
62. **Griffith, G. C. and Lin, D. T. Y.,** Severe heparin osteoporosis in pregnancy, *Postgrad. Med. J.*, 60, 424, 1984.
63. **Squires, J. W. and Pinch, L. W.,** Heparin-induced spinal fractures, *JAMA,* 22, 2417, 1979.
64. **Aarskog, D., Aksnes, L., Marhestadt Ulstein, M., and Sagen, N.,** Heparin induced inhibition of 1,25-dihidroxy vitamin D formation, *Am. J. Obstet. Gynecol.*, 148, 1141, 1984.
65. **De Swiet, M., Dorrington, W. P., Fidler, J., Horsman, A., Katz, D., Letsky, E., Peacock, M., and Wise, P. H.,** Prolonged heparin therapy in pregnancy causes bone demineralization, *Br. J. Obstet. Gynecol.*, 90, 1129, 1983.
66. **De Swiet, M.,** Thromboembolism, in Medical Disorders in Obstetric Practice, De Swiet, M., Ed., Blackwell Scientific, Oxford, 1984, 95.
67. **Samson, D., Stirling, Y., Wolf, L., Howarth, D., Seghatchian, M. J., and De Chazal, R.,** Management of planned pregnancy in a patient with congenital antithrombin III deficiency, *Br. J. Haematol.*, 56, 243, 1984.
68. **Teger-Nilsson, A., C.,** Antithrombin in infancy and childhood, *Acta Paediatr. Scand.*, 64, 624, 1975.
69. **Bjarke, B., Herin, P., and Blombäck, M.,** Neonatal aortic thrombosis, *Acta Paediatr. Scand.*, 63, 297, 1974.
70. **Peters, M.,** Intensive monitoring of coagulation and fibrinolysis in the first week of life, Thesis, Academic Medical, Amsterdam, 1984.
71. **Hellgren, M.,** Thromboembolism and pregnancy, Thesis, Karolinska Institute, Stockholm, 1981.
72. **McDonald, M. M., Hathaway, W. E., Reeve, E. B., and Leonard, B. D.,** Biochemical and functional study of antithrombin III in newborn infants, *Thromb. Haemostas.*, 47, 56, 1982.

73. **Anderson, O., Hevitt, P., Machin, S. J., Mackie, J., and Wilkinson, L.**, Therapy of thrombosis with antithrombin III deficiency, *Br. J. Haematol.*, 51, 326, 1982.
74. **Shapiro, S.**, Oral contraceptives — a time to take stock, *N. Engl. J. Med.*, 315, 450, 1986.
75. **Stadel, B. V.**, Oral contraceptives and cardiovascular disease, *N. Engl. J. Med.*, 305, 612, 1981.
76. **Inman, W. H. W., Vessey, M. P., Westerholm, B., and Eragelund, A.**, Thromboembolic disease and the steroidal content of oral contraceptives. A report to the Committee on Safety of Drugs, *Br. Med. J.*, 2, 203, 1970.
77. **Daniel, D. G., Campbell, H., and Tumbyll, A. C.**, Puerperal thromboembolism and supression of lactation, *Lancet*, 2, 287, 1967.
78. Boston Collaborative Drug Surveillance Program; Surgically confirmed gallbladder disease, venous thromboembolism, and breast tumors in relation to menopausal oestrogen therapy, *N. Engl. J. Med.*, 290, 15, 1974.
79. **Bonnar, J., Haddon, M., and Hunter, D. H.**, Coagulation system changes in postmenopausal women receiving oestrogen preparations, *Postgrad. Med. J.*, 52, 30, 1976.
80. **Von Kaulla, E., Droegmueller, W., and Von Kaulla, K. N.**, Conjugated oestrogens and hypercoagulability, *Am. J. Obstet. Gynecol.*, 122, 688, 1975.
81. **Stamatakis, J. D., Lawrence, D., and Kahhar, U. V.**, Surgery, venous thrombosis and anti-X_a, *Br. J. Surg.*, 64, 709, 1977.
82. **Beller, F. K. and Ebert, C.**, Effects of oral contraceptives on blood coagulation. A review, *Obstet. Gynecol. Surv.*, 40, 425, 1985.
83. **Notelovits, M.**, Oral contraception and coagulation, *Clin. Obstet. Gynecol.*, 28, 73, 1985.
84. **Bottiger, L. E., Boman, G., Eklund, G., and Westerholm, B.**, Oral contraceptives and thromboembolic disease: effect of lowering oestrogen content, *Lancet*, 1, 1097, 1981.
85. **Irey, N. S., Manion, W. C., and Taylor, H. B.**, Vascular lesions in women taking oral contraceptives, *Arch. Pathol.*, 89, 1, 1970.
86. **Irey, N. S. and Norris, H. J.**, Intimal vascular lesions associated with female reproductive steroids, *Arch. Pathol.*, 96, 227, 1973.
87. **Bonnar, J.**, Coagulation effects of oral contraception, *Am. J. Obstet. Gynecol.*, 157, 1042, 1987.
88. **von Kaulla, E. and von Kaulla, K. N.**, Oral contraceptives and low antithrombin III activity, *Lancet*, 1, 36, 1970.
89. **Fagerhol, M. K. and Abildgaard, U.**, Immunological studies on human antithrombin III. Influence of age, sex and use of oral contraceptives on serum concentration, *Scand. J. Haematol.*, 7, 10, 1970.
90. **Howie, P. W., Prentice, C. R. M., Mallinson, A. C., Horne, C. H. W., and McNicol, G. P.**, Effect of combined oestrogen-progestagen oral contraceptives, oestrogen and progestagen on antiplasmin and antithrombin activity, *Lancet*, 2, 1329, 1970.
91. **Rákóczi, I., Nagy, J., Szigetvári, I., Losonczy, H., Hadnagy, J., and Gáti, I.**, Oestrogen containing oral contraceptives and antithrombin III activity, *Acta Physiol. Acad. Sci. Hung.*, 45, 281, 1974.
92. **Poller, L.**, Oral contraceptives, blood clotting and thrombosis, *Br. Med. Bull.*, 34, 151, 1978.
93. **Notelovitz, M., Kitchens, C., and Coone, L.**, Low-dose oral contraceptive usage and coagulation, *Am. J. Obstet. Gynecol.*, 141, 71, 1981.
94. **Notelovitz, M., Kitchens, C., and Ware, M. D.**, Low-dose oral contraceptives and coagulation: comparison with high-dose oral contraceptives and intra-uterine devices, *Curr. Ther. Res.*, 33, 207, 1983.
95. **Sabra, A. and Bonnar, J.**, Haemostatic system changes induced by 50 ug and 30 ug estrogen/progestagen oral contraceptives, *J. Reprod. Med.*, 28, 85, 1983.
96. **Meade, T. W., Haines, A. P., and North, W. R. S.**, Haemostatic lipid and blood pressure profiles of women on oral contraceptives containing 50 ug or 30 ug oestrogen, *Lancet*, 2, 948, 1977.
97. **Rákóczi, I., Gerö, Gy., Demeter, J., and Gáti, I.**, Comparative metabolic effects of oral contraceptive preparations containing different progestagens, *Drug Res.*, 35, 630, 1985.
98. **Weenink, G. H., Kahlé, L. H., Lamping, R. J., Ten Cate, J. W., and Treffers, P. E.**, Antithrombin III on oral contraceptive users and during normotensive pregnancy, *Acta Obstet. Gynecol. Scand.*, 63, 57, 1984.
99. **Howie, P. W., Prentice, C. R. M., and McNicol, G. P.**, A method of antithrombin estimation using plasma defibrinated with ancroid, *Br. J. Haematol.*, 25, 101, 1973.
100. **Weenink, G. H., Ten Cate, J. W., Lamping, R. J., and Treffers, P. E.**, "Morning after pill" and antithrombin III, *Lancet*, 2, 1105, 1981.
101. **Conard, J., Cazenave, B., Samama, M., Hopellou, M. H., Zorn, J. R., and Neau, C.**, AT III content and antithrombin activity in oestrogen-progestagen and progesteron only treated women, *Thromb. Res.*, 18, 675, 1980.
102. **Fagerhol, M. K., Abildgaard, U., Bergsjo, P., and Jacobsen, J. H.**, Oral contraceptives and low antithrombin III concentration, *Lancet*, 1, 1175, 1970.
103. **Gjonnoess, H. and Fagerhol, M. K.**, Studies on plasma coagulation and fibrinolysis during oral contraception of various types, *Scand. J. Haematol.*, 12, 232, 1974.

104. **Kobayashi, N. and Takeda, Y.,** Effects of a large dose of oestradiol on antithrombin III metabolism in male and female dogs, *Eur. J. Clin. Invest.*, 7, 373, 1977.
105. **Walters, W. A. and Lim, Y. L.,** Haemodynamic changes in women taking oral contraceptives, *J. Obstet. Gynaecol. Br. Commonw.*, 77, 1007, 1970.
106. **Teger-Nilsson, A. C.,** Antithrombin III in infancy and childhood, *Acta Paediatr. Scand.*, 64, 624, 1975.
107. **Hathaway, W. E., Neumann, L. L., Borden, C. A., and Jacobson, L. J.,** Immunologic studies of antithrombin III in the newborn, *Thromb. Haemostas.*, 39, 624, 1978.
108. **Peters, M., Jansen, E., Ten Cate, J. W., Kahlé, L. H., Ockelford, P., and Breaderveld, C.,** Neonatal antithrombin III, *Br. J. Haematol.*, 58, 579, 1984.
109. **Andrew, M., Massicotte-Nolan, P., Mitchell, L., and Cassidy, K.,** Dysfunctional antithrombin III in sick premature infants, *Pediatr. Res.*, 19, 237, 1985.
110. **Biland, L. and Duckert, F.,** Coagulation factors of the newborn and his mother, *Thromb. Diath. Haemorrh.*, 29, 644, 1973.
111. **Cederholm-Williams, S. A., Spencer, J. A. D., and Wilkinson, A. R.,** Plasma levels of selected haemostatic factors in newborn babies, *Thromb. Res.*, 23, 555, 1981.
112. **McDonald, M. M., Hathaway, W. E., Reeve, E. B., and Leonard, B. D.,** Biochemical and functional study of antithrombin III in newborn infants, *Thromb. Haemostas.*, 47, 56, 1982.
113. **De Stefano, V., Leone, G., De Carolis, M. P., Ferrelli, R., De Carolis, S. D., Pagano, L., Tortorolo, G., and Bizzi, B.,** Antithrombin III in full-term and pre-term newborn infants. Three cases of neonatal diagnosis of AT III congenital defect, *Thromb. Haemostas.*, 57, 329, 1987.
114. **De Stefano, V., Di Donfrancesco, A., De Carolis, S., De Carolis, M. P., Moneta, E., and Leone, G.,** Neonatal diagnosis of antithrombin III congenital defect in a premature newborn, *Br. J. Haematol.*, 65, 117, 1987.
115. **Peters, M., Breederveld, C., Kahlé, L. H., and Ten Cate, J. W.,** Rapid microanalysis of coagulation parameters by automated chromogenic substrate methods. Application in neonatal patients, *Thromb. Res.*, 28, 773, 1982.
116. **Peters, M.,** Intensive monitoring of coagulation and fibrinolysis in the first week of life, Thesis, Amsterdam, 1984.
117. **Mahasandana, Ch. and Hathaway, W. E.,** Circulating anticoagulants in the newborn: relation to hypercoagulability and the idiopathic respiratory distress syndrome and hemorrhage. I. Coagulation studies, *Biol. Neonat.*, 17, 84, 1971.
118. **Hathaway, W. E., Mahasandana, Ch., and Makowski, E. L.,** Cord blood coagulation in infants of high risk pregnant women, *Am. J. Obstet. Gynaecol.*, 51, 121, 1974.
119. **Karmazsin, L., Balla, G., Misz, M., Beck, P., Nagy, P., and Rák, K.,** Antithrombin III levels in term and pre-term infants measured by rate nephelometry, *Acta Paediatr. Hung.*, 25, 119, 1984.
120. **Peters, M., Ten Cate, J. W., Breederveld, C., DeLeeuw, R., Emeis, J., and Koppe, J.,** Low antithrombin III levels in neonates with idiopatic respiratory distress syndrome: poor prognosis, *Pediatr. Res.*, 18, 273, 1984.
121. **Gobel, U., v.Voss, H., Jürgens, H., Petrich, C., Pothmann, R., Sprock, J., and Lemburg, P.,** Efficiency of heparin in the treatment of newborn infants with respiratory distress syndrome and disseminated intravascular coagulation, *Eur. J. Pediatr.*, 47, 133, 1980.
122. **Hambleton, G. and Aplleyard, W. J.,** Controlled trial of fresh frozen plasma in asphyxiated with hyaline membrane disease, *Arch. Dis. Child.*, 43, 116, 1968.
123. **Ambrus, C. A., Weintraub, D. H., Choi, Th. S., Eisenberg, B., Staub, H. P., Courey, N. G., Foote, R. J., Complerud, D., Moesch, R. W., Ray, M., Bross, I. D. J., Jung, O. S., Mink, I. B., and Ambrus, J. L.,** Plasminogen in the prevention of hyaline membrane disease, *Am. J. Dis. Child.*, 127, 189, 1974.
124. **Gross, G. P., Hathaway, W. E., and McGaughey, H. R.,** Hyperviscosity in the neonate, *J. Pediatr.*, 32, 1004, 1973.
125. **Hakanson, D. O. and Oh, W.,** Hyperviscosity in small for gestational age infants, *Biol. Neonat.*, 37, 109, 1980.
126. **Perlman, M. and Drilansky, A.,** Blood coagulation status of small for dates and postmature infants, *Arch. Dis. Child.*, 50, 424, 1975.
127. **Weissbach, G., Lenk, H., Vogtmann, C., Donula, H., and Bottcher, H.,** Gerinnungsparameter bei Neugebornen mit Symptomen der Dysmaturität, *Wiss. Z. Karl Marx Univ. Leipzig*, 25, 185, 1976.
128. **Peters, M., Ten Cate, J. W., Koo, L. H., and Breederveld, C.,** Persistent antithrombin III deficiency: risk factor for thromboembolic complications in neonates small for gestational age, *J. Pediatr.*, 105, 310, 1984.
129. **Büller, H. R., Bolwerk, C., and Ten Cate, J.,** Postoperative haemostatic profile in relation to gram negative septicaemia, *Crit. Care Med.*, 10, 311, 1982.
130. **Siegel, J. D. and McCracken, G. H.,** Sepsis neonatorum, *N. Engl. J. Med.*, 304, 642, 1982.
131. **Corrigan, J. J., Ariz, T., Jordan, Ch. M., and Bennet, B. B.,** Disseminated intravascular coagulation in septic shock, *Am. J. Dis. Child.*, 126, 629, 1973.

Chapter 4

THE GENETICS OF ANTITHROMBIN-III DEFICIENCY

Edward V. Prochownik

TABLE OF CONTENTS

I. TYPES OF AT-III DEFICIENCIES

For the purpose of understanding the pathophysiological basis of antithrombin III (AT-III) deficiencies, it is convenient to divide them into two broad categories: congenital or hereditary, and acquired. The latter category has been covered in Chapter 2 and little further will be said about it here except to reiterate that this condition may result from a variety of causes. In all cases, these result from factors which either decrease the synthesis of AT-III, such as hepatic diseases, or from factors which decrease the plasma half-life of the molecule, such as protein-losing enteropathies or nephropathies. In general, this condition is corrected as soon as the underlying disorder is effectively treated.[1]

Congenital or hereditary AT-III deficiencies are defined as those with a familial basis and which demonstrate an autosomal-dominant mode of transmission. Classically, these have been categorized as Type I, in which both AT-III antigen levels and activity are proportionally reduced, or Type II, in which normal or near normal antigen levels are associated with low activity.[2,3] As will become apparent later, each of these falls into distinct molecular categories. Theoretically, a congenital AT-III deficiency could result *de novo* from a germ line mutation and, thus, be associated with perfectly normal parental AT-III activity. In fact, at least two individuals have been described with chromosomal deletions resulting in AT-III deficiencies.[4]

The incidence of all inherited AT-III deficiencies has been variously estimated at between 1:2000 to 1:5000 in the general population. More recent studies, however, suggest that it is somewhat rarer than this.[3,5] It should be kept in mind that, since most families are identified because of a symptomatic propositus (*vide infra*), many individuals will go undetected. Therefore, the true incidence of the disorder is undoubtedly higher than suggested from published studies. Irrespective of its true frequency, it is apparent that AT-III deficiency is among the most common inherited coagulopathies.

II. EARLY STUDIES OF CONGENITAL AT-III DEFICIENCIES

A. TYPE I (QUANTITATIVE) DISORDERS

Since the original description of a hereditary AT-III deficiency by Egeberg in 1965,[6] numerous additional examples have been published.[2,3,7-9] Most families are identified because of a propositus who has experienced recurrent or severe thrombotic episodes, coupled with an unusually impressive family history of thromboembolic disease or descriptions of deaths due to "pneumonia" or "stroke." Biochemical investigations of such individuals reveals a remarkably homogeneous population of patients with a 50 to 70% reduction in plasma AT-III levels compared to normal, pooled, control populations. The evaluation of family members often reveals a similar reduction of AT-III levels, even among asymptomatic individuals. The functional activities of these individuals' AT-IIIs are entirely normal.

B. TYPE II (QUALITATIVE) DISORDERS

In 1974, Sas et al.[10] reported on a Hungarian family with a high incidence of venous thrombotic complications associated with normal levels of AT-III as determined by radial immunodiffusion studies. Despite normal antigen levels, AT-III activity, heparin cofactor activity, and anti-Xa activity were reduced. Subsequently, it was shown that this patient's plasma demonstrated two AT-III-specific precipitin peaks when examined by two-dimensional immunoelectrophoresis (in the presence of heparin). One peak was of normal electrophoretic mobility, while the other was of decreased mobility. Since these original publications, several other reports have appeared documenting other qualitative deficiencies (*vide infra*).[11-18]

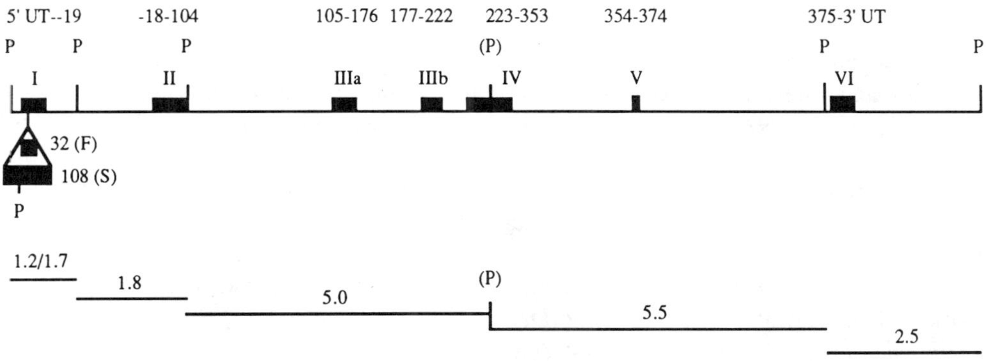

FIGURE 1. Map of the human AT-III gene. The gene consists of seven exons and six introns, distributed over approximately 16 kb. All PstI sites are shown. The polymorphic PstI site in exon IV is indicated by P. The fragments seen when PstI-digested genomic DNA is probed with a full-length cDNA are shown below the map. Note that, depending upon the presence or absence of the exon IV, PstI site fragments of 5.0 kb + 5.5 kb or 10.5 kb are seen. In exon I is shown diagramatically the two different insertion segments of 32 or 108 bp that are found in the 5′-untranslated (5′UT) region. The longer of these contains an internal PstI site. In this allele, exon I coding sequences reside on a 1.2 kb PstI genomic fragment. The allele containing the 32 bp insertion contains no internal PstI site. First exon coding sequences thus reside on a 1.7 kb Pst segment. Enzymes cutting at sites which flank these two insertions will generate fragments which differ in length by 76 bp. The numbers above the map refer to the codons found in the cDNA-18 and -19, and refer to codons of the signal peptide.

III. RESTRICTION FRAGMENT LENGTH POLYMORPHISMS (RFLPS) IN THE HUMAN AT-III GENE

The use of RFLPs has been of paramount importance in helping to determine the molecular basis of AT-III deficiencies. To date, two RFLPs have been identified. One of these results from a single, silent nucleotide change in the coding region of the gene, whereas the second is due to an insertion/deletion in the 5′-flanking region.

A. THE SILENT NUCLEOTIDE CHANGE

The first evidence for RFLPs in the AT-III gene was obtained by Prochownik et al. during the original cloning and characterization of AT-III cDNAs.[19] These investigators screened two human liver cDNA libraries derived from different individuals. They found that clones originating form one library contained no internal PstI restriction, whereas those obtained from the second library contained one such site. DNA sequencing through the relevant region indicated that this was due to a single base substitution in the third position of the Gln 305 codon (Figure 1). The sequence of this codon could be either CAG or CAA, which in either case still encodes Gln. Thus, the structure of the AT-III protein remains unchanged. Since the preceding amino acid at position 304 is Leu (CTG), individuals may possess either the sequence CTG CAG or CTG CAA. The former sequence is the recognition site for PstI, whereas the latter site fails to be recognized by this enzyme. The authors also presented evidence that the polymorphism is inherited in typical Mendelian fashion. Individuals were thus classified as −/− if both AT-III alleles were missing the PstI site, +/+ if both alleles contained the site, and +/− if one of each allele was present. In a subsequent publication, Prochownik et al. demonstrated the high frequency (approximately half of all alleles examined) of this RFLP.[20] That it is present to an equal degree in all racial groups examined implies that the RFLP is extremely ancient, presumably antedating the racial divergence of the human species.

B. INSERTION/DELETION IN THE 5′-FLANKING REGION

Bock and Levitan have described an unusual length polymorphism within the 5′ flanking region of the AT-III gene.[21] This results from the insertion of either a 32 bp or 108 bp sequence at an identical point, 345 bp upstream of the translational start site. The two sequences are entirely nonhomologous. This contrasts with most other length polymorphisms in which identical DNA sequences are inserted at variable positions in one allele relative to another.

Digestion of genomic DNA with enzymes whose recognition sites flank the polymorphic sequence generates allelic fragments differing from one another in length by 76 bp (Figure 1). Bock and Levitan have designated these different fragments as "F" (fast-migrating) or "S" (slow-migrating). The author has identified the same polymorphism using PstI digested DNAs probed with 5′-specific genomic DNA fragment. Interestingly, the 32 bp insertion which generates Bock and Levitan's F-fragment gives rise to a 1.77 kb PstI allele, whereas the 108 bp insertion which generates the S-fragment gives rise to 1.2 kb allele. This seeming contradiction results from the fact that the 108 bp insertion element contains within itself a PstI site, whereas the 32 bp element does not. Since the next 3′PstI site is the same in both alleles, PstI digestion of the S allele actually generates a DNA fragment that is smaller by 500 bp than that generated by the F allele.

C. STRUCTURE OF THE HUMAN AT-III GENE

A complete map of the AT-III gene has been derived by Prochownik et al.[22] and is a useful aid in conceptualizing the results of genetic analyses of AT-III-deficient families (Figure 1). The gene contains seven exons and six introns distributed over approximately 16 kb of DNA. Either four or five PstI fragments containing AT-III coding sequences are generated from individual alleles. The 5′ most fragment is the one containing the insertion polymorphism described above and migrates with a size of either 1.2 or 1.7 kb. 3′ to this is an invariant fragment 1.8 kb is size. This is followed by either a 10.5 kb fragment or by two fragments of 5.0 kb and 5.5 kb. This results from the fact that the polymorphic CG codon at the Gln 305 position lies at the 5.0/5. 5 kb fragment border. Finally, the 3′-most coding region resides on an invariant 2.5 kb fragment.

The presence of two frequent polymorphisms in the AT-III gene allows for the resolution of parental alleles in almost all individuals. Indeed, in a recent collaborative study with Bock, our laboratories have been successful in this regard in 14 of 15 cases.[23] This analysis makes it possible to determine the inheritance of the affected allele in AT-III deficiency as well as to document allelic deletion (*vide infra*).

IV. GENETIC ANALYSIS OF KINDREDS WITH TYPE I AT-III DEFICIENCIES

Using the analysis described above for the examination of individual parental alleles, Prochownik et al. were the first to demonstrate the molecular basis for Type I AT-III deficiencies.[20] In this study, only the polymorphism described in the previous section was used to resolve parental alleles. In one family, it was demonstrated that the affected father had a +/+ genotype, whereas the unaffected mother had a +/− genotype. An affected daughter was also a +/− heterozygote. If only the father is considered, it is possible to tentatively conclude that his AT-III deficiency is the result of mutation on a + allele. However, since he presumably contains two such alleles, as evidenced by his +/+ genotype, it is impossible to identify the mutant one. An alternate explanation would be that the father contains a complete deletion of one AT-III locus and is thus hemizygous. This issue can easily be resolved by consideration of the daughter's genotype (+/−). Since she could only have inherited the − allele from her mother, she must have inherited the + allele from her father. This + allele must, therefore, be the affected one, otherwise the daughter would not have an AT-III deficiency. This analysis indicates that the father is truly homozygous.

In addition, since the affected AT-III allele appears normal by restriction mapping, the mutation is not due to a large deletion or to rearrangement.

In the second family examined, the results were much different. Here, the kindred consisted of a normal father (+/− phenotype), an affected mother (an apparent −/− phenotype), and four affected sons. A consideraton of the possible inheritance patterns indicates that the only genotypes of the sons could be +/− (50%) and −/− (50%). However, two of the sons showed only + alleles, whereas the other two showed only − alleles. The only explanation for such an occurrence (other than that of nonpaternity, which was excluded by HLA-typing) is that the AT-III deficiency in this family is due to the complete deletion of one allele. The mother and each of her sons are therefore hemizygotes. The sons would be expected to always reflect only the allele inherited from their +/− normal father.

Subsequent to this study, we have analyzed a total of 15 kindreds using both polymorphic markers.[23] In all but one case, it has been possible to distinguish parental alleles. Our results indicate that in only one of these families is the deficiency the result of complete gene deletion; this family is the same as that originally described by Prochownik et al.[20] Affected individuals in all other families contained two grossly intact AT-III genes. We have concluded from these studies that the majority of Type I individuals probably contain mutations that cannot be detected by the resolution afforded by conventional Southern blot analysis.

One caveat should be born in mind when considering the above analyses. Since all of the families studied have consisted of members of only two generations, it is conceivable that the true defect in nondeletion families lies in a gene which controls plasma AT-III levels. Such a locus could be closely linked to that encoding AT-III or could reside on a different chromosome entirely. We cannot rigorously exclude such a possibility although we consider it unlikely. Proof that the defect lies within the AT-III locus would come from identifying a specific mutation within the allele predicted to be the affected one. The polymorphisms described above provide an unambiguous way of ensuring the isolation of such a defective allele for those whose intent is to identify AT-III mutations.

V. GENETIC ANALYSIS OF INDIVIDUALS WITH TYPE II AT-III DEFICIENCIES

Based on the experience gained from prior molecular analysis of mutations which inactivate various genetic loci, it is likely that Type I AT-III deficiencies occur as a result of small deletions or insertions, frameshift, and nonsense mutations within the AT-III protein-coding domain or mutational inactivation of critical noncoding segments such as promotors, enhancers, or splice junctions. In this sense, Type II mutations are of intrinsically greater interest as they result not from mutations which ultimately prevent the translation of AT-III protein, but from defects within the protein itself which causes its aberrant function.

For operational purposes, it is convenient to divide the AT-III protein into two major functional regions: the heparin-binding domain and the thrombin-binding domain. The former is located in the N-terminal end of the molecule with the Arg 47 moiety being particularly important.[24-26] The thrombin-binding domain is situated in the C-terminal end of the molecule where it has been shown that the Arg 393-Ser 394 region is critically important to this function.[27]

A. HEPARIN-BINDING MUTANTS

AT-III Toyama. Koide and coworkers have recently described an individual homozygous for a mutation affecting heparin binding.[25,28,29] The propositus was a 23-year-old female who suffered form recurrent episodes of peripheral vein thrombosis. Investigations of her AT-III level showed it to be normal as were the progressive AT-III and factor Xa inhibitory activities. Crossed immunoelectrophoresis in the presence of heparin showed no increase in AT-III mobility, suggesting not only that the basic defect involved the heparin-binding domain, but that the patient was homozygous for the defect. This was confirmed by an investigation of her parents who, although apparently unrelated, were each heterozygous for the heparin-binding defect.

The propositus' abnormal AT-III was purified by immunoabsorbent chromatography and subjected to cyanogen bromide cleavage. Eleven fragments were obtained that were indistinguishable from those seen following the cleavage of normal AT-III. One of these fragments generated an abnormal tryptic peptide pattern following HPLC chromatography. Edman degradation of the abnormal peptide revealed that it differed form normal by virtue of a substitution of Cys for Arg at position 47. The authors speculated that the charge alteration due to this substitution might be responsible for an altered heparin-binding capacity of the molecule due to a change in the ionic charge of this peptide.[29] While this analysis provided compelling evidence that the patient's heparin-binding abnormality was due to the described mutation, it did not constitute proof since the molecule was not sequenced in its entirety. Thus, it was formally possible that an additional mutation, perhaps at a distance from the Cys 47 residue, was equally responsible for contributing to the abnormal phenotype or even that the Cys 47 mutation was a protein polymorphism. These possibilities, however, seem very unlikely particularly in light of other heparin-binding mutants of AT-III that have been described (*vide infra*). A notable feature of this individual is that she constitutes the only known homozygote for AT-III deficiency. It is likely that virtually all other homozygous mutations are lethal at the embryonic or fetal stage. Of note is that an identical heterozygous mutation has been described in a French family by Duchange et al. and named "AT-III Tours."[17]

AT-III Rouen. Owen et al. have described an abnormal AT-III molecule that is similar to AT-III Toyama.[30] The propositus was a 40-year-old woman who was noted to have a reduced AT-III activity, but not an antigen, following admission to the hospital for an apparent cerebral vascular accident. Further investigation demonstrated that her plasma was heterozygous for an AT-III with a reduced heparin-binding capacity. Progressive AT-III and anti-factor Xa activities were normal. Agarose gel electrophoresis at pH 8.6 showed that AT-III Rouen migrated more slowly than normal, whereas its mobility was identical to that of normal AT-III at pH 6.0. *Staphylococcus aureus* V8 protease-generated peptide maps of the abnormally binding AT-III gave two well-separated tryptophan peptides, one of which was both electrophoretically and chromatographically altered in comparison to the homologous peptide from normal At-III. Amino acid analysis of this peptide demonstrated an Arg to His mutation at position 47. The results, particularly when interpreted in light of those obtained with AT-III Toyoma, provide strong evidence that the Arg 47 residue is an extremely critical one in determining heparin affinity of the AT-III molecule.

AT-III Basel. As in the case of AT-III Toyama and AT-III Rouen, AT-III Basel was first indentified in a patient with recurrent episodes of thrombophlebitis.[11,31,32] Like the other two molecules, AT-III Basel also demonstrated normal progressive AT-III activity while showing a reduced heparin affinity. Approximately 50 tryptic peptides were isolated, one of which, representing amino acid residues 40 to 60, had a mobility different from that of its normal counterpart. Sequencing of this peptide show a Pro to Leu substitution at position 41. The authors have speculated that, while the normal Pro 41 moiety is unlikely to be involved directly in heparin binding, the Leu substitution in AT-III Basel may destabilize the AT-III- heparin interaction by increasing helical structure and hydrophobicity.

In summary, the above investigations have provided evidence that distinct mutations in the N-terminal region of the AT-III molecule can exert profound effects on heparin-binding capability without altering other functions. Previous chemical modification studies on the actual AT-III protein have suggested that the heparin binding site is located in this region and is comprised of basic amino acids.[24-26] Trp 49 appears to be a particularly critical residue as its modification results in the loss of heparin binding. The clustering of mutations in the above described variants indicates that the region between residues 41 and 49 is likely to participate directly in heparin binding. Furthermore, these mutations have defined a minimal size of this domain.

B. THROMBIN-BINDING MUTANTS

AT-III Denver. Sambrano et al. and Stephens et al. have investigated an AT-III variant with abnormal thrombin-binding properties.[16,33] The propositus was a 16-year-old black female with a lower extremity deep vein thrombosis which occurred 2 months after the initiation of oral contraceptive therapy. AT-III antigen levels were within normal limits. Crossed immunoelectrophoresis studies performed both with and without heparin were normal. However, the purified AT-III fraction showed only half the normal amount of progressive thrombin neutralization and factor Xa activity. The propositus' nonreacting AT-III fraction, isolated by affinity chromatography, showed electrophoretic migration patterns characteristic of normal AT-III, but was unable to bind thrombin or factor Xa. Tryptic peptide analysis of the nonreacting species revealed a single aberrant peptide not seen in control samples. Sequencing of this peptide showed that it corresponded to residues 394 to 399 except for the replacement of Leu for Ser at position 394. Thus, the mutation in this variant falls within the actual active site of the molecule. As a result of this mutation, the rate constant for thrombin binding in the presence of heparin was reduced by a factor approximately 4000.

AT-III Utah. A large kindred in Utah with a familial predisposition to thrombosis has been studied by Bock and her coworkers.[14] Affected individuals in this family display reductions in both AT-III antigen as well as mutant molecules with aberrant electrophoretic properties. For example, when plasma from 11 individuals with reduced AT-III activities and antigens was analyzed by immunoblotting, the normally observed major and minor immunoreactive bands were reduced in intensity. A new species of somewhat increased mobility was observed. The relationship between AT-III deficiency and the structural gene was investigated by comparing segregation patterns of AT-III gene polymorphisms and the deficiency state. Maximum liklihood analysis indicated that, at least in this family, AT-III deficiency and AT-III gene were tightly linked. This finding argued against the theoretical possibility that deficiency was due to a distal mutation affecting AT-III levels in a more indirect fashion.

The finding of reductions in both activity and antigen in AT-III Utah was unlike that for any other previously reported mutation. This suggested the possiblity that two mutations might be responsible for the observed phenotype. However, in a subsequent report, this has proven not to be the case.[34] The workers have molecularly cloned an entire AT-III genomic locus from a deficient individual. PstI polymorphisms were used to distinguish the normal from mutant allele.[23] The entire coding region of the mutant allele was sequenced. The only change was seen in codon 407 where, as the result of a C to T transition, Pro was mutated to Leu. This site is 14 amino acids away from the Arg-Ser reactive center. Of note is that the mutated site is highly conserved among the various members of the serine protease inhibitor super family and has been detected in 12 of 13 serpins sequenced to date. The authors have presented two models to explain the possible effect of this mutation. In the first model, the mutation generates an inactive inhibitor molecule by altering the conformation of the active site. In the alternate model, the loss of the proline residue results in an incorrect folding of the polypeptide chain. Using the x-ray crystallographic model of α-1-antitrypsin as a paradigm for the three-dimensional structure of AT-III, these workers have postulated that Pro 407 plays a critical role in maintaining a separation between two beta sheets. These sheets normally form a core around which the remainder of the inhibitor is organized.

Alteration of this structure might be expected to not only disrupt binding of thrombin to the active site, but might also cause enough denaturation of the protein so as to significantly alter its half-life. Thus, the single amino acid change could explain both the quantitative and qualitative aspects of this unique AT-III protein.

AT-III Hamilton. Devraj-Kizuk et al. have investigated the molecular basis for a novel AT-III molecule in a French-Canadian family.[18] The propositus had been originally identified as a result of numerous deep vein and portal vein thrombotic events.[35] AT-III functional activities in this individual's plasma, using both thrombin and factor Xa as substrates, were reduced by approximately 50%, whereas immunoreactive AT-III levels consistently assayed within the normal range. The same functional aberrancies of AT-III were detected in the propositus' two children.

Using Southern blotting of PstI-digested genomic DNAs to resolve AT-III alleles, the workers determined that the abnormal AT-III molecule segregated with a −/1.7 kb allele (see Section III). This allele was molecularly cloned from a genomic library prepared from the propositus' leukocyte DNA. DNA sequences encompassing exon 6 of the AT-III gene were further subcloned into appropriate m13 vectors and subjected to dideoxy sequencing. The sequence obtained was entirely colinear with the normal AT-III coding sequence except for a single G→A transition in the first base of codon 382. This results in a Ala→Thr substitution. It is of interest that this mutation occurs in the first of a stretch of three alanine residues and is part of a larger sequence of ten amino acids, eight of which are highly hydrophobic. One explanation for the effect exerted by this mutation is that this hydrophobic region serves to "present" the more hydrophilic active site to the substrate. Disruption of the hydrophobic region may alter the accessibility of substrate to the active site and/or actually alter the conformation of the active site through more indirect processes.

As in the case of AT-III Utah, a distal mutation has been shown to adversely affect substrate binding. Whereas the Utah mutation lies 13 amino acids N-terminal to the active site, the Hamilton mutation lies 12 amino acids C-terminal to it. These two mutations thus serve to define, as in the case for the heparin-binding mutants described above, a minimal size for the substrate binding domain.

VI. NATURAL ALTERATION OF THE SUBSTRATE SPECIFICITY OF α_1-ANTITRYPSIN CAUSES CONVERSION TO AN AT-III-LIKE MOLECULE

A recent observation by Owen et al. has provided a naturally occurring example of the remarkable specificity of the AT-III binding site.[37] The subject of this study was a 14-year-old boy who had experienced a lifetime of intermittent hemorrhagic diatheses, all associated with disproportionately mild traumatic episodes. Detailed investigations revealed that his plasma contained a potent inhibitor of the thrombin-fibrinogen reaction which could not be activated with heparin. This inhibitor was found to be a protein with an electrophoretic mobility similar to that of α_1-antitrypsin (α_1-AT). The abnormal protein was not found in plasma from either of his parents or siblings, suggesting that it represented a *de novo* mutation.

The variant protein was isolated and shown by peptide mapping to correspond to α_1-AT. However, a single aberrant peptide was detected. Amino acid analysis showed that this peptide corresponded to the active site of α_1-AT and that it bore a mutation resulting in a substitution of an Arg for Met at position 358. This position corresponds to the active site for AT-III (Arg 393-Ser 394) and indeed, this substitution converts the Met 358-Ser 359-α_1-AT active site to the active site for AT-III. The variant was named α_1-AT Pittsburgh.

α_1-AT Pittsburgh showed considerable variation in plasma levels, behaving as an acute phase reactant in a manner similar to native α_1-AT; levels were elevated 3.6-fold when comparison was made between plasma samples obtained during a well period as opposed to an immediate posttraumatic period. This increase corresponded to elevations in other acute phase reactants.

Both α_1-AT Pittsburgh and normal α_1-AT were potent inhibitors of trypsin although no antielastase activity could be demonstrated for the variant. However, α_1-AT Pittsburgh was thirty times as active in its thrombin inhibitory activity. It was calculated, based on the activity and concentration of α_1-AT Pittsburgh, that the effective AT-III activity in the patient was equal to 21 U/ml. This compares to 15 U/ml in a fully heparinized patient. Based on these observations, it is easy to envision the pathophysiological basis of this boy's hemorrhagic diathesis: any traumatic event experienced by the patient resulted in an acute phase rise in α_1-AT Pittsburgh levels. This, combined with an otherwise normal level of AT-III resulted in superphysiological concentrations of AT-III activity and a resultant hemorrhagic tendency. These elegant investigations have underscored the importance of a single amino acid residue in determining the specificity of the serine protease inhibitors.

VII. A CLASSIFICATION OF CONGENITAL AT-III DEFICIENCIES

The various AT-IIII mutations described above now provide a molecular basis for the classification of AT-III deficiencies previously proposed by Nagy and Losonczy in 1979.[38] In their classification scheme, Type I deficiencies consist of what is probably a heterogeneous group of disorders with identical phenotypic consequences. Both AT-III antigens as well as functional activities are reduced proportionally. The defects causing these are probably similar to those causing thalassemias, that is missense, nonsense, and frameshift mutations, and small deletions and insertions either in the coding sequence or at splice donor/acceptor junctions. Promotor or enhancer mutations might also be responsible. Mutations distal to the AT-III structural gene might also play a role, conceivably by affecting genes whose products are concerned with AT-III mRNA or protein stability.

Type II deficiencies are a qualitative nature. AT-III antigen levels are within normal limits, but thrombin binding is defective. This presumably results from defects in or around the serine protease domain, as exemplified by AT-III's Denver and Hamilton. Heparin binding is left intact, but heparin cofactor activity as well as the progressive AT-III activity are reduced or nonexistent. Other variants of this type, yet to be fully characterized, include AT-IIIs Northwick Park, Trento, and Milano.[15,40,41]

Type III deficiencies affect the heparin-binding domain. In these cases, both heparin binding and heparin cofactor activity are reduced, whereas progressive AT-III activity is normal. Examples of this type of defect include AT-III's Tours, Toyama, and Rouen.[17,28] It should be mentioned that at least one other mutation has been described with an *increased* affinity for heparin: AT-III "Chicago." Such a mutation might thus be classified as a Type IIIB, whereas the first three, as well as other mutations yet to be sequenced (AT-III's Basel, Budapest, and Paris), could be called Type IIIA.[5,11,31,42]

We might postulate yet an additional type of mutation (Type IV). This would be exemplified by AT-III Utah in which both quantitative as well as qualitative disorders exist as a result of a single mutation. In this case, both antigen levels as well as thrombin-binding capacities are reduced.

Yet another disorder, reminiscent of AT-III Utah but distinctly different, was suggested by the work of Leone et al.[12] They identified a kindred with both a qualitative and quantitative deficiency (AT-III Roma). Abnormal AT-III mobility in heparin-agarose gels suggested that the former defect may involve the heparin-binding domain. Separate classifications of this variant (Table 1) must be deemed tentative, however, until the precise molecular defect has been identified.

TABLE 1
Classification of Congenital AT-III Deficiencies

Type	Antigen level	Heparin binding	Thrombin binding	Example
I	↓	↓	↓	All deficiencies associated with structurally normal AT-III molecules
II	nl	nl	↓	Denver, Hamilton
IIIA	nl	↓	nl	Toyama, Tours, Rouen
IIIB	nl	↑	nl	Chicago
IV[a]	↓	↓	↓ ↓	Utah
V[b]	↓	↓ ↓	↓	Roma

[a] In Class IV mutations, antigen levels and heparin binding are reduced proportionally. Thrombin binding is reduced even more due to an alteration of the binding site. This feature distinguishes this class from Type I mutations in which antigen levels, heparin binding, and thrombin binding are all reduced proportionally.

[b] In Class V mutations, antigen levels and thrombin binding are reduced proportionately. Heparin binding is reduced even further, presumably due to a point mutation in or near the N-terminal heparin-binding domain.

VIII. PROSPECTS FOR THE FUTURE

The characterization of naturally occurring AT-III mutants has allowed for a partial definition of the critical amino acid residues involved in heparin and thrombin-binding functions. It is expected that the basis for more of the previously described mutations will become known as modern methods of protein sequencing and molecular genetics are applied. In addition, the ability to express biologically active AT-III in E. coli and, more recently, in eukaryotic cells, combined with the powerful techniques of site-directed *in vitro* mutagenesis, should now permit an evaluation of the role of virtually any residue in the protein.[43,44] Certain residues will be of particular interest and will probably be among the first to be examined. Current techniques should permit investigators to obtain sufficient material to evaluate all of the critical functions of these newly engineered AT-III molecules.

A. THE HEPARIN-BINDING DOMAIN

The importance of amino acids Pro 41, Arg 47, and Trp 49 in heparin binding has already been emphasied. Other questions remain, however, as to what other residues might play a role in this activity and whether very conservative mutations can attenuate heparin binding without completely eliminating it. For example, Arg 47 is immediately preceded by another Arg at position 46. What is the role of this amino acid in determining the critical nature of its neighbor? Selective *in vitro* mutation of this residue, say to Gln (CGG → CAG), would provide insight into this question. Another question would be whether the mutation of Arg 47 to Lys or His would completely abolish activity. Both of these mutations would retain the overall basic nature of the region. The change to Lys would be fairly conservative while that to His potentially more disruptive to the overall secondary structure of the region.

B. THE THROMBIN-BINDING DOMAIN

The naturally occurring, mutation-generating AT-III Denver has confirmed the importance of the Arg 393-Ser 394 region, while AT-III's Hamilton and Utah have emphasized the importance of the surrounding structure in apparently maintaining the correct conformation for proper interaction with the thrombin substrate. The hydrophobic regions flanking the active site (residues 382 to 391 and residues 408 to 412) make attractive targets at which to aim initial efforts in establishing whether their presence is necessary for maintaining a correct exposure of the active site in relation to its substrate. Techniques of *in vitro* mutagenesis may now be applied by asking the converse of the experiments of nature that has occurred with α_1-antrypsin Pittsburgh; that is can the active site of AT-III be mutated to that of α_1-antitrypsin so as to generate a mutant AT-III molecule with substrate specificity for trypsin and elastase? Futhermore, would this new molecule be activated by heparin?

Clearly, the knowledge learned from naturally occurring AT-III mutations should now allow rapid progress in our understanding of the structure-function relationships of this most interesting molecule.

REFERENCES

1. **Prochownik, E. V.,** The treatment of antithrombin III deficiency, in *Current Therapy in Hematology/Oncology,* Brain, M. C. and Carbone, P. C., Eds., B. C. Decker, Toronto, 1985, 122.
2. **Sas, G., Peto, I., Banhegyi, D., Blasko, G., and Domjan, G.,** Heterogeneity of the "classical" antithrombin III deficiency, *Thromb. Haemost.,* 43, 133, 1980.
3. **Thaler, E. and Lechner, K.,** Antithrombin III deficiency and thromboembolism, *Clin. Haematol.,* 10, 369, 1981.
4. **Winter, J. H., Bennett, B., Watt, J. L., Brown, T., San Roman, C., Schinzel, A., King, J., and Cook, P. J. L.,** Confirmation of linkage between antithrombin III and Duffy blood group and assignment of ATIII to 1q22 → w25, *Ann. Hum. Genet.,* 46, 29, 1982.
5. **Rosenberg, R. D.,** Action and interacton of antithrombin and heparin, *N. Engl. J. Med.,* 16, 146, 1975.
6. **Egeberg, O.,** Inherited antithrombin III deficiency causing thrombophilia, *Thromb. Diath. Haemorrh.,* 13, 516, 1965.
7. **Filip, D. J., Eckstein, J. D., and Veltkamp, J. J.,** Hereditary antithrombin III deficiency and thromboembolic disease, *Am. J. Hematol.,* 2, 343, 1976.
8. **Johansson, L., Hedner, U., and Nilsson, I. M.,** Familial antithrombin III deficiency as pathogenesis of deep venous thrombosis, *Acta Med. Scand.,* 204, 491, 1978.
9. **Mackie, M., Bennett, B., Ogston, D., and Douglas, A. S.,** Familial thrombosis: inherited deficiency of antithrombin III, *Br. Med. J.,* 1, 136, 1978.
10. **Sas, G., Blasko, G., Banhegyi, D., Jako, J., and Palos, L. A.,** Abnormal antithrombin III (antithrombin III "Budapest") as a cause of familial thrombophilia, *Thromb. Diath. Haemorrh.,* 32, 105, 1974.
11. **Tran, T. H., Bounameaux, H., Bondeli, C., Honkanen, H., Marbet, G. A., and Duckert, F.,** Purification and partial characterization of a hereditary abnormal antithrombin III fraction of a patient with recurrent thrombophlebitits, *Thromb. Haemost.,* 44, 87, 1980.
12. **Leone, G., Cotumaccio, R., DeStefano, V., and Zunetti, L.,** Antithrombin III Roma: a familial quantitative-qualitative ATIII deficiency identifiable by crossed immunoelectrofocusing and by crossed immunoelectrophoresis, *Haematol. Pavia.,* 68, 765, 1983.
13. **Aiach, M., Nora, M., Fiessinger, J. N., Roncato, M., Francois, D., and Gelas, M. A.,** A functional abnormal antithrombin III (ATIII) deficiency: ATIII Charleville, *Thromb. Res.,* 39, 559, 1985.
14. **Bock S. C., Harris, J. F., Schwartz, C. E., Ward, J. H., Hershgold, E. J., and Skolnick, M. H.,** Hereditary thrombosis in a Utah kindred is caused by a dysfunctional antithrombin III gene, *Am. J. Hum. Genet.,* 37, 32, 1985.
15. **Howarth, D. J., Samson, D., Stirling, Y., and Seghatchian, M. J.,** Antithrombin III "Northwick Park": a variant antithrombin with normal affinity for heparin but reduced heparin factor activity, *Thromb. Haemost.,* 53, 314, 1985.
16. **Sambrano, J. E., Jacobson, L. J., Reeve, E. B., Manco-Johnson, M. J., and Hathaway, W. E.,** Abnormal antithrombin III with defective serine protease binding (antithrombin "Denver") *J. Clin. Invest.,* 77, 887, 1986.
17. **Duchange, N., Chasse, J. F., Cohen, G. N., and Zakin, M. M.,** Molecular characterization of the antithrombin III Tours deficiency, *Thromb. Res.,* 45, 115, 1987.
18. **Devraj-Kizuk, R., Prochownik, E. V., Carter, C. J., Chui, D. H. K., and Blajchman, M. A.,** Antithrombin III Hamilton: a gene with a point mutation (guanine to adenine) in codon 382 causing impaired serine protease reactivity, *Blood,* 72, 1518, 1988.

19. **Prochownik, E. V., Markham, A. F., and Orkin, S. H.,** Isolation of a cDNA clone for human antithrombin III, *J. Biol. Chem.*, 258, 8389, 1983.
20. **Prochownik, E. V., Antararakis, S., Bauer, K. A., Rosenberg, R. D., Fearon, E., and Orkin, S. H.,** Molecular heterogeneity of inherited antithrombin III deficiency, *N. Engl. J. Med.*, 308, 1549, 1983.
21. **Bock, S. C. and Levitan, D. J.,** Characterization of an unusual DNA length polymorphism 5′-to the human antithrombin III gene, *Nucl. Acids Res.*, 11, 8569, 1983.
22. **Prochownik, E. V., Bock, S. C., and Orkin, S. H.,** Intron structure of the human antithrombin III gene differs from that of other members of the serine protease inhibitor superfamily, *J. Biol. Chem.*, 260, 9608, 1985.
23. **Bock, S. C. and Prochownik, E. V.,** Molecular genetic survey of sixteen kindreds with hereditary antithrombin III deficiency, *Blood,* 70, 1273, 1987.
24. **Blackburn, M. N., Smith, R. L., Carson, J., and Sibley, C. C.,** The heparin-binding site of antithrombin III, *J. Biol. Chem.*, 259, 939, 1984.
25. **Koide, T., Odani, S., Takahashi, K., Ono, T., and Sakuragawa, N.,** Antithrombin III Toyama: replacement of arginine-47 by cysteine in hereditary abnormal antithrombin III that lacks heparin-binding ability, *Proc. Natl. Acad. Sci. U.S.A.*, 81, 289, 1984.
26. **Pecon, J. M. and Blackburn, M. N.,** Pyridoxylation of essential lysines in the heparin-binding site of antithrombin III, *J. Biol. Chem.*, 259, 935, 1984.
27. **Bjork, I., Jackson, C. M., Jornvall, H., Lavine, K. K., Nordling, K., and Salsgiver, W. J.,** The active site of antithrombin: release of the same proteolytically cleaved form of the inhibitor from complexes with factor IXa, factor Xa and thrombin, *J. Biol. Chem.*, 257, 2406, 1982.
28. **Sakuragawa, N., Takahashi, K., Kondo, S-I., and Koide, T.,** Antithrombin III Toyama: a hereditary abnormal antithrombin III of a patient with recurrent thrombophlebitis, *Thromb. Res.*, 31, 305, 1983.
29. **Koide, T., Odani, S., Takahashi, K., Ono, T., and Sakuragawa, N.,** Antithrombin III Toyama: replacement of arginine-47 by cysteine in hereditary abnormal antithrombin III that lacks heparin binding ability, *Proc. Natl. Acad. Sci. U.S.A.*, 81, 289, 1984.
30. **Owen, M. C., Borg, J. Y., Soria, C., Soria, J., Caen, J., and Carrell, R. W.,** Heparin binding defect in a new antithrombin III variant: Rouen, 47 Arg to His, *Blood,* 69, 1275, 1987.
31. **Tran, T. H., Bondeli, C., Marbet, G. A., and Duckert, F.,** Reactivity of a hereditary abnormal antithrombin III fraction in the inhibition of thrombin and factor Xa, *Thromb. Haemost.*, 44, 92, 1980.
32. **Chang, J-Y. and Tran, T. H.,** Antithrombin III Basel: identification of a pro-leu substitution in a hereditary abnormal antithrombin with impaired heparin cofactor activity, *J. Biol. Chem.*, 261, 1174, 1986.
33. **Stephens, A. W., Thalley, B. S., and Hins, C. H. W.,** Antithrombin III Denver, a ser to leu^{394} variant without protease inhibitory activity, *Thromb. Haemost.*, 54, 49, 1987.
34. **Bock, S. C., Marrinan, J. A., and Radziejewska, E.,** Antithrombin III Utah: Proline-407 to leucine mutation in a highly conserved region near the inhibitor reactive site, submitted for publication.
35. **Carter, C. J., Johnson, M., Brain, M. C., and Glynn, M. F. X.,** A new antithrombin III variant presenting as familial thrombophilia, *Blood,* 58, 231a, 1981.
36. **Sanger, F., Nicklen, S., and Coulson, A. R.,** DNA sequencing with chain-terminating inhibitors, *Proc. Natl. Acad. Sci. U.S.A.*, 74, 5463, 1977.
37. **Owen, M. C., Brennan, S. O., Lewis, J. H., and Carrell, R. W.,** Mutation of antitrypsin to antithrombin: α_1-antitrypsin Pittsburgh (358 Met → Arg), a fatal bleeding disorder, *N. Engl. Med.*, 309, 694, 1983.
38. **Nagy, I. and Losonczy, H.,** Three types of hereditary antithrombin III deficiency, *Thromb. Haemost.*, 44, 187, 1979.
39. **Bauer, K. A., Ashenburst, J. B., Chediak, J., and Rosenberg, R. D.,** Antithrombin "Chicago": a functionally abnormal molecule with increased heparin affinity causing familial thrombophilia, *Blood,* 62, 1242, 1983.
40. **Boyer, C., Tripodi, A., Wolf, M., Manucci, P. M., and Larrieu, M. J.,** A new familial variant of antithrombin III: Antithrombin III Milano, *Thromb. Haemost.*, 50, 51, 1983.
41. **Girolami, A., Rubertelli, M., Marafiotti, F., Zamboni, A., and Vicarioto, M. A.,** Crossed immunoelectrophoresis in the study of abnormal antithrombin III: behavior of ATIII Trento, *Br. J. Haematol.*, 55, 559, 1983.
42. **Wolf, M., Boyer, C., Lavergne, J. M., and Larrieu, M. J.,** A new familial variant of antithrombin III: Antithrombin III Paris, *Br. J. Haematol.*, 51, 285, 1982.
43. **Bock, S. C., Wion, K. L., Vehar, G. A., and Lawn, R. M.,** Cloning and expression of the cDNA for human antithrombin III, *Nucl. Acids Res.*, 10, 8113, 1982.
44. **Stephens, A. W., Siddiqui, A., and Hirs, C. H. W.,** Expression of functionally active human antithrombin III, *Proc. Natl. Acad. Sci. U.S.A.*, 84, 3886, 1987.

Chapter 5

PROPHYLACTIC AND THERAPEUTIC USE OF ANTITHROMBIN-III CONCENTRATES

Lisbet Javelin

TABLE OF CONTENTS

I. INTRODUCTION

Antithrombin III (AT-III) concentrates used for substitution therapy are produced from human plasma. Since the term antithrombin was introduced at the beginning of this century, several attempts to concentrate AT-III have been reported.[1,2] The two methods usually referred to as the first of practical use were presented in 1967 by Abildgaard and by Heimburger.[3,4] Further works were published by the same authors and by others in the following years.[5-7] However, the yields were poor.

A great improvement took place when AT-III purification by Heparin-Sepharose was introduced.[8] This method, modifictions of it, and alternative methods also based on adsorption to Heparin-Sepharose are today used for the production of AT-III concentrates for clinical use.[9,10]

The clinical research on AT-III concentrates from two plasma-fractionating companies was started in 1974.[11-12] During the following years, AT-III concentrates were tested in pharmacokinetic and clinical studies in many European countries. In 1981 and 1982, AT-III concentrates from the two above-mentioned companies were approved by the registration authorities in the respective country of origin, namely West Germany (Behringwerke AG) and Sweden (KabiVitrum AB).

AT-III concentrates are now commercially available from at least four international plasma-fractionating companies. In addition, AT-III concentrates are supplied by national Red and Green Cross Organizations.

A. QUALITY AND PACKAGES

Since the first batches of AT-III concentrates for clinical use were introduced, production methods have improved further and the quality of the products has increased. In addition, heat treatment in solution for 10 h at 60°C has been introduced.

Differences in quality between the main products earlier reported seem to have decreased, and the three main products are considered of high purity.[13-16] In one study, the specific activity of AT-III in concentrates from four producers was found to be between 3.67 and 4.73 IU/mg.[16] However, in at least one case, albumin for stabiliztion has been added before lyophilazation, i.e., the specific activity of that primary product was above 5 IU/mg.

The heparin content in the above-mentioned concentrates was found to be between 0.08 and 0.21 IU/ml. The products are readily soluble in sterile water. Vials of 500 IU, 1000 IU, and 1500 IU are available; however, not all producers supply all the three sizes.

B. SAFETY

There has been great interest in the virus safety of blood products in recent years, not only due to the reported transmission of the acquired immunodeficiency disease syndrome (AIDS) to patients with haemophilia, treated with factor VIII concentrates, but also due to the increased knowledge of the trasmission of hepatitis B and hepatitis non-A, non-B (NANB) by blood transfusions and blood products.

Several measures have been taken in order to diminish the risk of virus transmission by blood products. The following measures are of relevance for the AT-III concentrates.

All plasma donors are tested for hepatitis B surface antigens (HBsAg) and for antibodies to the Human Immunodeficiency Virus (HIV). In some countries, all donations are also screened for alanine aminotransferase (ALT) in order to diminish the risk of the transmission of NANB hepatitis.[17]

There is a virus reduction in conjunction with the fractionation and purification process of AT-III concentrates. However, the main procedure for virus in activation is heat treatment in solution for 10 h at 60°C. The efficacy of the virus inactivation by heat treatment of AT-III concentrates has been tested both *in vitro* and *in vivo*.[18-21]

Efficient and rapid inactivation of HIV added to AT-III concentrates has been reported in an *in vitro* study.[20] In a chimpanzee study, inactivation by heat treatment of a hepatitis B virus added to an AT-III concentrate was shown.[21] Virus safety of a heat-treated AT-III concentrate has also been shown in a study of 13 healthy volunteers.[19] Hepatitis has been reported in a few patients treated with nonheat-treated AT-III concentrates and concurrent blood transfusions in clinical trials.[22,23] However, there are no reports of virus transmission in patients treated only with AT-III concentrates, whether heat-treated or not.

Based on, among others, studies mentioned here and the absence of reports on virus transmission since registration, heat-treated AT-III concentrates are considered not to transfer virus infections, i.e., they are, with respect to hepatitis and HIV-infection, considered virus safe.

II. HUMAN PHARMACOLOGICAL STUDIES

When talking about human pharmacological studies of blood products, biological half-life and recovery *in vivo* are variables often referred to.

A. RECOVERY *IN VIVO*

The percentage *in vivo* recovery could be calculated as:

$$\frac{\text{Actual increase of AT-III (IU/ml)} \times 100}{\text{Theoretical increase of AT-III (IU/ml)}}$$

$$\text{Theoretical increase of AT-III (IU/ml)} = \frac{\text{Amount of AT-III concentration (IU) injected}}{\text{Plasma volume (ml)}}$$

Some authors use an alternative definition of recovery, namely the increase of plasma AT-III level after the administration of 1 IU AT-III concentrate per kg of body weight.

Human pharmacological studies on AT-III concentrates were performed by Tengborn.[24] An AT-III concentrate was given to two patients with hereditary AT-III deficiencies and two volunteers with normal AT-III levels in plasma in order to study catabolism and coagulation properties. One of the patients was on long-term warfarin treatment. In the other patient and the volunteers, the AT-III concentrate was studied both before and during treatment with warfarin. All the individuals were in good health during the investigation period. Using data from this study recovery *in vivo* has been estimated.

The recoveries *in vivo* in subjects not treated with warfarin were for the patient, 73%, and for the two control subjects, 104 and 95%. Recovery was complete in the control subjects and somewhat less in the patient. When warfarin was given concurrently, the recovery in the healthy volunteers was higher than expected. However, in the patient treated with warfarin over several years because of recurrent pulmonary embolism, the recovery was only 32%.

To sum up, the recovery of AT-III concentrate was complete or almost complete in healthy volunteers and in one patient with a hereditary antithrombin deficiency. Warfarin given concurrently seems to increase the recovery of AT-III in healthy volunteers.

In order to test whether heat treatment of an AT-III concentrate reduces the biological activity of the protein, pharmacokinetic studies also have been performed on a heat-treated product.[25] Using data from this study, recovery *in vivo* has been estimated and found to be 105, 70, 74, and 122%, respectively, in three patients and a control subject. The mean increase of plasma AT-III (tested by a funcitonal method) after the administration of, in the first case, one IU of nonheat-treated AT-III concentrate and, in the second case, one IU of heat-treated AT-III concentrate, was 1.7% of the normal plasma level (or 1.7 IU/ml) in both cases. Equivalent results, 1.6% and 1.5%, were obtained in clinical trials of AT-III concentrates.[22,23]

B. BIOLOGICAL HALF-LIFE

Most published reports on the biological half-lives of AT-III concentrates have been performed on nonheat-treated products.[24,26-29] Mannucci and Sas studied an AT-III concentrate in one and three patients, respectively, with hereditary AT-III deficiencies.[27,28] Collen studied labeled AT-III in 15 hospitalized patients.[26] Scully gave labeled AT-III to one patient with a hereditary AT-III deficiency and to one control subject.[29] Tengborn gave both labeled and unlabeled AT-III concentrates to two patients with hereditary AT-III deficiencies and to two healthy volunteers.

In these studies, the mean value of the biological half-life of the AT-III concentrate was 3.05 d. Altogether, 24 patients and healthy volunteers were tested 28 times. One of the patients with a hereditary antithrombin deficiency had an extremely low biological half-life of 1.08 d. That value was excluded. The range of the remaining 27 values was 2.05 to 4.80 d.

In three patients with venous thrombosis treated with heparin, half-life was decreased. However, concurrent treatment with warfarin in three other patients did not seem to increase the biological half-life of the AT-III concentrate as indicated in other studies.

In a study on a labeled, human-purified AT-III concentrate, the half-life did not differ significantly between six patients with hereditary AT-III deficiencies and six healthy control subjects. The mean half-lives were 66.9 and 61.4 h (2.78 and 2.56 d).[30]

Finally, in one study on heat-treated AT-III concentrate administrated to three patients and a control subject, the mean value of the biological half-life was 3.0 d.[25]

When deciding on the dosage of the AT-III concentrate, it is of the greatest importance to keep in mind that the half-life is related to clearance and that the consumption of AT-III is often increased in patients with acquired AT-III deficiencies. In other words, the biological half-life of an AT-III concentrate is strongly dependent on the actual clinical situation. Biological half-lives as low as 4 h have been reported in a group of patients in circulatory shock.[31]

Futhermore, AT-III is identical with heparin co-factor I. i.e., it is the factor in plasma that is necessary if heparin is to have any anticoagulant effect. In the presence of heparin, AT-III inhibits the various coagulation enzymes more rapidly. Thus, the biological half-life of AT-III is decreased during treatment with heparin.

III. HEREDITARY AT-III DEFICIENCY — CLINICAL EXPERIENCES

In 1964, Egeberg found two patients with low levels of AT-III. A 45-year-old woman and her 12-year-old son were admitted to Rikshospitalet, Oslo, Norway, because of recurrent thrombotic episodes.[32] Except for low levels of AT-III, no defects were found in the coagulation status. There was a high incidence of thrombotic disease in the family of the patients. In the affected members and some of their children, the levels of AT-III were found to be about 50% of the levels found in 30 normal subjects. The AT-III deficiency seemed to be associated with venous thromboembolic disease, and the inheritance of the defect seemed to be autosomal dominant.

In the last 20 years, Egeberg's findings have been confirmed by authors all over the world. The disorder has been described in almost every ethnic group. Hundreds of papers concerning hereditary AT-III deficiencies, case reports, and descriptions of pedigrees have been published. The reported families show a uniform pattern as regards inheritance and pathological picture.[33-40]

About half of the members of reported families have an AT-III deficiency. In some families, almost all the adults with an AT-III deficiency have suffered from thromboembolic disease.[41-43] In other families, about one half to two thirds of adult AT-III-deficient members have experienced thrombotic events.[44-48]

Venous thrombosis often occurs in young adults, but has also been reported in children.[29,49-51] The first thrombotic episode often occurs in connection with trauma, surgery, infection, or pregnancy. Many of the AT-III-deficient patients have suffered from pulmonary embolism; some cases of mesenteric venous thrombosis are also reported.[40,52-57]

In some families, the hereditary AT-III deficiency occurs together with other defects; for instance, hyperaggregability of platelets, hyperlipidemia, and reduced inducible fibrinolytic activity.[58-60] Neonatal aortic thrombosis in two babies to mothers with hereditary AT-III deficiencies has been diagnosed at autopsy.[61] Aortic thrombosis has been reported in adult patients.[62]

In patients with hereditary AT-III deficiencies, prophylaxis with heparin and oral anticoagulants has earlier been used. However, in some situations, conventional therapy has not been sufficient or has been precluded. The heparin effect is decreased at low levels of AT-III in plasma. Furthermore, as mentioned, the plasma level of AT-III decreases during heparin treatment and thus, the effect of heparin may be still more reduced. Warfarin or other presently available oral anticoagulants are contraindicated during pregnancy.[63] Both heparin and oral anticoagulants in high doses can cause bleeding complications in connection with surgery. Thus, an adjuvant drug would be of great value.

When an AT-III concentrate became available for clinical research and programs for the evaluation of its clinical effect had to be started, the hereditary AT-III deficiency was one of the indications of greatest interest.

The aim of the first clinical studies on AT-III concentrates in this indication was to investigate whether the intravenous administration of the concentrate could, without causing unacceptable adverse reactions:

- prevent thromboembolic disease if given prophylactically to patients with hereditary AT-III deficiencies before and during surgery, during pregnancy, delivery, and postpartum, and
- supplement and improve the conventional anticoagulant treatment of patients with hereditary AT-III deficiencies and acute thromboembolic events.

Published documentation on clinical studies on AT-III concentrates consists mainly of case reports and summaries of case reports. No controlled studies have been performed since the available number of comparable patients with hereditary AT-III deficiencies is limited. Furthermore, the high risk of thromboembolic events in patients with hereditary AT-III deficiencies is well-documented, and it would be unethical to perform a trial with a control group without thromboprophylaxis. Thus, historical control groups and information in the literature are often referred to when the results are evaluated.

Treatment with an AT-III concentrate in these respects is considered to be comparable to substitution therapy with other specific plasma proteins, such as coagulation factor VIII in hemophilias.

A. PREGNANCY

There is a high risk of thromboembolic events in conjunction with pregnancy in women with hereditary AT-III deficiencies. The incidence of thromboembolism during pregnancy was studied by Hellgren and co-workers.[64] All available Swedish and Norwegian women with diagnosed hereditary AT-III deficiencies were interviewed by the investigators, that is, not only patients treated in connection with thrombosis, but also their female relatives with hereditary AT-III deficiencies were included in the study. Twenty-nine women had suffered from thromboembolism in 32 (68%) of their 47 pregnancies. There were 24 thromboses (51%) during pregnancy and eight (17%) during puerperium.

The Scandinavian results were verified in a French study.[65] In that study, however, a higher frequency of thrombosis in the puerperium than during pregnancy was found. In 38 out of 50 pregnancies in 18 women, without prophylaxis against thromboembolism, the total frequency of thromboses was 55%. In 21 of the 38 pregnancies there were thromboses, 10 (25%) during pregnancy and 11 (30%) postpartum. Two pregnancies ended with abortions, both in connection with thrombosis.

In three families with hereditary AT-III deficiencies in the U.K., 15 out of 16 pregnancies were associated with thrombosis.[66]

The first report on treatment with AT-III concentrates in pregnant women with hereditary AT-III deficiencies was published in 1981.[67] Two patients belonging to a large family with a hereditary AT-III deficiency were treated with heparin and AT-III concentrates in conjunction with, in one case, a complicated labor and delivery, and in the other, an abortion. The reported observations showed that the effect of heparin and AT-III was more complex than so far assumed. The following year, Hellgren and co-workers could report their results from an uncontrolled clinical trial on eight women with hereditary AT-III deficiencies treated with an AT-III concentrate and heparin during nine pregnancies.[64]

As the results of this study have been of greatest importance for the subsequent treatment of pregnant women with hereditary AT-III deficiencies, the reported summary is quoted here, however, with minor revisions:

> Before prophylaxis was started, two out of nine pregnancies were already complicated by thromboembolism (TE) in two women with previous TE. One out of seven pregnancies was complicated by TE despite heparin prophylaxis, and another woman suffered from rethrombosis during therapeutic treatment with heparin. Both women with TE during heparin treatment had previous TE, and insufficient prolongation of the activated partial thromboplastin time (APTT) was registered at the time of TE.
>
> Four out of nine pregnancies were terminated by induced abortion. The reason for three of the abortions was high doses of radiation from angiography due to suspected mesenteric vein thrombosis in one woman and manifest TE in two women. One woman decided to have the pregnancy terminated owing to the risks entailed by continued pregnancy, and a spontaneous abortion occurred in one woman 2 weeks after acute TE. The remaining four pregnancies resulted in delivery in three women by the vaginal route and in one woman by Caesarean section. The latter was indicated by a genital herpes simplex infection.
>
> All four children were in good health and no complications were noted in the neonatal period. AT-III activity was determined in three children at birth and was found to be normal for gestational age; a mean 57% of normal plasma. In the fourth child, AT-III activity was normal at 6 months of age.
>
> Heparin was given as prophylaxis to six women during seven pregnancies and as treatment to three women with TE during pregnancy. The dosage of heparin was adjusted to give the desired APTT prolongation, which was attained even during very low AT-III levels and during the entire course of the treatment period. The AT-III level decreased to approximately 25% during s. c. heparin treatment. The heparin dosage required for adequate APTT effect was increased compared to conditions with normal AT-III levels.
>
> An AT-III concentrate was administered during abortion and delivery, or in connection with TE during the nine pregnancies. AT-III levels were normalized by doses varying between 2,000 and 5,000 IU per infusion and maintained ≥80% by repeated infusions of AT-III concentrate.

The AT-III plasma level and APTT during treatment with heparin and AT-III concentrate in connection with pregnancy and vaginal delivery is shown in Figure 1.

The dosage recommendation based on this study was followed during treatment of one patient who suffered from her first thrombosis as early as age 15. When she decided to start a pregnancy, warfarin was discontinued and subcutaneous heparin treatment twice daily was started. Contraception was stopped, and the patient conceived within 6 weeks. The pregnancy and labor were uncomplicated and resulted in the delivery of a healthy infant.[68]

Three sisters with an hereditary AT-III deficiency and reduced fibrinolytic activity, who had earlier suffered from severe thromboembolism, were given thromboprophylaxis with heparin and AT-III concentrates. The individual dosage was based on the plasma level of the beta-thromboglobulin (BTG). Two of the sisters received prophylaxis with s.c. heparin

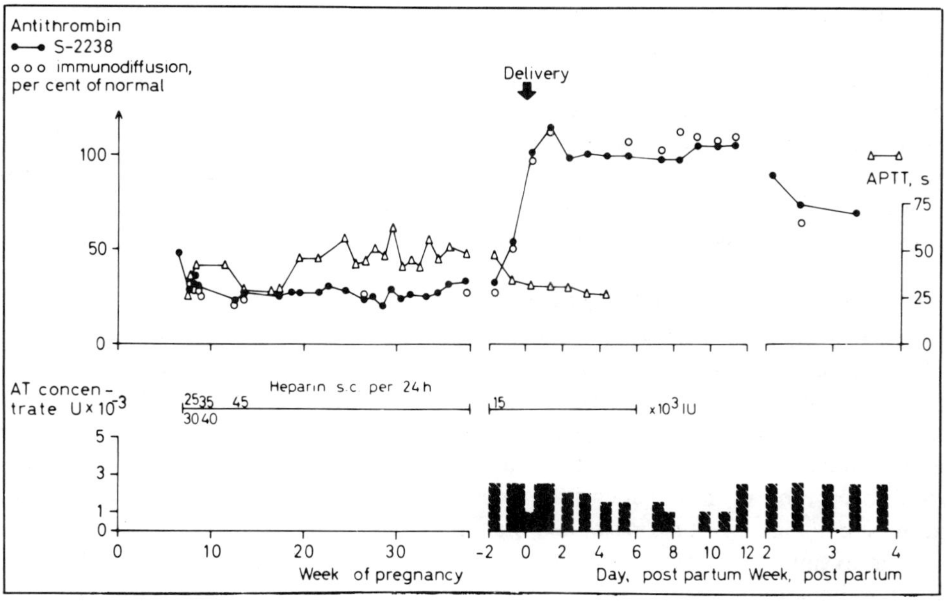

FIGURE 1. The AT-III level and APTT during treatment with heparin and an AT-III concentrate in connection with pregnancy and vaginal delivery. The AT-III level in connection with AT-III concentrates is shown daily before infusion. (From *Gynecol. Obstet. Invest.*)

from the first increase of BTG (around the 10th week of gestation) and 5000 IU of an AT-III concentrate from the onset of labor. The third sister received not only s.c. heparin, but also increasing doses of an AT-III concentrate from the 25th week of gestation. Her total dose of AT-III concentrate was 66,000 IU. The three pregnancies were uncomplicated.[60]

Another pregnant woman with a hereditary AT-III deficiency received an alternative prophylactic treatment. From the 22nd week of pregnancy, she was given AT-III concentrates in increasing doses from 3000 IU twice weekly to 4000 IU three times a week. Altogether, 181,500 IU of AT-III concentrates were administered, 149,500 IU during the last 18 weeks of pregnancy and 32,000 IU in conjunction with delivery and the following 11 d.[69] Summarizing, the authors suggest that treatment with an AT-III concentrate(s) may be an alternative to heparin during pregnancy.

This alternative would be expensive and is not recommended by others. However, in pregnant patients with hereditary AT-III deficiencies, in combination with further disorders such as reduced fibrinolytic activity, as mentioned above, or if these patients were suffering from deep venous thrombosis before prophylactic treatment was started, a combined therapy with s.c. heparin and an AT-III concentrate could be of value during parts of the pregnancies.[14,66] A successful therapy with heparin, AT-III concentrate, and antihypertensive drugs in a hereditary AT-III-deficient patient with severe pre-eclampsia is also reported.[70]

The recommendation stated by Hellgren et al. are referred to by others, but agreement is not complete.[33,36,71,72] However, there are only reports of successful thromboprophylaxis with AT-III concentrations in pregnancy, delivery, or postpartum. As mentioned before, the frequency of thromboembolic events in conjunction with pregnancy without any thromboprophylaxis in women with hereditary AT-III deficiencies is more than 50%.

B. SURGERY

The level of AT-III is decreased during surgery.[57,73-75] Consequently, patients with hereditary AT-III deficiencies run a very high risk of thromboembolic events in connection with surgery. Hereditary AT-III deficiencies are often first diagnosed in connection with operations, and the necessity for prophylactic treatment in these patients before surgery seems undoubted.[32,37,43,59,66,76]

The use of an AT-III concentrate as a thromboprophylactic agent is reported in conjunction with different surgical operations, like neurosurgery, tonsillectomy, removal of a metal plate on a fractured tibia, reparation of an indirect inguinal hernia, and laparatomy.[27,36,77-79] Doses of AT-III concentrates in order to normalize the AT-III level in plasma were administrated before surgery and during the following 3 to 5 postoperative days.[27,79] There were no thromboembolic complications in connection with the operations.

C. DEEP VENOUS THROMBOSIS AND PULMONARY EMBOLISM

Conventional treatment with intravenous infusions of heparin used to be the first therapy of choice in acute thrombosis in patients with hereditary AT-III deficiencies. However, heparin resistance has been observed in patients with AT-III deficiencies.[80,81] Treatment with an AT-III concentrate as a therapeutic agent in AT-III-deficient patients with deep venous thrombosis are reported since the late 1970s.[11,15,50,57,64,77,82,83] An AT-III concentrate has also been used in these patients as a complement to the conventional treatment with heparin, streptokinase or urokinase, and oral anticoagulants.

As an example, details of coagulation test values and treatment of a 26-year-old male with a thrombus in the left calf are given in Figure 2. The patient recovered and returned to his work within 2 weeks.[83]

Thrombosis has been diagnosed in infants and has been treated with an AT-III concentrate.[50]

D. FURTHER CLINICAL EXPERIENCES

Besides the published reports reviewed here of treatment with AT-III concentrates, there are unpublished documentation on clinicial studies. The experiences from treatment with AT-III concentrates produced by KabiVitrum AB in patients with hereditary AT-III deficiencies are summarized here. The experiences are derived from clinical research in eight European countries and routine treatments in Sweden and Norway. Thirty-nine patients have gone through 60 treatment sessions with an AT-III concentrate.

The results of the clinical research were originally given in patient record forms or in published reports, some of which were referred to earlier. Information from the routine treatments have been collected from hospital patient records, mainly by courtesy of Margareta Hellgren, M.D.; Lilian Tengborn, M.D.; and Ulrich Abildgaard, M.D. The 60 reports are grouped into four main indications:

- prophylaxis against thromboembolism in connection with pregnancy, delivery, and postpartum; most of the patients in this group were treated with an AT-III concentrate only in connection with delivery and postpartum (Table 1);
- prophylaxis against thromboembolism in connection with abortion, or abortion and sterilization (Table 2);
- prophylaxis against thromboembolism in connection with surgery (Table 3); and
- therapy in patients with deep venous thrombosis and pulmonary embolism (Table 4).

One patient was treated five times, three patients four times, eight patients twice, and the remaining 27 patients only once.

E. PROPHYLACTIC AGENT

In Tables 1, 2, and 3 the use of AT-III concentrates as prophylaxis against thromboembolism in 47 treatments is summarized. The high risk of thrombosis and details of prophylactic treatment during pregnancy, delivery, postpartum, or abortion are given in Tables 5 and 6. Twenty women were treated with an AT-III concentrate during delivery and postpartum.

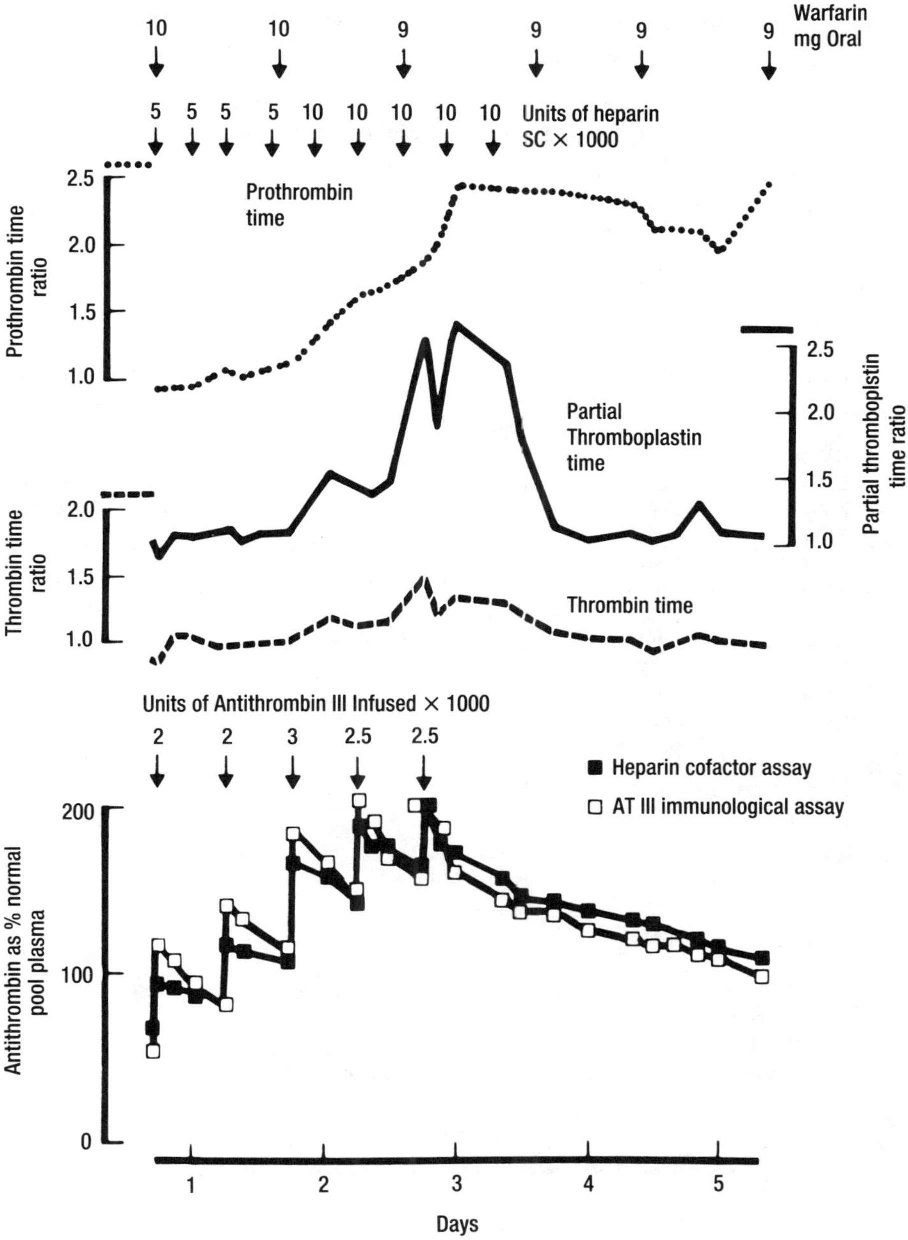

FIGURE 2. Coagulation, AT-III, and treatment parameters in an AT-III-deficient patient with acute venous thrombosis. (From *Clin. Lab. Haematol.*)

Twelve of them had suffered earlier from thromboembolism. Seven women were treated with an AT-III concentrate in connection with abortions. All of them had suffered from thromboembolism at least twice. Nine patients were treated with AT-III in connection with 13 operations. At least seven of them had suffered earlier from thromboembolism.

There is no doubt that the group of patients who were given an AT-III concentrate as a prophylaxis ran a very high risk of thrombosis. There was no thrombosis in connection with treatment with an AT-III concentrate or with an AT-III concentrate in combination with other anticoagulants.

These results, together with the experiences of others, form the basis for the use of AT-III concentrates as thromboprophylaxis in patients with hereditary AT-III deficiencies.

TABLE 1
Treatment with an AT-III Concentrate — Dosage and Duration[a]

Treatment No.	Treatment year	Total dose (IU)	Duration of therapy[b]	Dose/kg of body wt. (IU)	Remarks[c]
KV-06	1980	42,500	4.5 w	17-85	D, PP
KV-17	1980	4,000	2 d	24	D, PP
KV-18	1980	4,000	2 d	31	D, PP
KV-19	1984	4,000	2 d	32—35	D, PP
KV-21	1981	27,500	17 d	38—77	D, PP
KV-22	1980	20,000	10 d	36—72	CS, PP
KV-27	1978	5,900	7 d	6—34	D, PP
KV-31	1980	26,500	53 d	10—30	P, D
KV-36	1982	9,000	11 d	17—51	D, PP
KV-38	1983	2,500	2 d	—	D, PP
KV-39	1984	10,000	7 d	—	D, PP
KV-41	1982	25,000	13 d	42—83	CS, PP
KV-42	1985	15,000	7 d	40	CS, PP
KV-43	1986	7,000	2 d	45	D, PP
KV-44[1]	1983—84	149,500	18 w	50—70	P
KV-44[2]	1984	32,000	12 d	≤70	D, PP
KV-45[1]	1986	24,000	3 w	50	P
KV-45[2]	1986	18,000	9 d	50	D, PP
KV-46	1983	5,500	2 d	26-45	D, PP
KV-47	1986	4,000	2 d	24—30	D, PP
KV-48	1985	4,000	2 d	28—30	CS, PP
KV-51	1983—84	12,000	11 w	15—20	P
KV-52	1984	6,000	2 d	45	D, PP
KV-53	1982	5,000	3 d	20—35	D, PP
KV-54	1985	4,000	2 d	30—33	D, PP
KV-55	1987	19,500	7 d	—	D, PP
KV-56	1987	6,000	4 d	—	D, PP
KV-60	1981	3,000	1 d	—	D

[a] An AT-III concentrate as prophylaxis against thromboembolism in connection with pregnancy, delivery, or postpartum.
[b] (W) Week, (d) day.
[c] (P) Pregnancy, (D) delivery, (CS) Caesarean section, and (PP) postpartum.

TABLE 2
Treatment with an AT-III Concentrate — Dosage and Duration[a]

Treatment No.	Treatment Year	Total dose (IU)	Duration of therapy (d)	Dose/kg of body wt. (IU)	Remarks[b]
KV-04	1979	4,000	1	67	A
KV-10	1980	17,000	11	33—42	A
KV-12	1979	6,500	4	28—46	A
KV-13	1980	28,500	11	19—148	A S
KV-20	1980	7,500	4	42	M
KV-28	1978	2,000	2	7—27	A
KV-40	1982	7,500	4	39	A
KV-59	1981	5,000	1	—	A

[a] An AT-III concentrate as prophylaxis aginst thromboembolism after abortion.
[b] (A) Abortion, (M) miscarriage, and (S) sterilization.

TABLE 3
Treatment with an AT-III Concentrate — Dosage and Duration[a]

Treatment No.	Treatment Year	Total dose (IU)	Duration of therapy (d)	Dose/kg of body wt. (IU)	Remarks
KV-01	1980	16,000	6	47	Removal of metal plate, right ilia
KV-05	1979	5,000	2	33—50	Sterilization
KV-08	1984	10,000	8	9—36	Laparotomy
KV-09	1985	10,500	7	9—67	Ablatio mammae
KV-11	1984	5,000	3	25—33	Sterilization
KV-14	1983	7,000	3	40—60	Diathermy
KV-15	1985	4,500	2	30—60	Hand surgery
KV-16	1987	4,500	3	20—70	Extraction of six teeth
KV-23	1981	17,500	6	42—84	Laparotomy
KV-24	1980	14,000	7	31—63	Operation of varices
KV-25	1981	12,000	6	31—63	Operation of varices
KV-37	1982	6 × 50/kg bw	8	50	Gynaecological operation
KV-57	1981	9,000	12	25—38	Operation of varices

[a] An AT-III concentration as prophylaxis against thromboembolism after surgery.

TABLE 4
Treatment with an AT-III Concentrate — Dosage and Duration[a]

Treatment No.	Treatment Year	Total dose (IU)	Duration of therapy (d)	Dose/kg of body wt. (IU)	Remarks[b]
KV-02	1979	2,000	1	33	Thrombophleb.
KV-03	1979	2,000	1	33	Bilat. DVT
KV-07	1984	8,000—9,500	5	27—36	Bilat. DVT
KV-26	1980	2,250	3	33	Thrombosis
KV-29[1]	1978, Nov.	6,840	6	12—42	Thrombosis, PE
KV-29[2]	1978, Dec.	15,500	11	12—42	Thrombosis, PE
KV-30	1980	14,000	10	20—60	Thrombosis, PE
KV-32	1981	17,000	11	40—50	PE
KV-33	1981	12,000	3	25—61	DVT
KV-34	1981	8,000	3	13—70	DVT
KV-35	1981	2,000	3	20	Haematoma
KV-49	1983	12,000	12	15—35	Thrombosis
KV-50	1983	7,000	14	15—35	DVT
KV-58	1978	2,500	3	—	Thrombosis

[a] Therapy with an AT-III concentrate in patients with thrombophilia or bleeding
[b] The terminology of the reporting investigator has been used. (DVT) deep venous thrombosis and (PE) pulmonary embolism.

F. THERAPEUTIC AGENT

Five patients with hereditary AT-III deficiencies and acute thromboses were treated with heparin without the disappearance of soreness, swelling, and pain. However, the expected heparin effect was seen when the therapy was supplemented with an AT-III concentrate and when there was an obvious reduction of the acute signs of thrombosis. In these five patients, the effect of heparin was probably strongly reduced due to very low plasma levels of AT-III. The five patients were their own controls as they all were treated both with and without an AT-III concentrate.

In addition, a combined therapy of an AT-III concentrate, heparin, and oral anticoag-

TABLE 5A
Patients Treated with an AT-III Concentrate During Delivery and Postpartum — All Known Thromboembolic Events and All Known Pregnancies

		All known thromboembolic events		All known pregnancies[a]			
				Thromboembolic events			Prophylaxis during delivery and postpartum
Treatment No.	Patient	Year	Triggering event	Year	P	PP	
KV-06	A, 1944	1967	Oral contraceptives	1970	No	Yes	NO
		1970	Postpartum	1980	No	No	A, H
KV-17	B, 1949	None		1980	No	No	A, H, O
KV-18	C, 1953	None		1980	No	No	A, H
KV-19				1984	No	No	A, H, O
(KV-20)	D, 1948	1968	Oral contraceptives	1972	Yes	No	No
KV-21		1972	Pregnancy week 12	1980	Yes	Miscarriage	
		1980	Pregnancy week 6	1981	Yes	No	A, H, M
		1981	Pregnancy week 7				
KV-22	E, 1956	None		1980	No	No	A, H, M
KV-27	F, 1951	None		1970	No	No	A, H,
KV-31	G, 1950	1976		1980	No	No	A, H, O
KV-36	H, 1957	1973		1982	No	No	A, H
KV-38	I, 1962		Twice, once in connection with oral contraceptives	1983	No	No	A, H
KV-39	J, 1952	1974	Oral contraceptives	1984	No	No	A, H, O
		1985					

Note: Abbreviations: (P) pregnancy, (A) Antithrombin, (O) oral anticoagulants, (PP) postpartum, (H) heparin, and (M) Macrodex.

ulants was given to six patients during seven thromboembolic events. In five of the six patients, the expected heparin effect was seen. As heparin was not given without the supplementation of an AT-III concentrate in these patients, it is not possible to say if heparin would have been effective, even without administration of an AT-III concentrate. However, the combined therapy of an AT-III concentrate and heparin was effective both in these patients and in the five previously mentioned (Table 4).

G. CONCLUSION

Based on results in clinical research and routine treatments, it is concluded that patients with hereditary AT-III deficiencies will benefit from treatment with an AT-III concentrate as prophylaxis in connection with delivery, postpartum, and surgery, and as a therapeutic agent in thrombophilia.

IV. DOSAGE RECOMMENDATION — HEREDITARY AT-III DEFICIENCY

AT-III concentrates are indicated for the treatment of patients with hereditary AT-III deficiencies in connection with surgery and delivery, and when they suffer from thromboembolism. The dosage should be related to the actual AT-III level, so that after the first dose, the AT-III level should increase to about 120% of normal. Thereafter, it should be maintained at levels higher than 80%. Adult subjects require 30 to 50 IU of AT-III concentrate per kg body weight and day.

TABLE 5B
Patients Treated with an AT-III Concentrate During Delivery and Postpartum — All Known Thromboembolic Events and All Known Pregnancies

		All known thromboembolic events		All known pregnancies			
				Thromboembolic events			Prophylaxis during delivery and postpartum[a]
Treatment No.	Patient	Year	Triggering event	Year	P	PP	
KV-41	K, 1955	Yes		1982	No	No	A, H, M
KV-42	L, 1964	None		1985	No	No	A, H, M
KV-43	M, 1962	None		1986	No	No	A, H, M
KV-44	N, 1958	1975	Influenza	1984	No	No	A
KV-45				1986	No	No	A, H, M
KV-46	O, 1954	1981		1983	No	No	A, H, O
KV-47				1986	No	No	A, H, O
KV-48	P, 1955	1974	Oral contraceptives	1985	No	No	A, H, O
KV-49	Q, 1956	1983 Nov	Pregnancy	1980	No	No	—
KV-50		1983 Dec	Pregnancy				
KV-51							
KV-52				1983	Twice	No	A, H, O
KV-53	R, 1955	None		1982	No	No	A, H, O
KV-54				1985	No	No	A, H, O
KV-55	S, 1963	1986 May	Pregnancy				
		1986 Jun	Pregnancy	1986	Twice	No	A, H, O
KV-56	T, 1965	None		1987	No	NO	A, H, O

[a] Abbreviations: (P) pregnancy, (A) antithrombin, (O) oral anticoagulants, (PP) postpartum, (H) heparin, and (M) Macrodex.

A. PREGNANCY

Treatment with s.c. heparin is to be started as soon as a pregnancy is diagnosed. An initial dosage of 7500 to 10,000 IU twice a day is recommended. It is of the greatest importance to measure if the treatment with heparin results in an anticoagulant effect. An anti-Factor X_a concentration of 0.1 to 0.2 IU/ml of plasma or an APTT prolongation of 5 to 10 sec before injection (i.e., 12 h after previous injection) is recommended. (It has been discussed whether the previously mentioned anti-Factor X_a concentration or APTT prolongation would be sufficient 3 h after injection in patients who have not suffered from previous thromboembolic events.)

At delivery, the dosage of s.c. heparin has to be decreased to 5000 IU twice daily, but increased again to the same heparin effect as before on the first day postpartum and for 5 to 7 d. Heparin can be discontinued when oral anticoagulants, started the first day postpartum, are effective. Infusion of an AT-III concentrate 30 to 50 IU/kg body weight and day is to be started the day before induced delivery or on the day of delivery, and given so that the level increases to 100%. The treatment period should be 2 to 8 d postpartum until treatment with oral anticoagulants and heparin, or treatment with oral anticoagulants alone is effective. In the latter case, an AT-III concentrate has to be given for a longer period than in the former case.

B. SURGERY

Thromboprophylactic treatment before and after surgery could be given with AT-III concentrates alone for 2 to 8 d in doses of 30 to 50 IU/kg body weight and day, or in

TABLE 6
Patients Treated with an AT-III Concentrate During Abortion — All Known Thromboembolic Events and All Known Pregnancies

		All known thromboembolic events		All known pregnancies			
					Thromboembolic events		Prophylaxis during delivery and postpartum*
Treatment No.	Patient	Year	Triggering event	Year	P	PP	
KV-04	U 1955		Several times				
		1970	Pregnancy	1979	Yes	—	—
KV-10	V 1947	1968	Pregnancy (intrauterine death)	1968	No	Yes	—
		1970	Pregnancy (the baby died, aortic thrombosis)	—	—	—	—
KV-12	W 1944	1972	No event, but the baby died, aortic thrombosis)	1972	No	No	—
KV-13		1973	Pregnancy (twins, one died of asphyxia)	1973	Yes	No	H
		1979	Pregnancy	1979	Yes	—	—
		1980	Pregnancy	1980	Yes	—	—
KV-20	X 1948	1968	Oral contraceptives	1972	Yes	No	—
(KV-21)		1972	Pregnancy week 12	1980	Yes	Miscarriage	—
		1980	Pregnancy week 6	1981	Yes	No	A, H, M
		1981	Pregancy week 7	—	—	—	—
KV—28	Y 1958	1978	Four times associated with oral contraceptives or pregnancy	—	—	—	—
		1978	Pregnancy	1978	Yes	—	—
KV-40	Z 1956	1979	Bronchopneumonia	—	—	—	—
		1980	Oral contraceptives	—	—	—	—
		1982	(Before pregnancy)	1982	—	—	—
KV-59	III-15	1981	Pregnancy	1981	—	Yes	(Time not stated)
		1981	Pregnancy week 9	1981	Yes	—	—

* Abbreviations: (P) pregnancy, (A) Antithrombin, (O) oral anticoagulants, (PP) postpartum, (H) heparin, and (M) Macrodex.

combination with heparin or oral anticoagulants. The treatment depends on the type of surgery, local traditions, etc.

C. DEEP VENOUS THROMBOSIS

Patients with hereditary AT-III deficiencies and earlier thromboembolisms are to be treated with both heparin and AT-III concentrates; the latter in doses as mentioned earlier, that is 30 to 50 IU/kg body weight and day for 2 to 8 days.

V. ACQUIRED AT-III DEFICIENCY — CLINICAL EXPERIENCES

Several methods for the determination of AT-III activity in plasma and serum have been published. These assays have been of great importance for the knowledge of the metabolism and function of AT-III and for the knowledge of AT-III plasma levels in patients with coagulation disorders.

Decreased levels of AT-III, which is the most important inhibitor of the serine proteases in blood, have frequently been described in hospitalized patients. Thus, it has been presumed that treatment with AT-III concentrates could be of benefit also in the treatment of patients with an acquired deficiency of AT-III.

An acquired AT-III deficiency is detected in several clinical states and may be subclassified as:

- increased consumption, e.g., disseminated intravascular coagulation;
- decreased synthesis, e.g., liver disease;
- increased loss, e.g., renal disease; and
- drug induction, e.g., heparin, L-asparaginase, and oestrogens.

Published works on treatment with AT-III concentrates in acquired AT-III deficiencies are reviewed in this chapter. The conventional treatment of this type of patient is extremely complex and it should be stressed that the intention with this chapter is only to summarize experiences on the use of AT-III concentrates, not to discuss the entire therapy of the patients.

A. DISSEMINATED INTRAVASCULAR COAGULATION, RESPIRATORY DISTRESS SYNDROME, AND BACTERIAL INFECTION

Several authors,[84-89] have reported low levels of AT-III caused by increased consumption in intensive care patients. These patients are often found to have disseminated intravascular coagulation (DIC). DIC, also known as consumption coagulopathy, is a pathological syndrome which can be initiated in a great many diseases or clinical states. Multiple etiologies for DIC could be present in the individual patient. Not only the coagulation system, but also the fibrinolytic, the kallikrein-kinin, and complement systems are activated in DIC. The underlying causes may be classified according to the mechanisms which probably initiated blood coagulation:[90]

- Tissue injury (thromboplastin release), e.g., obstetrical complications, pregnancy complications, trauma, surgical complications, carcinoma, leukemia.
- Endothelial injury (Hageman factor activation), e.g., septicemia, surgery, trauma, large vessel catheterization.
- Platelet or red cell injury (phospholipid release), e.g., immunologic, hemolysis.
- Reticuleondothelial system injury, e.g., liver injury, splenectomy.

In septicemia, not only the endothelial injury but also the thromboplastin release from monocytes is of importance.[91]

If DIC is suspected or diagnosed, the underlying disease should be identified and treated. General intensive care, adequate ventilation support, and prevention from hypovolaemia are essential. However, it is also of great importance to normalize the coagulation. In this respect, AT-III concentrates have been given to patients with DIC in order to test if it has any beneficial effect on coagulation and morbidity. Four pilot studies on severely ill patients with DIC or signs of DIC published/presented in 1982 to 1984 are reviewed here.[23,31,92,93]

In three of these studies, 9, 15, and 21 patients were treated with AT-III concentrates in doses from 250 IU to 3500 IU/d. In the fourth publication, the number of patients and amount of AT-III concentrates were not stated.[93] The response to treatment with AT-III concentrates and other drugs in haemorrhagic diatheses and abnormal haemostasis were studied mostly by means of coagulation tests such as AT-III activity, platelet count, prothrombin time, prothrombin complex, and fibrinogen and fibrinogen degradation products. The number of tests differed slightly between investigators. These tests are hereafter referred to as coagulation tests.

In spite of differences in the trial plans, the results of the four studies were mainly in accordance with each other and are summarized in six points:

- The AT-III levels in plasma increased after the infusion of the AT-III concentrate.
- Coagulation test values were normalized or improved.
- In spite of normalized haemostasis, the patients did not survive due to the underlying disease.
- There were bleeding complications if heparin was concurrently given in too high doses.
- Treatment with the AT-III concentrate seemed to be of benefit to severely ill patients with curable diseases.
- The AT-III concentrate had to be dosed on an individual basis according to the AT-III level in plasma.

In a fifth study on 21 patients with DIC, treatment with an AT-III concentrate gave results of a similar kind to those in the previous mentioned studies.[94] The plasma levels of AT-III were normalized, the monomeric fibrin complexes decreased, and the progression of the DIC could be prevented. In patients with DIC, there is always, as mentioned earlier, an underlying disease or disorder. However, in addition, the underlying disorder as such or together with DIC could result in respiratory distress syndrome.

It has been reported that both radiological and coagulation studies are of importance in patients suffering from adult respiratory distress syndrome (ARDS).[95] Two out of three patients with ARDS due to multiple trauma or sepsis were treated with heparin and an AT-III concentrate; the third patient was treated with heparin and plasma only. Normalization of the coagulation by a relevant therapy such as heparin and/or AT-III concentrate is of importance for the recovery of the patients.

DIC may also occur in children, most frequently caused by a bacterial infection or severe respiratory distress syndrome.[96,97] In a report on six children (1 month to 5 years old) with DIC, the result of treatment with heparin and an AT-III concentrate was evaluated.[96] The concentrate was given in doses of 250 IU every 8 h for 1 to 3 days. DIC was successfully treated with heparin and an AT-III concentrate in five cases. However, one 2-year-old girl with a clinical diagnosis of Reye's syndrome died because of hepatic failure complicated by pulmonary atelectasis. The investigators found the treatment with heparin and an AT-III concentrate to be a reasonable therapy for DIC in these children.

Treatment with heparin and an AT-III concentrate was described in ten newborns with DIC. A clear improvement in the coagulation status was observed in eight children, all of whom survived. Two infants died due to their underlying septicemia.[97] The efficiency of treatment with an AT-III concentrate versus heparin has also been studied in newborn infants with respiratory distress syndrome. However, the number of patients was limited and the result are difficult to evaluate.[98]

Bjorvatn and co-workers reported promising results of their treatment program for patients suffering from meningococci septicemia.[99] The conventional treatment, including benzylpenicillin, methylprednisolone, and an AT-III concentrate, was used in three patients supplemented with plasmapheresis and leucopheresis, and, in one case, with blood exchange. All recovered without sequelae. Successful treatment with an AT-III concentrate was also reported in two patients with acute bacterial meningits.

A controlled study by Blauhut and co-workers confirmed the results of the pilot studies.[100] They studied 51 patients suffering from shock and DIC due to multiple trauma, septicemia, or hepatic coma. Each patient was randomized to one of three treatment groups. The first group received heparin in an intravenous dose of 3000 IU, followed by 250 IU/h, the second group was treated with infusions of an AT-III concentrate with the aim of keeping the AT-III activity in plasma around 100% (1 IU/ml), and the third group received combined therapy of an AT-III concentrate and heparin. The duration of DIC was significantly shortened in the patients treated with the AT-III concentrate. The administration of heparin did not improve the effect of the AT-III concentrate in this group of patients.

The investigators concluded that substitution of AT-III concentrates in patients with shock and DIC permitted a better control of the alterations of the clotting system. However, differences in mortality were not identified between the groups.

B. PRE-ECLAMPSIA AND COAGULATION PROBLEMS DURING PREGNANCY

In seven out of eight case reports published in English before 1983 on treatment with an AT-III concentrate in DIC, the patient was treated in conjunction with pregnancy, namely acute fatty liver (3), pre-eclampsia (2), postpartum haemolytic uraemic syndrome (1), myelodysplastic syndrome (pre-leukemia) during pregnancy (1), and in the eighth case, tampon-related toxic shock syndrome.[101-108] An AT-III concentrate was given in total doses of 2000 IU to 45,500 IU during 1 d to 6 weeks. All patients survived in spite of, in some cases, very poor prognoses, and the treatment was regarded as successful. The investigator found it impossible to say whether treatment with the AT-III concentrate influenced the clinical course in only one case.[107]

In 1984, Hellgren and co-workers reported the result of treatment with an AT-III concentrate in fourteen women with obstetric complications and acquired AT-III deficiencies. Eleven of the patients suffered from pre-eclampsia, three had liver disorders, and nephrotic syndrome was diagnosed in one case.[109] All patients survived, and the normalization of coagulation test values was obtained in all women postpartum. The summary of the treatment and the changes in coagulation test values of one of the patients are given in Figure 3. The authors recommend treatment with an AT-III concentrate in this type of patients.

The clinical use of an AT-III concentrate in patients with obstetrical complications and DIC is also reported by others. In a Japanese study, treatment with an AT-III concentrate was compared with a synthetic protease inhibitor.[110] The author found the effect of an AT-III concentrate to surpass that of the synthetic drug, but there were many excluded patients, and the results are difficult to evaluate. Finally, in one presentation on four patients with fatty liver of pregnancy, the authors concluded that treatment with an AT-III concentrate was effective in the management of abnormal hemostasis.[111]

C. SURGERY

As previously mentioned, the level of AT-III is decreased during surgery.[57,73-75] Infusions of an AT-III concentrate given to eight out of 16 patients with fractures of the neck of the femur were reported in 1979. No differences were seen between the groups, except in the AT-III plasma levels. The concentrate was given in low doses, and the report is of historical interest only.[112]

In another study, 45 out of 90 cardiopulmonary bypass patients were given one dose of 1500 IU of an AT-III concentrate in a prospective controlled study. There was a tendency towards decreased postoperative ventilation support in the treated group. The patients had a shorter stay in the intensive care ward than patients in the control group.[113]

AT-III concentrates are, in a few countries, used in connection with major surgery. Results have been reported at meetings, but the clinical effect, if any, is not scientifically shown.

D. LIVER CIRRHOSIS

In a steady state, the liver synthesis of plasma proteins, e.g., AT-III and fibrogen, is equal to the rate of degradation. In liver disease, the synthesis is decreased. Low levels of AT-III in plasma are reported in patients with liver cirrhosis.[114] When a patient with liver

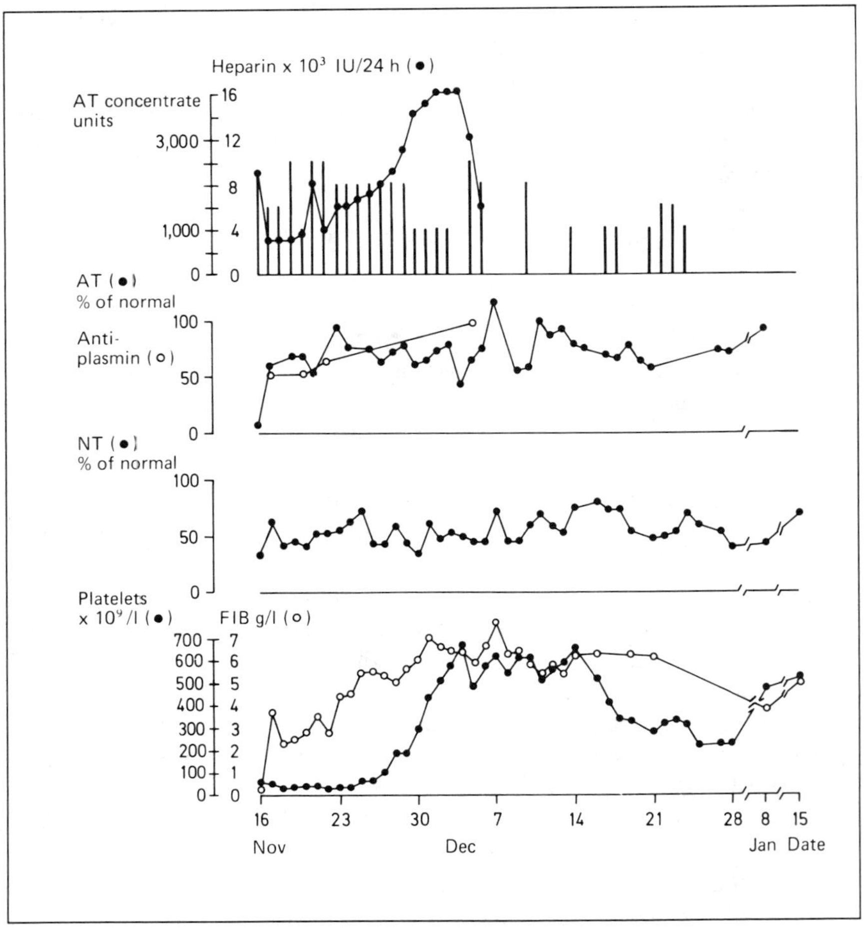

FIGURE 3. Severe acquired AT-III deficiency in late pregnancy. The changes in platelet count, fibrinogen (FIB), prothrombin complex (NT), α_2-antiplasmin, and antithrombin III (AT-III) during treatment with heparin and an AT-III concentrate. The AT-III level prior to infusion of the AT-III concentrate is presented. (From *Gynecol. Obstet. Invest.*)

disease bleeds, it may be due to the impaired synthesis of coagulation factors, thrombocytopenia, or DIC.

The first two patients treated with an AT-III concentrate suffered from liver disease.[11,12] These patients were treated in 1974. Four years later, Schipper and co-workers reported promising results.[115] Three patients with liver disease, DIC, and severe hemorrhagic diatheses were treated with an AT-III concentrate in total doses of about 2000 IU to 6600 IU. The plasma AT-III increased to normal levels, other coagulation test values improved, and bleeding was controlled. Schipper and co-workers then designed a pilot study in order to examine the effect of the selective correction of plasma AT-III activity on the increased turnover of fibrinogen, which occurs in patients with liver cirrhosis.[116]

The study confirmed the presence of an increased turnover of I-125-fibrinogen in patients with liver cirrhosis. Selected correction of the acquired AT-III deficiency with an AT-III concentrate induced a normalization of the turnover of I-125-fibrinogen. The authors summarize that the observations indicate that decreased levels of AT-III in plasma contribute to the increased I-125-fibrinogen turnover in patients with cirrhosis.

E. PERITONEOVENOUS SHUNT OPERATION

In three pilot studies,[117-119] patients with liver cirrhosis were given an AT-III concentrate in order to prevent DIC after peritoneovenous (LeVeen) shunt operations. In Boyer's study, five patients were given one dose of 40 IU of an AT-III concentrate per kg body weight immediately before surgery. These patients were compared with eight patients in a control group.[117] In untreated patients, there was a significant decrease in platelet count, and factor V and fibrinogen level associated with a significant increase in fibrinogen degradation products. In patients treated with an AT-III concentrate, there was only a slight change in the platelet count and factor V or fibrinogen level, and a moderate increase in fibrinogen degradation products. The author concluded that infusion of an AT-III concentrate prevented the occurrence of DIC in these patients.

Büller and co-workers gave their five patients a loading dose of 2000 IU of an AT-III concentrate, followed by a continuous intravenous infusion in order to maintain AT-III plasma levels of about 100%.[118] They started with studies of two patients without treatment with an AT-III concentrate and continued with five patients treated with an AT-III concentrate. The results of the first two patients in the AT-III group were promising, but the third patient developed fulminant DIC and suffered from bleedings. The two following patients died from cardiac arrest and septicemia and bleeding, respectively. The authors concluded that peritoneovenous shunting caused clinically significant coagulation abnormalities. The data of patients receiving an AT-III concentrate suggested that this regimen did not prevent DIC and bleeding in all cases.

Five out of ten patients with alcoholic liver cirrhosis were treated with AT-III concentrates. The severity of DIC was tempered but not prevented; only 20 IU/kg body weight was infused.[119] Thus, treatment with an AT-III concentrate in a peritoneovenous shunt operation is not properly evaluated. However, it is still an indication of interest.

H. NEPHROTIC SYNDROME, RENAL INSUFFICIENCY, AND HAEMOLYTIC UREMIC SYNDROME

a. Haemolytic Uremic Syndrome

In patients with nephrotic syndrome, albumin and other plasma proteins, e.g., AT-III, are lost into the urine. The nephrotic syndrome could be complicated by deep venous thrombosis and thromboembolic episodes. Among 15 patients with various degrees of proteinuria, five had AT-III levels below the normal range.[120] AT-III levels were also studied in 48 patients with proteinuria. Nine of these patients had clinical signs of thrombosis, including four with renal vein thrombosis. In eight of these nine patients, AT-III concentrations were below 70% of the level in normal human plasma.[121] In analogy to a hereditary AT-III deficiency, an acquired AT-III deficiency, due to renal loss, should be considered to be an essential etiology for the thrombophilia of nephrotic patients.[120] Thus, treatment with AT-III concentrates in nephrotic patients suffering from DVT is recommended by some investigators.[122] Twenty patients with dialysis-dependent renal insufficiencies were treated with an AT-III concentrate in connection with haemodialysis.[123]

The authors summarize their results as follows:

> Six patients with acute renal failure and disseminated intravascular coagulation were able to undergo dialysis using only 750 to 1000 IU heparin per hour after normalization of AT-III without complications. In three patients, thrombosing of the extracorporeal system had occurred despite increasing doses of heparin, only after 1500 IU of AT-III subsequent haemodialysis could be performed without thrombosis. Dialysis was performed with continous substitution if the AT-III-heparin-complex in six patients was prone to hemorrhage. Of the AT-III-heparin complex, 250 to 500 IU were sufficient and proved as safe. In five patients, repeated thrombosing of the hemofilter per day had occurred during continous arteriovenous hemofiltration. After AT-III administration, hemofilters could be left *in situ* for 18 to 46 h.

In one of the case reports on an acquired AT-III deficiency referred to previously, hemolytic uremic syndrome (HUS) was diagnosed.[101] This syndrome is also seen in children. Roth and co-workers reported the result of treatment of nine children with HUS and in ages from 3 months to 12 years.[124]

Plasma AT-III levels were determined on admission to the hospital and during the clinical course. In seven patients, plasma AT-III levels were decreased and did not rise after plasmapheresis with fresh frozen plasma and replacement therapy with an AT-III concentrate was started. After correction of the deficiency, about 50 IU/kg body weight and day was needed. However, for the first 24 to 30 h, an AT-III concentrate in higher doses was necessary to increase the AT-III plasma level to 1 IU/ml. The outcome with regard to renal function was complicated in only one of the seven patients, and the author summarized that the patients with HUS and AT-III levels less than 70% may benefit from therapy with an AT-III concentrate as an adjuvant symptomatic drug.

G. DRUG INDUCTION

The plasma AT-III level is decreased after treatment with some drugs, e.g., heparin, oestrogens, and tamoxifen.[125-132]

Drug induction has to be taken into consideration during treatment of patients with low levels of AT-III. In 13 children with acute lymphoblastic leukemia, substitution with an AT-III concentrate resulted in correction of the pathological alterations of the coagulation system induced by therapy with L-asparaginase.[133] In addition, in patients with decreased plasma levels of AT-III, heparin treatment was reported to give a poor anticoagulant response, and it was proposed to give patients substitution therapy with an AT-III concentrate rather than increasing the heparin dosage.[134]

H. DISCUSSION AND CONCLUSION

Experiences of treatment with AT-III concentrates in acquired deficiencies published to date have been reviewed. Most reports consist only of the results from one or a few cases; there are in addition some small pilot studies and one controlled clinical trial on 51 patients.[100] Most of the investigators have found treatment with an AT-III concentrate of value in acquired deficiencies. They have observed the normalization of coagulation test values as well as clinical signs of improvement. However, investigators are aware of the fact that the clinical effects of AT-III concentrates in acquired deficiencies are not yet scientifically shown in controlled randomized clinical trials.

Further studies are requested. Some investigators have spent a lot of time trying to find proper designs for clinical trials in acquired AT-III deficiencies. A number of problems arise, e.g., how to find comparable patients and how to find enough patients during a reasonable time. Finally, would it be ethical to start clinical trials with control groups when the effect of substitution with an AT-III concentrate so far has been promising? It has been estimated that at least 250 to 300 patients must be involved if the trial is to be meaningful, that is, able to show differences between groups with and without AT-III therapy.

Some years ago, many doctors did not want to include severely ill patients with acquired deficiencies into trials for ethical reasons. However, in recent years, controlled randomized clinical trials have been approved by health authorities in some countries and further studies are planned. Thus, knowledge on treatment with AT-III concentrates will increase during the coming years.

To summarize, in almost all reported cases, plasma coagulation test values improved after substitutions with an AT-III concentrate and, in most cases, clinical effects were observed. However, clinical effects of AT-III concentrates have not been shown in controlled clinical trials.

Treatment with an AT-III concentrate seems to be of benefit in severely ill patients with acquired AT-III deficiencies and coagulopathies. Thus, treatment with an AT-III concentrate is recommended[135] in order to normalize the coagulation and to make it possible to treat the underlying disease. If the underlying disease is incurable, treatment with an AT-III concentrate cannot prevent a bad outcome, but it could improve the patient's general condition.

VI. DOSAGE RECOMMENDATION — ACQUIRED AT-III DEFICIENCY

AT-III concentrates are indicated for treatment of severely ill patients with acquired AT-III deficiencies:

- patients with DIC due to trauma, sepsis, or complicated pregnancies
- patients with deep venous thrombosis and low plasma levels of AT-III
- patients with acute hepatic failure and bleedings

AT-III concentrate should be dosed on an individual basis, related to the actual AT-III level in plasma. This is to be normalized (i.e., brought up to 100% or 1 IU/ml), and an AT-III concentration exceeding 80% of the concentration of active AT-III present in normal plasma is to be aimed at during the entire course of therapy.

The dose in IU could, as recommended by Blauhut and co-workers, be calculated according to the following formula:

$$(100 - \text{measured AT-III level in }\%) \times \text{kg body weight}$$

The level of AT-III in plasma ought to be monitored during the whole treatment period. In acute states, determinations shall be performed at least twice a day. The treatment should be continued until normalized hemostasis.

REFERENCES

1. **Morawitz, P.,** Die Chemie der Blutgerinnung, *Ergeb. Physiol.*, 4, 307, 1905.
2. **Hensen, A. and Loeliger, E. A.,** Antithrombin III. Its metabolism and its function in blood coagulation, *Thromb. Diath. Haemorrh.* 9, (Suppl. 1), 1, 1963.
3. **Abildgaard, U.,** Purification of two progressive antithrombins of human plasma, *Scand. J. Clin. Lab. Invest.*, 19, 190, 1967.
4. **Heimburger, N.,** First Int. Symp. Tissue Factors in the Hemostasis of the Coagulation-Fibrinolysis System, Firenze, 1967, 353.
5. **Abildgaard, U.,** Highly purified antithrombin III with heparin cofactor activity prepared by disc electrophoresis, *Scand. J. Clin. Invest.*, 21, 89, 1968.
6. **Heimburger, N., Haupt, H., and Schwick, H. G.,** Proteinase inhibitors of human plasma, in Proc. Int. Res. Conf. on Proteinase Inhibitors, Munich, 1970.
7. **Rosenberg, R. D. and Damus, P. S.,** The purification and mechanism of action of human antithrombin-heparin cofactor, *J. Biol. Chem.*, 248, 6490, 1973.
8. **Miller-Andersson, M., Borg, H., and Andersson, L.-O.,** Purification of antithrombin III by affinity chromatography, *Thromb. Res.*, 5, 439, 1974.
9. **Thaler, E. and Schmer, G.,** A simple two-step isolation procedure for human and bovine antithrombin II/III (heparin cofactor): a comparison of two methods, *Br. J. Haematol.*, 31, 233, 1975.
10. **Wicherhauser, M., Williams, C., and Mercer, J.,** Development of large scale fractionation methods. VII. Preparation of antithrombin III concentrate, *Vox Sang.*, 36, 281, 1979.
11. **Schramm, W.,** Erfahrungen mit der Substitution von Antithrombin III-Konzentraten bei angeborenen und erworbenen Mangelzuständen, *Behring Inst. Mitt.*, 73, 66, 1983.
12. **Abildgaard, U.,** Personal communication, 1988.
13. **Barrowcliffe, T. W., Eggleton, C. A., and Mahmoud, M.,** Studies of the heterogeneity of antithrombin III concentrates, *Br. J. Haematol.*, 55, 37, 1983.
14. **Handeland, G. F. and Abildgaard, U.,** *In vivo* recovery of antithrombin concentrates, *Thromb. Res.*, 39, 133, 1985.
15. **Vinazzer, H.,** Clinical use of antithrombin III concentrates, *Vox Sang.*, 53, 193, 1987.
16. **Budde, U.,** Antithrombin-III-Konzentrat. Eine vergleichende Untersuchung, *Krankenhauspharmazie*, 8, 454, 1987.

17. **Lacher, D. A.,** Alanine aminotransferase and posttransfusion hepatitis, *J. Am. Med. Assoc.*, 257, 1048, 1987.
18. **Von Karges, H. E., Fuhge, P., and Heimburger, N.,** Eigenschaften und Virussicherheit eines pasteurisierten Antithrombin III-Konzentrates, *Arzneim. Forsch.*, 37, 756, 1987.
19. **Clemens, R.,** Virus safety of a pasteurized antithrombin III concentrate, *Arzneim. Forsch.*, 37, 759, 1987.
20. **Einarsson, M., Perenius, L., McDougal, J. S., and Cort, S. P.,** Heat inactivation of human immuno deficiency virus (HIV) in solutions of antithrombin III, submitted for publication.
21. **Tabor, E., Murano, G., Snoy, P., and Gerety, R. J.,** Inactivation of hepatitis B virus by heat in antithrombin III stabilized with citrate, *Thromb. Res.*, 22, 233, 1981.
22. **Schramm, W. and Marx, R.,** Congenital and acquired antithrombin III deficiency, clinical symptoms and therapy with antithrombin III concentrate, *Ann. Univ. Sarav. Med.*, Suppl. 3, 137, 1983.
23. **Hellgren, M., Javelin, L., Hägnevik, K., Blombäck, M., and Medén-Britth, G.,** Antithrombin III concentrate as adjuvant in DIC treatment — a pilot study in 9 severely ill patients, *Thromb. Res.*, 35, 459, 1984.
24. **Tengborn, L., Frohm, B., Nilsson, L. E., and Nilsson, I. M.,** Antithrombin III concentrate: its catabolism in health and in antithrombin III deficiency, *Scand. J. Clin. Lab. Invest.*, 41, 469, 1981.
25. **Tengborn, L., Frohm, B., Nilsson, L.-E., Johansson, L., and Andersson, L.-O.,** Properties and catabolism of heat treated antithrombin III concentrate, *Thromb. Res.*, 48, 701, 1987.
26. **Collen, D., Schetz, J., De Cock, F., Holmer, E., and Verstraete, M.,** Metabolism of antithrombin III (heparin cofactor) in man: effects of venous thrombosis and of heparin administration, *Eur. J. Clin. Invest.*, 7, 27, 1977.
27. **Mannucci, P. M., Boyer, C., Wolf, M., Tripodi, A., and Larrieu, M. J.,** Treatment of congenital antithrombin III deficiency with concentrates, *Br. J. Haematol.*, 50, 531, 1982.
28. **Sas, G.,** Congenital and acquired defects of antithrombin III, *Ric. Clin. Lab.*, 14, 491, 1984.
29. **Scully, M. F., De Haas, H., Chan, P., and Kakkar, V. V.,** Hereditary antithrombin-III deficiency in an English family, *Br. J. Haematol.*, 47, 235, 1981.
30. **Knot, E. A. R., De Jong, E., Ren Cate, J. W., Iburg, A. H. C., Henny, Ch. P., Bruin, T., and Stibbe, J.,** Purified radiolabeled antithrombin III metabolism in three families with hereditary AT III deficiency: application of a three-compartment model, *Blood*, 67, 93, 1986.
31. **Blauhut, B., Necek, S., Vinazzer, H., and Bergmann, H.,** Substitution therapy with an antithrombin III concentrate in shock and DIC, *Thromb. Res.*, 27, 271, 1982.
32. **Egeberg, O.,** Inherited antithrombin deficiency causing thrombophilia, *Thromb. Diath. Haemorrh.*, 3, 516, 1965.
33. **Winter, J. H. and Douglas, A. S.,** Familial venous thrombosis, *Postgrad. Med.*, J., 59, 677, 1983.
34. **Michiels, J. J. and Van Vliet, H. H. D. M.,** Hereditary antithrombin III deficiency and venous thrombosis, *Neth. J. Med.*, 27, 226, 1984.
35. **Thaler, E. and Lechner, K.,** Antithrombin III deficiency and thromboembolism, *Clin. Haematol.*, 10, 369, 1981.
36. **Miller, N., Hultin, M. B., Gounder, M., and Zarrabi, M. H.,** Hereditary antithrombin III deficiency: case report and review of recent therapeutic advances., *Am. J. Haematol.*, 21, 215, 1986.
37. **Halal, F., Quenneville, G., Laurin, S., and Loulou, G.,** Clinical and genetic aspects of antithrombin III deficiency, *Am. J. Med. Genet.*, 14, 737, 1983.
38. **Gallus, A. S.,** Antithrombin III deficiency: clinical relevance and replacement therapy, *Dev. Biol. Stand.*, 67, 59, 1987.
39. **Tilsner, V.,** Antithrombin III. Bedeutung, Diagnostik und Therapie, *Med. Welt*, 36, 534, 1985.
40. **Cosgriff, T. M., Bishop, D. T., Hershgold, E. J., Skolnick, M. H., Martin, B. A., Baty, B. J., and Carlson, K. S.,** Familial antithrombin III deficiency: its natural history, genetics, diagnosis and treatment, *Medicine*, 62, 209, 1983.
41. **Von Kaulla, E. and Von Kaulla, K. N.,** Deficiency of antithrombin III activity associated with hereditary thrombosis tendency, *J. Med.*, 3, 349, 1972.
42. **Mackie, M., Bennett, B., Ogston, D., and Douglas, A. S.,** Familial thrombosis: inherited deficiency of antithrombin III, *Br. Med. J.*, 1, 136, 1978.
43. **Marciniak, E., Farley, C. H., and Desimone, P. A.,** Familial thrombosis due to antithrombin III deficiency, *Blood*, 43, 219, 1974.
44. **Johansson, L., Hedner, U., and Nilsson, I. M.,** Familial antithrombin III deficiencies as pathogenesis of deep venous thrombosis, *Acta Med. Scand.*, 204, 491, 1978.
45. **Van der Meer, J., Stoepman-Van Dalen, E. A., and Jansen, J. M.,** Antithrombin-III deficiency in a Dutch family, *J. Clin. Pathol.*, 26, 532, 1973.
46. **Nagy, I., Losonczy, H., Szaksz, I., Temesi, C., and Hergert, K.,** An analysis of clinical and laboratory data in patients with congenital antithrombin III (AT III) deficiency, *Acta Med. Acad. Sci. Hung.*, 36, 53, 1979.

47. **Stathakis, N. E., Papayannis, A. G., Antonopoulos, M., and Gardikas, C.,** Familial thrombosis due to antithrombin III deficiency in a Greek family, *Acta Haematol.*, 57, 47, 1977.
48. **Thout, C., Marion, D., and Boucher, H.,** Congenital antithrombin III deficiency: a study of a family from Quebec, *Union Med. Can.*, 57, 673, 1977.
49. **Leone, G., Valori, V. M., Storti, S., and Myers, T. J.,** Inferior vena cava thrombosis in a child with familial antithrombin III deficiency., *Thromb. Haemost.*, 1, 74, 1980.
50. **Schander, K., Niesen, M., Rehm, A., Budde, U., and Müller, N.,** Diagnose und Therapie eines kongenitalen Antithrombin-III-Mangels in der Neonatalperiode, in Fibrinolyse, Thrombose, Húmostase, Deutsch, E. and Lechner, K., Eds., Schattauer Verlag, Stuttgart, 1980, 483.
51. **Vomberg, P. P., Breederveld, C., Fleury, P., and Arts, W. F. M.,** Cerebral thromboembolism due to antithrombin III deficiency in two children, *Neuropediatrics*, 18, 42, 1987.
52. **Arko, F. R., Jewell, C. T., Dainer, P., and Macleod, W. A.,** Primary mesenteric vein thrombosis associated with antithrombin III deficiency, *J. Am. Med. Assoc.*, 242, 2324, 1979.
53. **Dayan, L., Donadio, D., David, E., and Huguet, M.,** Maladie thrombo-embolique familiale recidivante par deficit congenital en anti-thrombine III, *Nouv. Presse Med.*, 7, 3229, 1978.
54. **Fontcuberta, J., De Diego, I., Felez, J., Borrell, M., Elez, I., and Rutlant, M. L.,** Estudio clinico biologico de tres nuevas familias afectas de deficit congenito de AT-III. Utilizacion en un caso de concentrados de AT-III purificada., *Biol. Clin. Hematol.*, 4, 145, 1982.
55. **Gruenberg, J. C., Smallridge, R. C., and Rosenberg, R. D.,** Inherited antithrombin-III deficiency causing mesenteric venous infarction: a new clinical entity, *Ann. Surg.*, 1981, 791, 1975.
56. **Peters, T. G., Lewis, J. D., Filip, D. J., and Morris, L.,** Antithrombin III deficiency causing post-splenectomy mesenteric venous thrombosis coincident with thrombocytopenia, *Ann. Surg.*, 185, 229, 1977.
57. **Wilson, C., Walker, I. D., Davidson, J. F., and Imrie, C. W.,** Mesenteric venous thrombosis and antithrombin III deficiency, *J. Clin. Pathol.*, 40, 906, 1987.
58. **Matsuo, T., Ohki, Y., Kondo, S., and Matsuo, O.,** Familial antithrombin III deficiency in a Japanese family, *Thromb. Res.*, 16, 815, 1979.
59. **Gyde, O., Littler, W. A., and Stableforth, D. E.,** Familial antithrombin III deficiency, *Br. Med. J.*, 1, 508, 1978.
60. **Schoch, U., Zanetti, E., and Von Felten, A.,** Thromboembolieprophylaxe während der Schwangerschaft bei drei Schwestern mit kongenitalem Antithrombin III-Mangel und vermindert stimulierbarer Fibrionlyse. *Schweiz. Med. Wochshr.*, 117, 1807, 1987.
61. **Bjarke, B., Herin, P., and Blombäck, M.,** Neonatal aortic thrombosis. A possible clinical manifestation of congenital antithrombin III deficiency, *Acta Paediatr. Scand.*, 63, 297, 1974.
62. **Shapiro, M. E., Rodvien, R., Bauer, K. A., and Salzman, E. W.,** Acute aortic thrombosis in antithrombin III deficiency, *J. Am. Med. Assoc.*, 245, 1759, 1981.
63. **Hall, J. G., Pauli, R. M., and Wilson, K. M.,** Maternal and fetal sequelae of anticoagulation during pregnancy, *Am. J. Med.*, 68, 122, 1980.
64. **Hellgren, M., Tengborn, L., and Abildgaard, U.,** Pregnancy in women with congenital antithrombin III deficiency: experience of treatment with heparin and antithrombin, *Gynecol. Obstet. Invest.*, 14, 127, 1982.
65. **Conard, J., Horellou, M. H., Van Dreden, P., and Samama, M.,** Pregnancy and congenital deficiency in antithrombin III or protein C, *Thromb. Haemost.*, 58, 39, 1987.
66. **Winter, J. H., Fenech, A., Ridley, W., Bennett, B., Cumming, A. M., Mackie, M., and Douglas, A. S.,** Familial antithrombin III deficiency, *Quarter. J. Med.*, 204, 373, 1982.
67. **Brandt, P.,** Observations during the treatment of antithrombin III deficient women with heparin and antithrombin concentrate during pregnancy, parturition, and abortion, *Thromb. Res.*, 22, 15, 1981.
68. **Samson, D., Stirling, Y., Woolf, L., Howarth, D., Seghatchian, M. J., and De Chazal, R.,** Management of planned pregnancy in a patient with congenital antithrombin III deficiency, *Br. J. Haematol.*, 56, 243, 1984.
69. **Tengborn, L. and Bengtsson, T.,** Antithrombin III concentrate. Thromboprophylaxis during pregnancy in a patient with congenital antithrombin III deficiency, *Acta Obstet. Gynecol. Scand.*, 65, 375, 1986.
70. **Massignon, D., Pegaz-Fiornet, M., and Coeur, P.,** Therapy carried out in pregnancy in a patient with congenital antithrombin III deficiency and complicated by preeclamptic toxaemia. Congenital antithrombin III deficiency and pregnancy, *J. Gynecol. Obstet. Biol. Reprod.*, 15, 299, 1986.
71. **Letsky, E. A.,** Coagulation Problems During Pregnancy, Churchill Livingstone, London, 1985, 51.
72. **Michiels, J. J., Stibbe, J., Vellenga, E., and Van Vliet, H. H. D. M.,** Prophylaxis of thrombosis in antithrombin III deficient women during pregnancy and delivery, *Eur. J. Obstet. Gynecol. Reprod. Biol.*, 18, 149, 1984.
73. **Olsson, P.,** Variations in antithrombin activity in plasma after major surgery, *Acta Chir. Scand.*, 126, 24, 1963.
74. **Collins, G. J., Barber, J. A., Zajtchuk, R., Vanek, D., and Malogne, L. A.,** The effects of operative stress on the coagulation profile, *Am. J. Surg.*, 133, 612, 1977.

75. **Andersson, T. R., Berner, N. S., Larsen, M. L., Ødegard, O. R., and Abildgaard, U.,** Plasma heparin cofactor II, protein C and antithrombin in elective surgery, *Acta Chir. Scand.*, 153, 291, 1987.
76. **Zucker, M. L., Metz, J., and Gomperts, E. D.,** Inherited antithrombin III deficiency as a cause of multiple venous thrombosis, *S. Afr. Med. J.*, 49, 1425, 1975.
77. **Thaler, E., Niesser, H., Kleinberger, G., and Gassmer, A.,** Antithrombin III replacement therapy in patients with congenital and acquired antithrombin III deficiency, *Thromb. Haemostas.*, 42, 327, 1979.
78. **Müller, N., Budde, U., Schander, K., Niesen, M., and Etzel, F.,** Preoperative substitutive therapy in a family with congenital antithrombin III deficiency, *Blut,* 40, 70, 1980.
79. **Hambley, H., Davidson, J. F., Walker, I. D., and Menzies, T.,** Prophylactic use of antithrombin III concentrate following surgery in congenital antithrombin III deficiency, *Clin. Lab. Haematol.*, 9, 27, 1987.
80. **Marciniak, E. and Gockerman, J. P.,** Heparin-induced decrease in circulating antithrombin III, *Lancet,* 2, 581, 1977.
81. **Nielsen, L. E., Bell, W. R., Borkon, A. M., and Neill, C. A.,** Extensive thrombus formation with heparin resistance during extracorporeal circulation, *Arch. Intern. Med.*, 147, 149, 1987.
82. **Fischer, A.-M., Gazenzel, C., Dautzenberg, M.-D., Benhammo, J., Béguin, S., and Vergoz, D.,** A new case of abnormal antithrombin III (AT III): biological characteristics and thromboembolic accidents management, *Thromb. Haemost.*, 50, 358, 1983.
83. **Winter, J. H., Fenech, A., Mackie, M., Bennett, B., and Douglas, A. S.,** Treatment of venous thrombosis in antithrombin III deficient patients with concentrates of antithrombin III, *Clin. Lab. Haematol.*, 4, 101, 1982.
84. **Bick, R. L.,** Clinical relevance of antithrombin III, *Sem. Thromb. Hemost.*, 8, 276, 1982.
85. **Ten Cate, J. W.,** Antithrombin III: clinical significance, *Acta Chir. Scand.*, 509, 101, 1982.
86. **Damus, P. S. and Wallace, G. A.,** Immunologic measurement of antithrombin III-heparin cofactor and alpha 2-macroglobulin in disseminated intravascular coagulation and hepatic failure coagulopathy, *Thromb. Res.*, 6, 27, 1975.
87. **Hellgren, M., Egberg, N., and Eklund, J.,** Blood coagulation and fibrinolytic factors and their inhibitors in critically ill patients, *Intensive Care Med.*, 10, 23, 1984.
88. **Smith-Erichsen, N., Aasen, A. O., Gallimore, M. J., and Amundsen, E.,** Studies of components of the coagulation systems in normal individuals and septic shock patients, *Circ. Shock,* 9, 491, 1982.
89. **Thaler, E.,** Disseminierte intravaskuläre Gerinnung: antithrombin III und Heparin, *Folia Haematol.*, 104, 740, 1977.
90. **Minna, J. D.,** Disseminated Intravascular Coagulation in man, Charles C. Thomas, Springfield, IL, 1974.
91. **Österud, B. and Björklid, E.,** Human factor VII associated with endotoxin stimulated monocytes in whole blood, *Biochem. Biophys. Res. Commun.*, 108, 620, 1982.
92. **Sakata, Y., Yoshida, N., Matsuda, M., and Aoki, N.,** Treatment of DIC with antithrombin III concentrates, *Bibl. Haematol. Basel,* 49, 307, 1983.
93. **Breddin, H. K., Kirchmaier, C. M., and Bender, N.,** Antithrombin III deficiency and antithrombin III-substitution in intensive care patients, in Proc. VIII Int. Congr. Thromb., Istanbul, 1984, 26.
94. **Von Waltraud, E., Töpfer, G., Dornheim, G., Seifert, A., Schmidt, L. A., Senger, C., Funke, U., and Schulze, M.,** Antithrombin III-Substitution bei Verbrauchskoagulopathie, *Klin. Med.*, 42, 1319, 1987.
95. **Von Svendsen, J., Jespersen, J., and Skjøldt, T.,** Adult respiratory distress syndrome, *Fortschr. Röntgenstr.*, 145, 205, 1986.
96. **Hanada, T., Abe, T., and Takita, H.,** Antithrombin III concentrates for treatment of disseminated intravascular coagulation in children, *Am. J. Pediatr. Hematol. Oncol.*, 7, 3, 1985.
97. **Von Kries, R., Stannigel, H., and Göbel, U.,** Anticoagulant therapy by continous heparin-antithrombin III infusion in newborns with disseminated intravascular coagulation, *Eur. J. Pediatr.*, 144, 191, 1985.
98. **Potron, G., Leroux, B., Droulle, C., Santepne, B., and Poynard, A.,** Efficiency of antithrombin treatment in newborn infants with respiratory distress syndrome, *Thromb. Haemost.*, 50, 48, 1983.
99. **Bjorvatn, B., Bjertnaes, L., Fadnes, H. O., Flaegstad, T., Gutteberg, T. J., Kristiansen, B. E., Pape, J., Rekvig, O. P., Osterud, B., and Aanderud, L.,** Meningococcal septicaemia treated with combined plasmapheresis and leucapheresis or with blood exchange, *Br. Med. J.*, 288, 439, 1984.
100. **Blauhut, B., Kramar, H., Vinazzer, H., and Bergmann, N. H.,** Substitution of antithrombin III in shock and DIC: a randomized study, *Thromb. Res.*, 39, 81, 1985.
101. **Brandt, P., Jespersen, J., and Gregersen, G.,** Post-partum haemolytic-uraemic syndrome treated with antithrombin III, *Nephron,* 27, 15, 1981.
102. **Büller, H. R., Weenik, A. H., Treffers, P. E., Kahlé, L. H., Otten, H. A., and Ten Cate, J. W.,** Severe antithrombin III deficiency in a patient with pre-eclampsia. Observations on the effect of human AT III concentrate transfusion, *Scand. J. Haematol.*, 25, 81, 1980.
103. **Haak, H. L., Stolk, J. C., Gratama, J. W., Van Hulsteyn, H., and Briet, E.,** Use of antithrombin concentrate in stable diffuse intravascular coagulation, *Acta Haematol.*, 68, 28, 1982.

104. **Hellgren, M., Hägnevik, K., Robbe, H., Björk, O., Blombäck, M., and Eklund, J.,** Severe acquired antithrombin III deficiency in relation to hepatic and renal insufficiency and intrauterine fetal death in late pregnancy, *Gynecol. Obstet. Invest.*, 16, 107, 1983.

105. **Jespersen, J., Rasmussen, N. R., and Toftgaard, C.,** Observations during the treatment with antithrombin-III concentrate of a case of tampon-related toxic shock syndrome and disseminated intravascular coagulation. Discrepancies between functional and immunologic determinations of antithrombin, *Thromb. Res.*, 26, 457, 1982.

106. **Laursen, B., Mortensen, J. Z., Frost, L., and Hansen, K. B.,** Disseminated intravascular coagulation in hepatic failure treated with antithrombin III, *Thromb. Res.*, 22, 701, 1981.

107. **Mosvold, J., Abildgaard, U., Jenssen, H., and Andersen, R.,** Low antithrombin III in acute hepatic failure at term, *Scand. J. Haematol.*, 29, 48, 1982.

108. **Weenink, G. H., Büller, H. R., Ten Cate, J. W., Smorenberg-Schoorl, M. E., Schutte, M. F., and Treffers, P. E.,** Severely impaired hemostasis in a pre-eclamptic patient successfully treated with human AT III concentrate and platelet transfusion, in Studies on Antithrombin III and Human Antithrombin III Concentrate Transfusion, Büller, H. R., Ed., Thesis, Wilhelmina Gasthuis, Amsterdam, 1980.

109. **Hellgren, M., Robbe, H., Hägnevik, K., and Faxelius, G.,** Antithrombin as adjuvant in the treatment of acquired antithrombin deficiency during pregnancy and delivery, IV World Congr. Int. Soc. The Study of Hypertension in Pregnancy, Amsterdam, 1984; Abstr. 152.

110. **Maki, M., Terao, T., Ikenoue, T., Takemura, T,. Sekiba, K., Shirakawa, K., and Soma, H.,** Clinical evaluation of antithrombin III concentrate for disseminated intravascular coagulation in obstetrics. Well-controlled multicenter trial, *Gynecol. Obstet. Invest.*, 23, 230, 1987.

111. **McGehee, W. G., Paul, R. H., and Feinstein, D. I.,** Antithrombin III concentrate in the management of patients with acute fatty liver of pregnancy, *Blood,* 66, 282a, 1985.

112. **Medén-Britth, G. and Teien, A. N.,** Infusion of purified antithrombin III to patients with fracture of the neck of the femur, *Eur. Surg. Res.*, 2, 289, 1979.

113. **Kesteven, P. J., Ahmed, A., Williams, B. T., and Savidge, G. F.,** Antithrombin III concentrates in cardiopulmonary bypass, *Thromb. Haemost.*, 54, 89, 1985.

114. **Biland, L., Duckert, F., Prisender, S., and Nyman, D.,** Quantitative estimation of coagulation factors in liver disease. The diagnostic value of Factor XIII, Factor V and plasminogen, *Thromb. Haemost.*, 39, 646, 1978.

115. **Schipper, H. G., Kahlé, L. H., Jenkins, C. S., and Ten Cate, J. W.,** Antithrombin III-transfusion in disseminated intravascular coagulation, *Lancet,* 1, 854, 1978.

116. **Schipper, H. G. and Ten Cate, J. W.,** Antithrombin III transfusion in patients with hepatic cirrhosis, *Br. J. Haematol.*, 52, 25, 1982.

117. **Boyer, C., Wolf, M., Lavergne, J. M., Haiat, A., Declere, A., Franco, D., and Larrieu, M. J.,** Prevention of disseminated intravascular coagulation after LeVeen peritoneovenous shunts by infusions of AT III concentrate, in Proc. Sixth Int. Congr. on Thrombosis of the Mediterranean League against Thromboembolic Disease, Monte Carlo, 1980.

118. **Büller, H. R. and Ten Cate, J. W.,** Antithrombin III infusion in patients undergoing peritoneovenous shunt operation: failure in the prevention of disseminated intravascular coagulation, *Thromb. Haemost.*, 49, 128, 1983.

119. **Korninger, C., Klepetko, W., Miholic, J., Schwarz, C., and Lechner, K.,** Randomized trial of antithrombin III versus placebo in patients undergoing peritoneovenous shunt operation, *Thromb. Haemost.*, 58, 426, 1987.

120. **Thaler, E., Balzar, E., Kopsa, H., and Pinggera, W. F.,** Acquired antithrombin III deficiency in patients with glomerular proteinuria, *Haemostasis,* 7, 257, 1978.

121. **Kauffman, R. H., Veltkamp, J. J., Van Tilburg, N. H., and Van Es, L. A.,** Acquired antithrombin III deficiency and thrombosis in the nephrotic syndrome, *Am. J. Med.*, 65, 607, 1978.

122. **Schramm, W.,** Thromboembolie die klinische Bedeutung des Antithrombin III, *Internist,* 25, 88, 1984.

123. **Schrader, J., Köstering, H., Kramer, P., and Scheler, F.,** Antithrombin-III-Substitution bei dialyspflichtiger Niereninsuffizienz, *Deutsch. Med. Wochenschr.*, 107, 1847, 1982.

124. **Roth, B., Von Lilien, T., Busch, B., Gillor, A., and Bulla, M.,** Deficiency of antithrombin III in children with hemolytic-uremic syndrome, *Eur. J. Pediatr.*, 142, 16, 1984.

125. **Blombäck, B., Blombäck, M., Lagergren, H., and Olsson, P.,** The heparin cofactor activity in plasma and its relation to the anticoagulant effect of intravenously injected heparin, *Acta Physiol. Scand.*, 58, 306, 1963.

126. **Conard, J., Barbier, P., and Samama, M.,** Automated amidolytic method for AT III determination, *Thromb. Haemost.*, 42, 1350, 1979.

127. **Pitney, W. R., Phadke, K. P., and Dean, S.,** Antithrombin III deficiency during asparaginase therapy, *Lancet,* 1, 493, 1980.

128. **Alkjaersig, N., Fletcher, A., and Burstein, R.,** Association between oral contraceptive use and thromboembolism: a new approach to its investigation based on plasma fibrinogen chromatography, *Am. J. Obstet. Gynecol.*, 199, 1975.
129. **Bounameaux, H., Duckert, F., Walter, M., and Bounameaux, Y.,** The determination of antithrombin III. Comparison of six methods. Effect of oral contraceptive therapy, *Thromb. Haemost.*, 39, 607, 1978.
130. **Sagar, S., Thomas, D. P., Stamatakis, J. D., and Kakkar, V. V.,** Oral contraceptives, antithrombin III activity and postoperative deep-vein thrombosis, *Lancet*, 1, 509, 1976.
131. **Buchanan, G. R. and Holtkamp, C. A.,** Reduced antithrombin III levels during L-asparaginase therapy, *Med. Pediatr. Oncol.*, 8, 7, 1980.
132. **Jordan, V. C., Fritz, N. F., and Tormey, D. C.,** Long-term adjuvant therapy with tamoxifen: effects on sex hormone binding globulin and antithrombin III, *Cancer Res.*, 47, 4517, 1987.
133. **Zaunschirm, A. and Muntean,** Correction of hemostatic inbalance induced by L-asparaginase therapy in children with acute lymphoblastic leukemia, *Pediatr. Haematol. Oncol.*, 3, 19, 1986.
134. **Wenzel, E., Von Blohm, G., Hellstern, P., and Miyashita, C.,** Importance of acquired AT III deficiency and monitoring of AT III substitution therapy, Abstract, VIII Int. Congr. on Thromb., Istanbul, 1984.
135. **Vinazzer, H.,** Clinical use of antithrombin III concentrates, *Vox Sang.*, 53, 193, 1987.

Chapter 6

HEPARIN COFACTOR II: STRUCTURE, FUNCTION, AND CLINICAL IMPORTANCE

Helmut Vinazzer

TABLE OF CONTENTS

I. INTRODUCTION

In 1967, a heparin cofactor activity was described in addition to antithrombin III (AT-III), which had a slower electrophoretic mobility at pH 8.6.[1] A better separation of the two activities could be obtained by a different author at pH 7.4.[2] The protein with a faster anodal migration (apparently AT-III) was active also in the absence of heparin and diminished during the process of coagulation. The other thrombin inhibitor migrated more slowly to the anode and required heparin for the inactivation of thrombin. A similar observation was made in 1974 when the two substances with antithrombin activities were separated by DEAE cellulose chromatography.[3,4] An apparently identical substance was found independently by two authors and was called antithrombin binding moderately (ATBM) and Heparin cofactor II (HC II), respectively.[5,6] This substance was isolated and was thoroughly examined by different research groups.

II. ISOLATION AND IDENTIFICATION OF HC II

One group observed that during the purification of AT-III, only about 70% of the total antithrombin activity was bound to a heparin-sepharose column.[5] When the conditions were changed to a lower ionic strength of the equilibration buffer, two separate peaks of AT activity could be identified. When the concentration of the buffer used for equilibration of the heparin-sepharose and for the sample application was reduced to 10 mmol/1 phosphate at pH 7.8, two distinct peaks with AT activity were found after elution with a phosphate-NaCl gradient. The first one which eluted at a low salt concentration was different from AT-III. This second antithrombin was isolated from Cohn fraction IV by adsorption to aluminum hydroxyde, elution, fractionation of the eluates by ammonium sulphate precipitation, and chromatography on a heparin-sepharose column. The two AT activities were again eluted from the column at different ionic strengths. The fractions containing the second AT were precipitated with ammonium sulphate and redissolved in Tris pH 8.0.

When polyacrylamide gel electrophoresis was carried out on the two AT activities, a heterogenous glycoside moiety was found which was removed by treatment with endoglucosidase D. The remaining protein had a molecular weight of about 70 kD as determined in this system. The purified substance was also used to raise sheep antibodies against this human protein. The sheep antiserum obtained did not cross-react with AT-III, but showed a strong precipitation with the other AT. The purified protein had practically no influence on the inactivation of thrombin. In this respect, it clearly had a behavior different from AT-III. When heparin was added to the reaction mixture, thrombin inactivation occurred depending on the concentration of heparin and on the duration of incubation. A final heparin concentration of 3.17 IU/ml in the reaction mixture was found to have a maximum effect after 20 min preincubation time. In contrast, AT-III had a maximum effect after 5 min incubation with 0.018 IU/ml heparin. Since the new protein only bound moderately to heparin when compared with AT-III binding, the substance was called antithrombin binding moderately (ATBM) by the authors. When the interaction of ATBM with different serine proteases was examined and compared with that of AT-III, it was found that in the presence of heparin, ATBM only inactivated thrombin, but not factor Xa, plasmin, or trypsin. The inactivation of human thrombin was considerably more pronounced than the inactivation of bovine thrombin. Assays of ATBM and AT-III in different plasma samples showed that up to 40% of the total antithrombin activity was a consequence of the action of ATBM.

On purified ATBM, the amino acid composition was determined and compared with AT-III.[7] Though there were many similarities, it was evident that ATBM contained about twice as much histidine and tryptophan as AT-III. Amino acid sequencing of both proteins was carried out near the N-terminal end, and the first 24 amino acids were determined as follows:

ATBM: Gly-Ser-Lys-Gly-Pro-Leu-Asp-Gln-Leu-Glu-Lys-Gly-
AT-III: His-Gly-Ser-Pro-Val-Asp-Ile-Cys-Thr-Ala-Lys-Pro-
ATBM: Gly-Glu-Thr-Ala-Gln-Ser-Ala-Asp-Pro-Gln-Trp-Glu . . .
AT-III: Arg-Asp-Ile-Pro-Met-Asn-Pro-Met-Cys-Ile-Tyr-Arg . . .

Therefore, the N-terminal amino acid sequence of ATBM has no similarities to that of AT-III. ATBM was also found to contain more polar and acidic amino acid residues than the corresponding N-terminal sequence of AT-III.

A different approach was carried out by another group of authors.[8] Purification of the protein from plasma was achieved by fractionation with polyethylene glycol 6000 after adsorption with Al $(OH)_3$ and elution. This was followed by chromatography on QAE-Sephadex A-50, on heparin-sepharose 4B, and on Sephadex G-150. After elution with 280 mmol/l NaCl, AT-III was removed by immunoadsorption. The purified second antithrombin (HC II) had a molecular weight of 66.5 KD on SDS-PAGE and of 62.1 KD in the ultracentrifuge. Antibodies against HC II were raised in rabbits and were made monospecific by immunoadsorption on HC II-free plasma linked to Sepharose 4B.

An almost identical protein was obtained in the following way: total RNA was isolated from human liver biopsy material. After purification, RNA was used for cloning cDNA, which was then synthesized using *E. coli* HB101. From the cDNA library which was thereby obtained, a 2.1-kb cDNA clone was isolated which represented a protease inhibitor and which was called human Leuserpin 2 (hLS2). The purified substance was a single chain protein which consisted of 480 amino acids. Sequencing of this protein was carried out and was compared with the amino acid sequences of AT-III, HC II (ATBM), antitrypsin, and antichymotrypsin. There was a total identity of the first 24 amino acids at the N-terminal end of hLS2m ATBM and HC II. Comparison with the 36 amino acids of HC II at the COOH-terminal end resulted in these identities:

445 450 455
HC II: Ser-Thr-Gln-Val-Arg-Phe-Thr-Val-Asp-ARg-Pro-Phe-Leu-Phe-
hLS2: Ser-Thr-Gln-Val-ARg-Phe-Thr-Val-Asp-Arg-Pro-Phe-Leu-Phe-
460 465 470
HC II: Leu-Ile-Tyr-Glu-His-Pro-Thr-Ser-Thr-Leu-Leu-Phe-Met-Gly-
hLS2: Leu-Ile-Tyr-Glu-His-Arg-Thr-Ser-Cys-Leu-Leu-Phe-Met-Gly-
475 480
HC II: Arg-Val-Ala-Asn-Pro-Ser-Arg-Gln
hLS2: Arg-Val-Ala-Asn-Pro-Ser-Arg-Ser

Out of the 36 amino acids determined at the COOH-terminal end, 33 were identical with HC II/ATBM. There was a serine residue at the reactive site in position 445 of both inhibitors. An important difference, however, was a cystein residue in position 467 of hLS2, while a threonine residue was in the same position of HC II. Since cystein residues can form disulfide bridges which may be of importance for the activation by heparin, this difference may also have functional consequences. On the other hand, the possibility of an allele of HC II cannot be excluded as long as the complete amino acid sequence of HC II is not yet known and the question as to whether HC II also has an internal disulfide bond is still open. It could also be that HC II and hLS2 derive from different loci, which is also the case in other members of the alpha-interferon gene family.

As far as can be seen from the data presently available, HC II and ATBM are identical, and hLS2 may be either closely related to HC II or could also be an allele.

The heparin-binding site of HC II was examined by a different technique and was compared with that of AT-III.[10] Spleen cells from mice immunized against human AT-III were fused with SP-2 myeloma cells. An IgG monoclonal antibody derived from clone 109-F6 by limited dilution selectively inhibited the expression of purified AT-III/heparin cofactor activity in a heparin-catalyzed-binding assay for thrombin inhibition. The activity of human plasma AT-III was similarly inhibited by this antibody. After derivatization of the AT-III molecule by a tryptophane modifying reagent (dimethyl sulfonium bromide), the molecule did not react with the antibody any longer. When AT-III deficient plasma was added to this system, the antibody inhibited the activity of HC II, indicating structural homology at the heparin-binding site of the two inhibitors.

III. PROPERTIES AND ACTIVATION OF HC II

When the stability of HC II was examined, it was found to be stable for 2 weeks at 4°C and for 3 days at 37°C, but was destroyed within 10 min at 56°C.[11] During coagulation, little HC II was consumed and about 92% of the plasma activity was found in serum, whereas 40 to 50% of the AT-III activity is consumed during coagulation. The addition of heparin had little effect on the consumption of HC II, but increased the consumption of AT-III. Dermatan sulphate had no effect on the consumption of AT-III, but caused a considerable increase of the HC II consumption during coagulation. In cases of DIC, the HC II levels were as low as the AT-III levels which was ascribed to intravascular consumption probably accelerated by glycosaminoglycans of the vascular wall.

The turnover rate of HC II was determined in baboons and was compared with that of AT-III.[12] For this purpose, purified human AT-III and HC II were labeled with ^{131}I and ^{125}I, respectively, and were injected into nine animals. A placebo group was compared with two groups which, in addition received heparin (500 IU/kg) or Pentosan polysulfate (5 mg/kg). The half-life in the placebo group was between 1.95 and 2.33 d for AT-III, and between 1.96 and 2.21 d for HC II. There was no significant difference in the half-life when the animals had received heparin or Pentosan polysulfate (PPS). The same authors also examined the turnover of HC II in healthy volunteers.[13] Purified HC II was labeled with ^{125}I and was injected into three volunteers. Measurements of radioactivity showed a maximum after 2 min and rapid loss of about 10% of the activity within the first hour. This was followed by a slow process of equilibration within 2 d. The fast initial decrease was thought to be due to the presence of a third compartment, possibly the vascular endothelium, or to impurities which could, however, not be detected in plasma. The half-life of HC II was found to be 2.53 d and was, therefore, somewhat longer that the half-life of human HC II in baboons. A bulk of 92 to 95% of the entire radioactivity was found to migrate with HC II when SDS-PAGE analysis was applied. The activity was seen in a single protein band with an apparent molecular weight of 72 KD.

Inactivation of HC II was found to occur in the presence of activated polymorphnuclear leucocytes.[14] When these cells were activated by phorbol myristate acetate, they rapidly inactivated HC II. This process was depending on the concentration of leucocytes in the mixture. The half-life of HC II was between 1 min and 5 min. Resting polymorphnuclear leucocytes were considerably less active than activated cells. Inactivation occurred by proteolysis as could be determined by SDS-PAGE. HC II of 76 KD was first degraded into a 62 KD peptide which still retained full activity. This was further degraded into a series of peptides of 54 KD which were inactive. When HC II was labeled with ^{125}I, there was no radioactivity in bands with a molecular weight higher than 76 KD, indicating that complexes between HC II and the proteolytic substance from leucocytes do not form. Activated leucocytes also degraded AT-III, but more slowly than HC II. In the presence of heparin, HC II was partially protected from degradation, but AT-III was more rapidly inactivated. Dermatan sulphate did not influence the rate of inactivation of HC II or AT-III. It was assumed that *in vivo* HC II is only active in the vicinity of glycosaminoglycans (GAGs). In the case of local inflammation, decaying polymorphnuclear leukocytes can inhibit HC II and could, thereby, possibly add to the formation of local thrombosis.

A similar degradation of HC II was found when the substance was exposed to Proteinase I from Echis carinatus venom.[15] In this case, there was also a primary formation of an intermediary protein of a molecular weight of 62 KD with full activity, followed by further degradation to inactive 54 KD fragments. This work could show that leucine was at the reactive site of HC II, probably in position 25. Crude *Echis carinatus* venom inactivated HC II only in the presence of calcium.[16] The initial rate of inactivation increased proportionally with the addition of heparin. There was no inactivation and no influence of heparin when calcium was absent. When the fraction Proteinase I was used instead of the crude venom, there occurred also inactivation of HC II, but this process was not influenced by heparin. It was, therefore, assumed that two different proteinases in the venom can inactivate HC II.

Activation of HC II was carried out by different methods. Some authors used unfractioned standard heparin. In an experimental model, AT-III deficiency was simulated by the immunodepletion of human plasma (containing HC II, but no AT-III), which was mixed in different relations with defibrinated plasma containing both inhibitors.[17] Different concentrations of heparin ranging from 0.05 IU/ml to 0.125 IU/ml were added, and the inhibition of 0.75 NIH units of thrombin was measured. It was found that all the thrombin was inhibited in defibrinated plasma as well as in AT-III-deficient plasma. When, however, defibrinated plasma was diluted with buffer instead of AT-III deficient plasma, there was a progressive decrease of thrombin inhibition. This showed that at low concentrations of thrombin and heparin, HC II is a potent thrombin inhibitor.

In a different experiment, various fractions of standard heparin were prepared and were examined for their ability to activate AT-III and HC II.[18] Low-affinity (LA) and high-affinity (HA) heparin fractions were obtained by chromatography on heparin sepharose. In the presence of purified AT-III, the HA fraction was fifteen fold more active than the LA fraction, but in the presence of purified HC II, the activity was the same. When heparin was fractioned according to its molecular weight, the activities of both inhibitors increased with an increase of the molecular weight. However, at a molecular weight of less than 6 KD, there was no increase of the antithrombin activity of AT-III but a weak activation of HC II. It was assumed that AT-III and HC II do not compete for the same molecular species of standard heparin.

In another trial, heparin and fractions of different molecular weights showed a concentration-dependent stimulation of AT-III and HC II.[19] At a concentration of 0.3×10^{-6} mol/l heparin and fractions of molecular weights below 16.5 KD, a peak stimulation of HC II was found. The maximum rate of the peak decreased with decreasing molecular weight. HMW heparin fractions showed a twofold higher peak at a tenfold lower concentration. A pentasaccharide with a high affinity for AT-III had no influence on the activation of HC II. It was concluded that a higher molecular weight of heparin has a higher binding affinity for the inhibitor.

The influence of the ionic strength and pH was also examined.[20] For these test series, standard heparin of an average molecular weight of 16 KD was used. The affinity of HC II for heparin was greatest at a pH between 7.0 and 8.0, and decreased at pH 6.0. The optimum ionic strength was 0.40, and there was less HC II binding to thrombin when the ionic strength was increased to 0.80. The activation of HC II could also be carried out with heparinoids and with different natural GAGs. Already in 1976, the observation was made that Dermatan sulphate (DS), a GAG of the vascular endothelium, had an inhibitory effect on the amidolytic activity of thrombin, but not of factor Xa.[21] At concentrations which had an effect on the prolongation of the activated partial thromboplastin time (APTT), no acceleration of the AT III activity was found. It was, therefore, assumed that the anticoagulant effect of DS is not mediated via AT-III and differs in this respect from the anticoagulant activity of heparin. By another group, DS was fractioned according to its molecular size by gel chromatography on ultrogel AC 44; the fractions were characterized by sulphur content and by molecular weight.[22] Furthermore, methyl esters of the unfractioned DS were prepared by activation of the carboxyl groups and reaction with methanol. The HC II activity was increasing with increasing molecular weights and was abolished by esterification of the carboxyl groups. HC II activation by a heparinoid containing DS (ORG 10172) was also tested.[23] This substance also increased HC II activity, but not to the same extent as heparin or DS. In this experiment, a nonlinear decrease of activity was observed with increasing ionic strength. The potentiating action of heparin, of various heparin fractions, of DS, and of ORG 10172 on AT-III and on HC II was also examined.[24] In these tests, the inhibition of thrombin generation *in vitro* was studied. It was found that heparin, LMW heparin, Fragmin,® and HA ORG 10172 potentiate AT-III stronger than HC II. A reverse activation was observed with DS and with LA ORG 10172. Nonfractioned ORG 10172 had a low AT activity which was mainly mediated via HC II. Competition of heparin and other GAGs with immobilized heparin was examined.[25] It was found that there was a dependence of binding capacity on size, degree of sulphation, and backbone structure of the GAGs. Unfractioned heparin inhibited the binding of AT-III to immobilized heparin. This inhibition was destroyed by N-desulphation. LMW heparins and heparin sulphate also contain AT-III binding sequences, but at a lower rate than heparin. The affinity of HC II increased with heparin chain length. Binding was largely mediated by sulphate residues. HC II bound to HS and DS with a lower affinity than to heparin, while binding of HC II to dextran sulphate was mainly dependent on the molecular weight. The affinity of HC II for a sulphated polymer appeared to be dependent on the chain length and on the density of sulphation.

Other experiments with dextran sulphate and chondroitin polysulphates resulted in activation of both AT-III and HC II, whilst DS only activated HC II.[26] When another heparinoid, pentosan polysulphate (PPS), was studied, normal plasma and AT-III-depleted plasma were mixed with PPS and, for comparison, also with heparin and DS, respectively.[27] In the heparin samples of normal plasma, about 90% of the thrombin inactivating power was lost by AT-III depletion. After activation with DS, the thrombin inhibiting activity diminished only by 17% and after activation with PPS, by 23%. It was, therefore, assumed that the inactivation of thrombin by the addition of PPS to plasma is mainly achieved by the activation of HC II. This could also be shown after purification of HC II. The pure substance was activated by PPS, and the degree of thrombin inhibition was depending on the concentration of PPS and reached an optimum at 30 μg/ml. Inhibition of thrombin by HC II was found to increase up to 760-fold with heparin and up to 1280-fold with PPS.

PPS was also fractioned into molecules of different sizes.[28] The unfractioned heparinoid had an average molecular weight of 4.5 KD. A HMW fraction of PPS had considerably more activating power on HC II than unfractioned PPS, whilst a LMW fraction was inactive. It was assumed that the antithrombin activity of PPS occurs to 80% via HC II and only to 20% via AT-III. This action of PPS was also shown by a different method.[29] Purified HC II was labeled with ^{125}I and added to plasma as a tracer; thereupon PPS was added and thrombin was generated by contact activation and calcium chloride. By this method, the complexes between thrombin and HC II could be quantitated when an SDS-PAGE was carried out. This method was extremely sensitive to low concentrations of PPS. The amount of 0.1 μg/ml, could still be determined which is ten times lower than the lowest possible concentration of PPS, which can be found by an APTT test.

It was also observed that commercially available DS frequently contains a minimal amount of heparin which activates AT-III in plasma. Thereby, an activity could be ascribed to HC II which, in reality, is an AT-III activation.[30] A concentration as small as 5×10^{-5} IU/ml heparin per μg of DS increases the thrombin inhibiting activity of plasma by 50%.

This amount of heparin is undetectable in a routine coagulation test and can only be measured by its anti-Xa activity. It is, therefore, recommended to examine commercial DS for anti-Xa potentiating activity which would interfere with experiments on HC II.

Another substance which exclusively activates HC II is phosvitin, a phosphoglycoprotein.[31] At an optimum concentration of 30 μg/ml, this protein enhances HC II activity about 1600-fold at pH 8.0. However, there are other polynucleotides which accelerate the HC II-thrombin reaction to a lesser degree. Activation can also be obtained by polyphosphate anions of a chain length between 5 and 100. Protamine-polyphosphate anions have lost the activity of HC II enhancement. None of these polyphosphates was effective in enhancing the reaction between thrombin and AT-III.

A physiological inhibition of the HC II activation could be observed too.[32] Histidine rich glycoprotein (HRG) has a strong affinity to heparin and interferes with the binding between heparin and AT-III. HRG also inhibits the activation of HC II by heparin as well as by DS. However, for the latter inhibition, a considerably higher concentration of HRG is required. It is assumed that HRG and antithrombin compete for heparin, but that the affinity of HRG to heparin is higher than its affinity to DS.

Inactivation of thrombin by activated HC II also depends on the species from which thrombin was obtained. By the aid of amidolytic tests, the observation was made that in cases of congenital AT-III deficiencies, about 20% higher residual AT-III activities were found when human thrombin was used instead of bovine thrombin.[33] This was thought to be due to a faster inactivation of human thrombin by HC II which, in this case, interfered with the AT-III assay. The same observation was also made by a different group.[34] This phenomenon was further elucidated after the immunoadsorption of human plasma which resulted in samples free of AT-III and HC II, respectively.[35] With these samples, the inactivation of human and bovine thrombin was studied. Human thrombin was found to undergo faster inactivation than bovine thrombin when HC II was activated by heparin. After an incubation time of 30 sec, 20% of the total antithrombin activity was achieved through HC II when human thrombin was used, but only 7% of the activity when bovine thrombin was in the reaction mixture.

The inactivation of thrombin by activated AT-III and HC II was also examined via the thrombin-platelet reaction.[36] After incubation of thrombin with AT-III or HC II in the presence of heparin, the amidolytic activity as well as platelet secretion were inhibited. There was also an inhibition of thrombin-induced platelet aggregation when thrombin was incubated with heparin, PPS, or DS in the presence of AT-III and HC II. When HC II was removed from this system, DS could not inhibit thrombin-induced platelet aggregation. Inhibition of serotonin release was achieved by heparin plus either AT-III or HC II, or by DS and HC II. PPS had a slight inhibitory effect on the release when AT-III and thrombin were present, but had a strong effect when HC II was a partner of the reaction.

From the present knowledge about HC II, the characteristics which could be determined of this protein are summarized in Table 1.

IV. ASSAYS OF HC II

There exist two main principles of HC II assays. By immunologic methods, such as rocket immunoelectrophoresis, using a monospecific antiserum against HC II, the concentration can be determined.[37] The method is specific, sensitive, and relatively simple. A certain disadvantage is the fact that immunologic methods only determine the concentration of the protein, but give no information about its physiologic activity. By this method, the normal concentration of HC II was between 61 and 82 μg/ml, and was, therefore, about one third of the normal concentration of AT-III.[13] Assays of HC II activity can be carried out by amidolytic methods. In all these methods, HC II is activated either by heparin or by

TABLE 1
Characteristics of HC II

1. HC II is a single-chain glycoprotein with a molecular weight of about 76 KD.
2. It consists of 480 amino acids.
3. The active site is between Lys 444 and Ser 445.
4. The concentration in plasma is 70 ± 10 μg/ml.
5. The activity in healthy persons varies between 60% and 180%.
6. The half-life in circulation is 60 h.
7. Its production occurs in the liver.
8. HC II requires activation by heparin or by GAGs.
9. Active HC II exclusively inhibits thrombin.
10. After activation, the reaction with thrombin is progressive.
11. HC II is not consumed during normal coagulation.
12. It is stable at 37°C for 3 d, but is destroyed at 56°C in 10 min.
13. It is rapidly degraded by activated polymorphnuclear leucocytes.
14. HC II is also destroyed by Echis carinatus venom.
15. Its physiological action is probably thrombin inhibition directly at the vessel wall after activation with DS from the endothelium.

DS. Thrombin is added to the reaction mixture and the residual thrombin activity is measured by the aid of a chromogenic substrate. In contrast to immunologic procedures, amidolytic methods measure the activity of HC II. The main problem of this type of assay was the simultaneous presence of AT-III in plasma. Any activation of AT-III would interfere with the validity of the assay. For this reason, two different types of assay methods were developed.

Since DS exclusively activates HC II and has no influence on AT-III activation, a method was developed which used DS as an activator.[38] The test plasma was diluted 1 in 100 with a dilution buffer of pH 8.0 and 50 mg/l DS was added. The thrombin inhibition of this mixture was measured with the substrate Chromozym TH. This method required an incubation time of 20 min. Though there was no activation of AT-III, an interference of non-activated AT-III in the reaction mixture was assumed. The results were compared with an identical procedure carried out with AT-III-depleted plasma. Comparison between the two methods showed that with activation by DS and without removal of AT-III, an overestimation of approximately 16% HC II resulted. The authors, therefore, removed AT-III from plasma by immunoaffinity chromatography against human AT-III linked to Sepharose 4B. After immunodepletion, the activity obtained with heparin and DS was identical. When human thrombin was used, the optimum incubation time with heparin activated HC II was 5 min compared to 20 min with DS. Furthermore, the authors found that 1% AT-III left in the reaction mixture resulted in an overestimation of the HC II activity of 3.3%. Since AT-III as well as HC II bind to thrombin at a molar ratio of 1:1, the experiment showed that the molar concentration of AT-III is 3.3 times higher than the concentration of HC II, which is in good agreement with the results of other authors.[13] For these reasons, assays of HC II were performed by these investigators after the heparin activation of AT-III depleted plasma. The optimum heparin concentration was 2.9 IU/ml. The normal range of HC II in 40 healthy persons was from 70% to 150%.

In series of experiments, the assay of HC II was simplified still further.[39] The principle was again an amidolytic assay of residual thrombin after the heparin activation of AT-III-depleted plasma. Depletion was, however, carried out by direct admixture of an IgG fraction from goats immunized against human AT-III. In a preliminary test of anti-Xa activity, it could be shown that 40μl of the antibody completely inhibited Xa inactivation of 50 μl-heparinized plasma. AT-III was fully inactivated after 60-sec incubation of plasma with the antibody at room temperature. There was no precipitation of the AT-III-antibody complex. By this method, the step of immunoadsorption on anti-AT-III sepharose could be omitted, which is an advantage for routine test. In contrast to heparin-activated AT-III, the inactivation

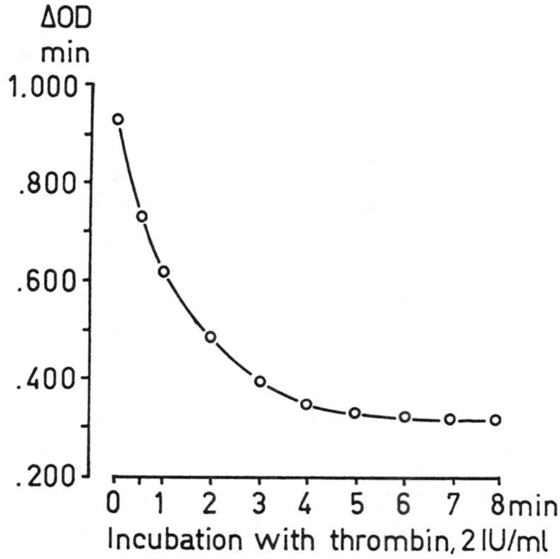

FIGURE 1. The inactivation of thrombin by HC II in the presence of heparin. The residual thrombin activities were measured by a chromogenic substrate (S-2238).

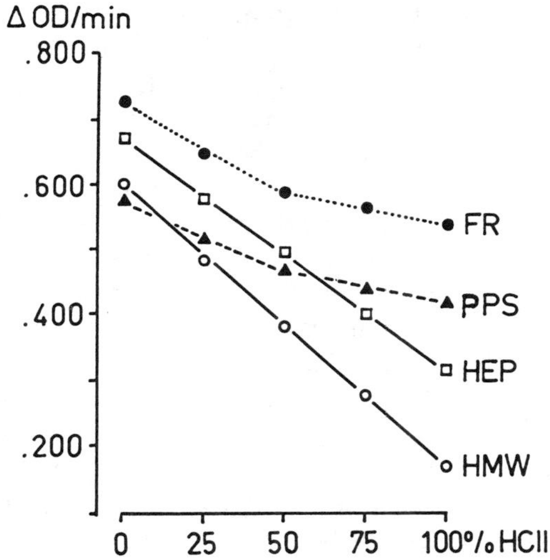

FIGURE 2. Activation of HC II by different heparin fractions and analoges. The experiments were performed as described in the test: Fragmin (●·····●) Pentosan Polysulphate (▲——▲), unfractioned heparin (-□—□-), and HMW heparin (-o—o—).

of thrombin by heparin-activated HC II is progressive. When bovine thrombin is used, an optimum inactivation is achieved after an incubation time of 5 min (Figure 1).

With this method, the influence of different heparin fractions and PPS was also examined (Figure 2). The figure shows that the highest activation of HC II was obtained with a HMW heparin fraction of an average molecular weight of 20 KD, followed by unfractioned heparin. When different concentrations of HC II were examined, there was a linear reaction between 0 and 100% HC II with standard heparin as well as with HMW heparin. A LMW heparin fragment (Fragmin®) showed a much weaker activation of HC II and was not linear. PPS showed a similar reaction as Fragmin, which was also not linear. For this reason, standard heparin was used in all further tests which were carried out in the following way: (All reagents were from the Antithrombin III kit by KABI, Stockholm. The anti-AT-III IgG was also a gift from KABI). The procedure of the method is shown in Table 2.

TABLE 2
Amidolytic Assay of HC II

1.	Citrate plasma, 50 μl
2.	AT III antibody, 50 μl
3.	Incubation at room temperature, 180 sec
4.	Buffer plus heparin (3 IU/ml), 900 μl
5.	Transfer into cuvette at 37°C, 200 μl
6.	Thrombin, bovine (2 IU/ml), 200 μl
7.	Incubation at 37°C, 300 sec
8.	S-2238 with polybrene, 200 μl
9.	Determine difference OD/min at 405 nm

The calibration curve was made with a plasma pool of 20 healthy individuals from which a series of further dilutions was carried out. With this method, the normal activities of HC II in 100 healthy persons was between 68% and 177% and, therefore, also showed a rather wide range as described earlier.

V. CLINICAL RESULTS OF HC II ASSAYS

After the detection of HC II and its properties, the clinical importance of this inhibitor was still unknown. Assays of HC II in different diseases, however, demonstrated that some acquired alterations of this protein existed. In 82 patients with chronic renal failure, there were normal AT-III activities, but significantly lower HC II activities than in normal persons.[40] There was a distinct difference between two groups of 12 patients each. One group had an average HC II activity of 63%, the other one of 96% before dialysis. These 24 patients were selected for further studies. Alterations of AT-III and HC II following dialysis were compared with the results obtained immediately before dialysis. Total protein was also determined in order to be able to compensate for hemoconcentration. Thereby, it was found that there was a moderate but significant drop of AT-III which was attributed to a loss by complexing of this inhibitor with heparin. On the other hand, there was a significant increase of HC II in the group which had a low HC II activity before dialysis. In the group with normal HC II, there was only a trend of an increase after dialysis. It was also noted that patients with a low HC II needed more heparin than patients with normal HC II. It was assumed that the low HC II in some patients was a consequence of the binding of HC II-heparin complexes to the endothelial cells, especially since such binding of heparin is known.[41] The increase of HC II after dialysis was thought to be due to the liberation from the endothelium.

In normal individuals, 15 cases of hereditary AT-III deficiencies and 15 cases of deep vein thromboses (DVT) HC II was found to be within a normal range which was between 63% and 132%[42] However, in eight cases of liver cirrhosis examined by the same authors, there was a diminution of HC II activity corresponding to the diminution of AT-III. A diminution of the HC II activity in liver cirrhosis was also described by other authors.[38,39] A very low HC II was found in a patient with septic shock which was even considerably lower than the AT-III activity of this patient, while in other cases of DIC, the diminution of HC II and AT-III were at the same level.[38]

The first cases of congenital HC II deficiencies were described in 1985. In one patient who had suffered cerebral thrombosis 2 years prior to the tests, there was a HC II activity of 47% and a concentration of 48%. It could, however, not be determined whether this HC II deficiency caused or contributed to the thrombotic episode since this patient also had a greatly prolonged euglobulin lysis time after venous occlusion, which is a well-known risk factor for thrombosis.[43] Another author examined 120 patients after episodes of DVT.[44] HC II was normal in all except one. In this patient, recurrent DVT had occurred since the age of 32. Further thrombosis could be avoided by oral anticoagulants. This patient had a HC II activity and concentration of around 56% at repeated occasions. The patient's father also had recurrent thrombosis, but died 4 years before the tests were carried out. One daughter of the patient at the age of 14 also had a HC II level between 47% and 63% at different occasions, but was clinically asymptomatic.

Out of 379 blood donors examined for HC II activity, HC II deficiencies were found in three.[45] In two of these, familial deficiencies were observed. In a total of five individuals with HC II deficiencies, there was a history of DVT in only one of them. In deceased family members, frequent episodes of thrombosis had occurred. Plasma samples of these five individuals were activated with DS and crossed immunoelectrophoresis was carried out. In the members of one family, an abnormal precipitation pattern with two distinct arcs was observed. It was assumed that in this family, molecular heterogeneity of HC II existed. No further cases of HC II deficiencies were found by these authors when 70 individuals with histories of thrombosis were screened. Another author found only one case of HC II deficiency after screening 870 patients suffering from thrombotic events.[46]

In series of tests, the following observations were made:[39] in 15 out of 268 patients with unexplained recurrent DVT, activities of HC II of less than 67% were found. In five of these patients with activities between 44% and 56% at different occasions, there was also familial HC II deficiency. Out of 14 family members examined, six had HC II activities of less than 55%, but only one of them had a history of thrombosis. Furthermore, in 18 out of 583 patients with cerebral thromboembolic manifestations, HC II deficiencies were detected, and the activities were between 44% and 59% at different occasions. In ten of these patients, a total of 21 family members could be examined, and in eight cases, there was familial HC II deficiency. Fourteen family members also had HC II levels of less than 60%, and there was a history of thrombosis in four of them. Therefore, in a total of 33 individuals with heterozygous HC II deficiencies, only 18 had thrombotic manifestations. It must be added that in six of the ten patients with familial HC II deficiency, there was also a greatly increased spontaneous platelet aggregation which is also a known risk factor for arterial thrombosis. A careful survey of cases of HC II deficiency was carried out in 121 healthy individuals and 277 patients with unexplained DVT.[47] In healthy persons, the range of distribution of HC II activities was also rather wide and was between 60% and 187%. The mean HC II activity was slightly higher in females than in males (108 vs. 101%). HC II was found to increase with age from an average 89% in the third decade to 124% in the fifth decade. It was recommended to suspect familial HC II deficiency only when the level is below 60%, when liver disease as well as DIC can be excluded, and AT-III, Protein C, and Protein S are in the normal range. Out of the 277 cases with DVT, there were three patients with HC II deficiency. In one of the families of these patients, there were six further cases of HC II deficiency, but there was no history of thrombosis. In the second family, one 17-year-old patient suffered from postoperative thrombosis and had a HC II deficiency. This was not found in any other family member, but there was a history of frequent thrombosis. This was explained by the detection of a familial Protein S deficiency from which also the patient suffered. In the third family, the proband had a history of DVT since the age of 18 years. There was no history of thrombosis in his family, but his daughter also had a heterozygous HC II deficiency. Altogether in nine individuals of three different families, HC II deficiencies were observed. Three of them had thromboembolic disease; one also had a congenital Protein S deficiency. It was, therefore, questioned whether a heterozygous HC II deficiency is a risk factor for thrombosis. From these data and also from data of other authors, it was concluded that there was not enough evidence that a heterozygous HC II deficiency is necessarily associated with thrombotic disease. It may, however, be an additional risk for the development of thrombosis. When the cases of heterozygous HC II deficiencies are surveyed and when the occurrence of thrombosis and

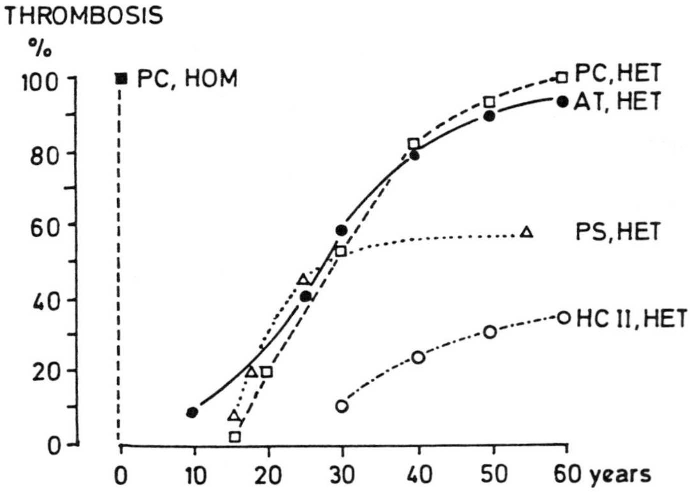

FIGURE 3. Occurrence of thrombosis in various inhibitor deficiencies in relation to age: PC HOM (homozygous Protein C deficiency) (■—■), PC HET (heterozygous Protein C deficiency) (□—□), AT HET (heterozygous Antithrombin III deficiency) (●—●), PS HET (heterozygous Protein S deficiency) (△·······△), and HC II HET (heterozygous Heparin Cofactor II deficiency) (·-○-·-○-·).

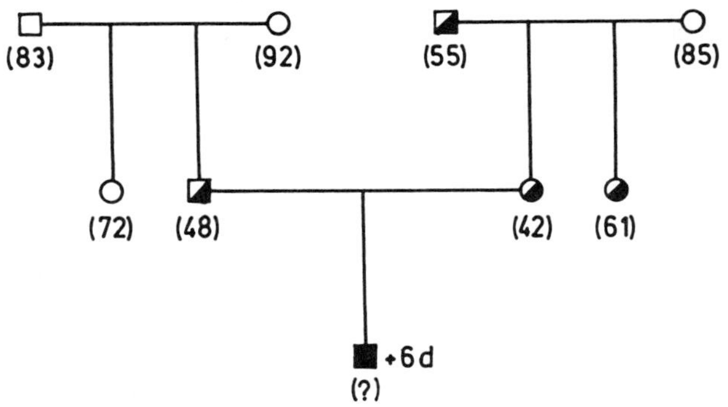

FIGURE 4. Family tree of a Heparin Cofactor II deficiency: (□) male, (◪) heterozygous male, (○) female, (◐) heterozygous female, (■) homozygous male baby died at 6th day. HC II activities are shown in brackets as percentage of normal.

the age of onset are compared with other deficiencies of inhibitors of the clotting system, a striking difference results (Figure 3).

It is clear from this figure that the occurrence of thrombotic disease in patients with HC II deficiencies is considerably less frequent than in other deficiencies and that the first manifestation of thrombosis is about 15 to 20 years later. All cases of HC II deficiencies described until now were heterozygous with residual activities of around 50%. No homozygous patients have been reported until now. A probable case of a homozygous HC II deficiency shall be described in brief. The patient was a male baby who suffered from anuria 2 d after birth and who died from uremia at the age of 6 d. Only the authopsy findings revealed the true cause of death. There was a massive thrombosis of the thoracic and abdominal aorta with a complete occlusion of the renal arteries, and a massive thrombosis of the umbilical vein, vena cava, and hepatic veins. Only after this report by the pathologist, the baby's family underwent test series for a possible familial defect. Both parents, all grandparents as well as a sister of the father and a sister of the mother, were examined (Figure 4).

There was a heterozygous HC II deficiency in both parents of the baby as well as in the mother's father and sister. Other risk factors such as AT-III, Protein C, Protein S, Plasminogen, Antiplasmin, and t-PA availability (by the venous occlusion test) were examined and were within the normal ranges. There is a high probability that the baby suffered from a homozygous HC II deficiency, but since a blood sample of the baby could not be obtained, there is no definite proof of this assumption. Out of the four family members with the heterozygous HC II deficiency, there was only a history of unexplained thrombosis in the mother's sister.

From all the data presently available, it can be assumed that a heterozygous HC II deficiency is a mild risk factor for thrombotic disease and probably requires an additional risk for the manifestation of thrombosis. In a few cases that developed thrombosis, further recurrences could be controlled by oral anticoagulants. It should, however, be known that DS is inactive in a HC II deficiency and that heparinoids for therapeutic use, which contain mainly DS, may be without effect in patients with HC II deficiencies. A definite case of a homozygous HC II deficiency still has to be found, but it can be assumed that such a case may be associated with a considerable thrombotic tendency.

REFERENCES

1. **Porter, B., Porter, M. C., and Shanberge, J. N.,** Heparin cofactor and plasma antithrombin in relation to the mechanism of inactivation of thrombin by heparin, *Clin. Chim. Acta,* 17, 189, 1967.
2. **Ganrot, P. O.,** Electrophoretic separation of two thrombin inhibitors in plasma and serum, *Scand. J. Clin. Lab. Invest.,* 24, 11, 1969.
3. **Birginshaw, G. F. and Shanberge, J. N.,** Identification of two distinct heparin cofactors in human plasma. I. Separation and partial purification, *Arch. Biochem. Biophys.,* 161, 683, 1974.
4. **Birginshaw, G. F. and Shanberge, J. N.,** Identification of two distinct heparin cofactors in human plasma. II. Inhibition of thrombin and activated factor X, *Thromb. Res.,* 4, 463, 1974.
5. **Wunderwald, P., Schrenk, W. J., and Port, H.,** Antithrombin BM from human plasma: an antithrombin binding moderately to heparin, *Thromb. Res.,* 25, 177, 1982.
6. **Tollefsen, D. M., Majerus, D. W., and Blank, M. K.,** Heparin cofactor II: purification and properties of a heparin dependent inhibitor of thrombin in human plasma, *J. Biol. Chem.,* 257, 2162, 1982.
7. **Witt, I., Kaiser, C., Schrenk, W. J., and Wunderwald, P.,** Amino acid composition and N-terminal sequence of Antithrombin BM, *Thromb. Res.,* 32, 513, 1983.
8. **Tran, T. H., Lämmle, B., Zbinden, B., and Duckert, F.,** Heparin cofactor II: purification and antibody production, *Thromb. Haemostas,* 55, 19, 1986.
9. **Ragg, H.,** A new member of the plasma protease inhibitor gene family, *Nucl. Acids Res.,* 14(2), 1, 1986.
10. **Barry, J. M., Penner, J. A., Hassouna, H. I.,** Monoclonal antibodies to probe the structural homology of the heparin binding sites on the heparin-dependent blood coagulation proteins, *Thromb. Haemostas.,* 54 (Abstr.), 25, 1985.
11. **Andersson, T. B.,** Consumption of heparin cofactor II (DS cofactor) and antithrombin during coagulation, *Thromb. Res.,* 46, 355, 1987.
12. **Sié, P., Lansen, L., Lacheretz, F., Verschuere, B., and Boneu, B.,** Comparative turn-over of heparin cofactor II and antithrombin III in baboons, *Thromb. Haemostas.,* 56, 302, 1986.
13. **Sié, P., Dupouy, D., Pichon, J., and Boneu, B.,** Turnover study of heparin cofactor II in healthy man, *Thromb. Haemostas.,* 54, 635, 1985.
14. **Sié, P., Dupouy, D., Dol, F., and Boneu, B.,** Inactivation of heparin cofactor II by polymorphnuclear leucocytes, *Thromb. Res.,* 47, 657, 1987.
15. **Griffith, M. J., Noyes, C. M., Tyndall, J. A., and Church, F. C.,** Structural evidence for leucine at the reactive site of heparin cofactor II, *Biochemistry,* 24, 6777, 1985.
16. **Griffith, M. J., Tyndall, J. A., Noyes, C. M., and Church, F. C.,** Enzymatic inactivation of heparin cofactor II by a proteinase (Proteinase I) isolated from echis carinatus venom, *Thromb. Res.,* 39, 659, 1985.
17. **Morgan, C. H. and Hassouna, H. I.,** The effect of varying concentrations of heparin and antithrombin III on the inactivation of thrombin in plasma by heparin cofactor II, *Thromb. Haemostas.,* 54 (Abstr.), 31, 1985.

18. **Sié, Gabaig, A. M., Dupouy, D., Choay, J., Lormeau, J. C., and Petitou, M.,** Structural requirements of heparin for the catalysis of thrombin inhibition by antithrombin III and heparin cofactor II, *Thromb. Haemostas.*, 54 (Abstr.), 111, 1985.
19. **Scully, M. F., Ellis, V., and Kakkar, V. V.,** Comparison of the molecular mass dependency of heparin stimulation of heparin cofactor II-thrombin interaction to antithrombin III-thrombin interaction, *Thromb. Res.*, 46, 491, 1987.
20. **Visser, A., Verhamme, I. M. A., Meuleman, D. G., and Van Dedem, G. W. K.,** An indirect kinetic method for estimating the affinity between heparin and heparin cofactor II, *Thromb. Haemostas.*, 58 (Abstr.), 423, 1987.
21. **Teien, A. N., Abildgaard, U., and Höök, M.,** The anticoagulant effect of heparan sulfate and dermatan sulfate, *Thromb. Res.*, 8, 859, 1976.
22. **Mardiguian, J., Corgier, M., and Jouany, M.,** Structure activity relationships of dermatan sulphate: effect of molecular size and carboxyl group esterification on heparin cofactor II activation, *Thromb. Haemostas.*, 58 (Abstr.), 423, 1987.
23. **Verhamme, I. M. A. and Van Dedem, G. W. K.,** Effect of the buffer composition and the presence of ORG 10172 and some GAG's on the inhibition of alpha-thrombin by heparin cofactor II, *Thromb. Haemostas.*, 58 (Abstr.), 422, 1987.
24. **Van Dinther, T. G., Hol, F., and Meuleman, D. G.,** Effect of various heparinoids on heparin cofactor II-mediated antithrombin activity and inhibition of thrombin generation *in vitro, Thromb. Haemostas.*, 58 (Abstr.), 423, 1987.
25. **Dawes, J. and Pepper, D. S.,** A comparison of the binding of antithrombin III and heparin cofactor II to heparins, naturally occurring GAG's and other sulfated polymers, *Thromb. Haemostas.*, 58 (Abstr.), 7, 1987.
26. **Yamagishi, R., Niwa, M., Kondo, S., Sakuragawa, N., and Koide, T.,** Purification and biological property of heparin cofactor II: activation of heparin cofactor II and antithrombin III by dextran sulfate and various glycosaminoglycans, *Thromb. Res.*, 36, 633, 1984.
27. **Scully, M. F. and Kakkar, V. V.,** Identification of heparin cofactor II as the principal plasma cofactor for the antithrombin activity of pentosan polysulphate, *Thromb. Res.*, 36, 187, 1984.
28. **Scully, M. F., Ellis, V., and Kakkar, V. V.,** Pentosan Polysulphate: activation of heparin cofactor II or antithrombin III according to molecular weight fractionation, *Thromb. Res.*, 41, 489, 1986.
29. **Dol, F., Sié, P., Dupouy, D., and Boneu, B.,** Effect of pentosan polysulphate administration in man on the formation of covalent complexes between heparin cofactor II and thrombin generated in plasma by contact activation, *Thromb. Haemostas.*, 56, 295, 1986.
30. **Tapon-Bretaudiere, J., Fischer, A. M., Millien, C., and Bros, A.,** Heparin cofactor II assay: importance and control of the noncontamination by heparin of dermatan sulphate, *Thromb. Haemostas.*, 58 (Abstr.), 422, 1987.
31. **Church, F. C., Treanor, R. E., and Whinna, H. C.,** Activation of heparin cofactor II by phosvitin, a phosphoglycoprotein and other phosphate containing polyanions, *Thromb. Haemostas.*, 58 (Abstr.), 293, 1987.
32. **Niwa, M., Yamagishi, R., Kondo, S., Sakuragawa, N., and Koide, T.,** Histidine-rich glycoprotein inhibits the antithrombin activity of heparin cofactor II in the presence of heparin or dermatan sulfate, *Thromb. Res.*, 37, 237, 1985.
33. **Friberger, P., Egberg, N., Holmer, E., Hellgren, M., and Blombäck, M.,** Antithrombin assay: the use of human or bovine thrombin and the observation of a second heparin cofactor, *Thromb. Res.*, 25, 433, 1982.
34. **Conard, J., Bara, L., Horellou, M. and Samama, M.,** Bovine or human thrombin in amidolytic antithrombin III assays: influence of heparin cofactor II, *Thromb. Res.*, 41, 873, 1986.
35. **Tran, T. H., Zbinden, B., Lämmle, B., Duckert, F.,** Influence of heparin cofactor II on the determination of antithrombin III, *Thromb. Haemostas.*, 54 (Abstr.), 204, 1985.
36. **Sié, P., Fernandez, F., Caranobe, C., Gabaig, A. M., and Boneu, B.,** Inhibition of thrombin-induced platelet aggregation and serotonine release by antithrombin III and heparin cofactor II in the presence of standard heparin, dermatan sulphate and pentosan polysulphate, *Thromb, Res.*, 35, 231, 1984.
37. **Sié, P., Dupouy, D., Pichon, J., and Boneu, P.,** Constitutional heparin cofactor II deficiency associated to recurrent venous thrombosis, *Lancet*, 2, 414, 1985.
38. **Tran, T. H. and Duckert, F.,** Heparin cofactor II determination: levels in normals and patients with hereditary antithrombin III deficiency and disseminated intravascular coagulation, *Thromb. Haemostas.*, 52, 112, 1984.
39. **Vinazzer, H. and Pangraz, U.,** Heparin cofactor II: a simple assay method and results of its clinical application, *Thromb. Res.*, 48, 153, 1987.
40. **Toulon, P., Jacquot, C., Capron, L., Frydman, M. O., Vignon, D., and Aiach, M.,** Antithrombin III and heparin cofactor II in patients with chronic renal failure undergoing regular hemodialysis, *Thromb. Haemostas.*, 57, 263, 1987.

41. **Sié, P., Ofosu, F., Fernandez, F., Buchanan, M. R., Petitou, M., and Boneu, B.,** Respective role of antithrombin III and heparin cofactor II in the *in vitro* anticoagulant effect of heparin and various sulphated polysaccharides, *Br. J. Haematol,* in press.
42. **Abildgaard, U. and Lie, M.,** Assay of dermatan sulfate cofactor (Heparin cofactor II) activity in human plasma, *Thromb. Res.,* 35, 257, 1984.
43. **Tran, T. H., Zbinden, B., Marbet, G. A. and Duckert, F.,** Congenital heparin cofactor II deficiency in a patient with cerebral thrombosis, *Thromb. Haemostas.,* 54 (Abstr.), 49, 1985.
44. **Sié, P., Dupouy, D., and Boneu, B.,** Constitutional heparin cofactor II deficiency in a patient with recurrent venous thrombosis, *Thromb. Haemostas.,* 54 (Abstr.), 49, 1985.
45. **Andersson, T. R., Larsen, M. L., and Abildgaard, U.,** Molecular heterogeneity of familial heparin cofactor II deficiency, *Thromb. Haemostas.,* 58 (Abstr.), 293, 1987.
46. **Scharrer, I.,** Untersuchungsprogramm bei Verdacht auf Thrombophilie, *Ellipse,* 9, 93, 1986.
47. **Bertina, R. M., Van der Linden, I. K., Engesser, L., Muller, H. P., and Brommer, E. J. P.,** Hereditary heparin cofactor II deficiency and the risk of development of thrombosis, *Thromb. Haemostas.,* 57, 196, 1987.

Chapter 7

α_2-MACROGLOBULIN AND α_1-PROTEINASE INHIBITOR

György Blaskó and Géza Sas

TABLE OF CONTENTS

I. α_2-MACROGLOBULIN — INTRODUCTION

Two entirely dissimilar groups of proteins are labeled as proteinase inhibitors. One of these is the macroglobulins, high molecular weight proteins, apparently found in the plasma of all mammals. They are exemplified by α_2-macroglobulin (α_2M), which has a molecular weight of 718,000 to 725,000. These macroglobulins combine with proteolytic enzymes, but the proteolytic activity towards large molecular-weight protein substrates is only decreased or lost. The main representatives of the second group of proteinase inhibitors are antithrombin-III and heparin cofactor II, both causing a complete loss of enzymatic activity towards high as well as low molecular weight substrates.[1]

α_2M was isolated from human serum by Schultze and coworkers in 1955.[2] Müller-Eberhard et al.[3] isolated α_2M clearly from IgM (because they have a like sedimentation constant). It was purified several years before discovering its enzyme-binding and -inhibiting properties. Since this time, extensive discussions regarding this inhibitor have been included in several books and was one of the main topics of the 23rd Meeting on Protides of Biological Fluids.

II. THE PURIFICATION OF α_2M

The conventional methods for the purification of α_2M are excellently reviewed by Bourillon and Razafimahaleo, but these have a disadvantage in common, i.e., activation of the coagulation factors as well as the complement system, resulting in the formation of large amounts of enzyme-α_2M complexes.[4-7] These included gel-filtration and ion-exchange chromatography on DEAE-cellulose.[8,9] The use of polyethyleneglycol (mol. wt. = 6000) for precipitation and finally, the use of affinity chromatography of the gel-filtered material on Cibacron-blue Sepharose and/or Affi-gell Blue (BioRad) resulted in an improvement in yield and purification.[10-12] An immunoadsorbent chromatography, utilizing rabbit anti-human-α_2M-conjugated Sepharose 4B has also been described.[13] It is very suitable for producing small quantities giving a yield of 90%.

A. PHYSICAL AND CHEMICAL PROPERTIES OF α_2M

The sedimentation constant, S_{20w}, is 17.3 to 19.6. α_2M can be precipitated by 25% ethanol, 1.2 to 1.8 *M* $(NH_4)_2SO$, 0.6 *M* perchloric acid, and 0.15 *M* TCA. The isoelectric point of the purified inhibitor is at 5.4. It denaturates easily at 56°C, and its trypsin-binding capacity is lost below pH 3.0. Absorbance at 280 nm of its 1% solution is between 8.1 to 8.7. Aliphatic amines have been shown to inactivate α_2M. Other, less important characteristics are summarized in References 10, 11, and 14. Its plasma concentration in adults is about 2.5 mg/ml.

III. THE STRUCTURE OF α_2-MACROGLOBULIN

α_2-Macroglobulin is a dimer of dimers and is composed of four identical polypeptide chains having a molecular weight of 180,000 Da each. The identical subunits contain 1451 amino acid residues. The complete amino acid sequence of α_2M has been determined and reported by Sottrup-Jensen et al. in Reference 15 and their previous publications. They have found 11 intrachain disulfide bridges. Eight glucosamine-based digosaccharide groups are attached to asparagines. The disulfide bridges form seven minor and four major wrinkles in the molecule. At Cys-447, a probably interchain disulfide forms a bond with another subunit.

They proved that a β-SH group of Cys-949 is thiol, esterified to the γ-carbonyl group of Glx-952, thus forming an activable reactive site which plays an important role in reactions with nucleophiles. The transglutaminase crosslinking site is constituted by Gln-670 and Gln-671. They clarified the location of some possible internal homologous sequences, too. α_2-Macroglobulin is probably evolutionarily related to the complement component C3 and C4, based on partial sequence homologies.

Welinder et al.[16] predicted the elements of the secondary structure in α_2M and showed the hydropathic character along the amino acid sequence. Hence, they could precisely distinguish between the buried and exposed peptide segments. α_2M has an alternating pattern of β-strands and turns. The circular dichroism spectra and data mentioned above showed that the tertiary structure of the C3b complement component is very similar to that of the α_2M monomer. They predicted the immunogenic peptide part of the molecule and suggested an approximately 100-residue hydrophobic core region, which could constitute parts of the tentatively assigned consecutive activation cleavage and thiol ester domains. This core might be responsible for the rearrangement transfer between the highly exposed bait region and partly buried thiol ester site. Sottrup-Hensen et al.[17] characterized a receptor-binding domain region in α_2M by digestion with papain. ^{1}H NMR studies of Arakawa et al.[18] showed conclusively that the bait region of native α_2M is highly flexible and exposed to the solvent. This flexibility is responsible for the susceptibility of the bait region to a proteolytic attack (see details below). Each subunit contains this "bait" region, which is highly susceptible for proteolysis. It will be discussed later in detail, when this region is split by proteinases. A conformational change occurs in the inhibitor, resulting in a reversible binding of the enzyme without blocking the proteinase-active site.[19] This phenomenon is termed "trapping." α_2M binds a broad spectrum of enzymes by a 2:1 to 1:1 molar ratio. Localization of the two protease-binding sites in the inhibitor was elucidated earlier.[20]

Covalent binding of the proteinase to α_2M is not necessary for the irreversible inhibition; however, such a bond may be formed by the reaction of a lysine residue of the enzyme with a reactive thiol-ester of the macroglobulin. This thiol-ester may be cleaved by small amines, like methylamine, in the absence of enzymes, too. Interestingly the change in the conformation of α_2M after the reaction with methylamine is very similar to that observed after the reaction with proteinases.[19] This region of the inhibitor is located in a hydrophobic environment, similar to that of transglutaminases. It is very questionable how this thiol-ester is formed throughout the protein-folding process after the ribosomal synthesis of the protein. The importance of a suitable-oriented glutamine residue in this interaction was also discussed.[21]

The receptor-recognition site of α_2M has partially been elucidated: it is a separate structure, not related to the bait region and internal thioester.[17,21] Its importance is unique in the rapid elimination of the complexed α_2M by fibroblasts and macrophages.

A. EVOLUTION OF α_2M

Based on their papain-binding properties, a variety of vertebrate plasmas were shown to contain this inhibitor, giving similar molecular weights on polyacrylamide gel electrophoresis (PAGE). In mammals, birds, and amphibians, an α_2M, similar to that in humans, has been shown, but interestingly, the migration of the papain-binding protein of fish showed the presence of only half a molecule of α_2M.[22] The investigation of α_2M originating from plaice showed that the plaice protein is a homologue of human α_2M. The long history of evolution, the partial homologies with complements C3 and C4, and the fact that no complete deficiency or abnormality has ever been described in human beings raises many questions.

B. GENETIC POLYMORPHISM

Three genetic forms of α_2M polymorphism have been described in man. The first was shown to be sex-linked: the antigen(s) appeared with a higher incidence among women than men in four different populations. The polymorphism was designated ''Xm,'' where ''X'' indicated the X-linked mode of inheritance and ''m'' indicated that the antigen was a macroglobulin.[23] The second, an Xm-independent polymorphism, was described in Japan.[24] The genetic locus was not closely linked to that of the haptoglobin. The third one was described by Gallango and Castilo in the Venezuelan Mestizo population, based on immunoelectrophoretic techniques.[25]

C. MICROHETEROGENEITY OF α_2M

It was an early observation that the electrophoretic mobility of α_2M differs in various subpopulations of the molecule. Saunders and co-workers separated five forms of α_2M, demonstrating that the slower migrating forms were capable of binding trypsin, whereas the rapidly moving forms were not. These latter forms were shown to be the complexed forms of the inhibitor.[26] The change in the sialic acid content as well as changes in other carbohydrate moieties result in a change of the isoelectric point. The differences in enzyme binding, amino acid composition, and carbohydrate content are the basis for microheterogeneity.[27]

IV. THE DISTRIBUTION AND FATE OF NATIVE AND COMPLEXED α_2M

The plasma concentration of α_2M is 2 to 4 mg/ml and it is unique among proteinase inhibitors in its ability to inhibit endopeptidases of any class and nearly any specificity.[28] The complexed form of α_2M is cleared very rapidly; the half-life time is about 10 min in man.[1] Thus, essentially all injected proteinases are cleared by the α_2M pathway.

As far as the site of synthesis of α_2M is concerned, it is in the hepatic tissue and its antigenicity can be demonstrated right from the 29th day of embryonic life.

α_2M has been identified in various body fluids, including normal joint fluid, peritoneal fluids, etc. In acute and chronic inflammations, numerous authors demonstrated it in the synovial fluid, pleural fluid, etc. It is important to note that in inflammatory processes, α_2M appears mainly in its complexed form, not capable of binding native and active enzymes, i.e., it has already been saturated by enzymes.

α_2M was found as a surface antigen of both human and murine B lymphocytes [chronic lymphocytic leukemia (CLL) patients have more α_2M on the surface of their lymphocytes]. Their presence on the membrane is not a result of absorption. Tunstal and James demonstrated an evidence of α_2M synthesis by B lymphocytes.[30] It can also be associated with platelet membranes. Mosher and Wing demonstrated that human-cultured fibroblasts (WI-38) synthesize and secrete α_2M.[31]

Earlier, it was thought that the complexed forms of α_2M are taken up very rapidly by the reticuloendothelial system, particularly by Kupfer cells. Gliemann and Davidsen had shown that the trypsin-α_2M complex was taken up by isolated hepatocytes, too.[32] They characterized a high-affinity receptor for this complex in the hepatocytes, which mediates the internalization and degradation of the complex. The binding is reversible to the complex and a negative cooperativity seems to be involved. If the binding occurs at body temperature, cooling to 4°C results in the liberation of 50% of the complex in its intact form, whereas the other half will be degraded.[33] The rate of internalization is very rapid at 37°C, k_{int} about 3×10^{-1}/min.

The half-life of the native, intact α_2M in human beings is about 56 h, whereas the half-lives of the complexes are less than 12 min (2 to 4 min).[33,61]

α_2M derived from animal sources shows immunological and functional homologies to human α_2M i.e., cross reactions have been described. On the analogy of human α_2M, bovine α_2M binds trypsin; plasmin and thrombin, however, fails to inhibit or bind bovine kallikrein (human α_2M inhibits kallikrein).[34]

V. THE INTERACTION OF α_2M WITH PROTEINASES

The following features are characteristic of the interaction of α_2M with proteinases:

1. Only active enzymes react.
2. Finally, the enzyme gets bound irreversibly to the inhibitor.
3. If the inhibitor has been saturated with one proteinase, it subsequently becomes incapable of binding to another one.
4. The reactions of the bound enzyme are sterically hindered.[35]

A. ENZYMES BEING TARGETS FOR α_2M ACTIONS

Proteinases from all the four catalytic classes, i.e., carboxyl-, thiol-, serine-, and metal-proteinases have been shown to react with α_2M.[36] These enzymes may originate from various sources, e.g., bacterial, plant, or animal species. Zymogens of proteinases, such as plasminogen or prothrombin, do not form complexes with this inhibitor. Compiled from the excellent review of Harpel and Rosenberg, the following enzymes are known to be bound to and inhibited by α_2-macroglobulin:[14]

1. Serine proteinases: native and acetylated bovine trypsin, human trypsin, chymotrypsin, human and bovine plasmin, human thrombin, kallikrein and urokinase, human and porcine leukocyte elastase, neutral proteinases from Staphylococcus aureus, Proteus vulgaris and Trichophyton mentagrophytes, Arvin (a coagulant enzyme of a Malayan pit viper), etc.
2. Thiol proteinases: human cathepsin B_1, papain, ficin and bromelain
3. Carboxy-peptides: human cathepsin D
4. Metal proteinases: thermolysin, clostridiopeptidase A and collagenases from various human and animal skins and connective tissues, aspartate aminotransferase, etc. For details, see References 37 to 46.

Exopeptidases and nonproteolytic hydrolases do not react with α_2M. The rate of reaction of proteinases with α_2M varies highly between enzymes. As it will be discussed later, trypsin and chymotrypsin react very rapidly, plasmin less rapidly, and thrombin and kallikrein rather slowly.

B. THE ENZYME-INHIBITOR INTERACTION

1. Irreversible Binding

Proteinases which react with and are inhibited by α_2M should be active: the presence of any competing substrate or substance would decrease the rate of these reactions.[45] The enzymes are irreversibly bound to the inhibitor, i.e., the inhibitor may be saturated on its enzyme recognition site(s), and the enzyme may get released from the complex only after denaturation. Barrett and Starkey demonstrated that the enzyme bound to the inhibitor does not remain catalitically active as active site-directed inactivation of the bound enzyme molecule does not result in its release.[36] The enzyme molecule cannot be transferred from α_2M to other inhibitors, but in an opposite direction, i.e., from soya-bean trypsin inhibitor to α_2M, a transfer is possible.

2. Presaturation of the Inhibitor

Despite the big variety of enzymes in specificity and characteristics, all the proteinases bind to α_2M in the same way. The presaturation of α_2M with one enzyme prevents the subsequent binding of another. Sakamoto et al.[48] demonstrated that the pretreatment of α_2M with trypsin, a serine-enzyme, prevented the binding of the metal-enzyme collagenase. α_2M has a definite number of binding sites available for all the complexing enzymes. It was very difficult to determine the binding sites of the inhibitor since we had to know simultaneously the concentrations of the active form of the enzyme as well as the inhibitor. Most data report that either one or two molecules of proteinases are bound per molecule of α_2M.[35] There is considerable evidence that α_2M contains two independent functional domains. The variation in the number of bound molecules seems to be in connection with the molecular weight of the enzymes; plasmin having the maximum size at which the 2:1 stoichiometry occurs. Inhibitable collagenases, including vertebrate collagenases, of less than 70,000 in molecular weight react α_2M, whereas larger collagenases having molecular weights greater than 100,000 are not inhibited.[19] The maximum M_r for an inhibitable proteinase appears to be about 90,000.

3. Steric Hindrance

The enzymes bound to α_2M generally retain their activity towards small molecular weight substrates, whereas activity towards large substrates is greatly reduced or lost.[19,49] The steric blockade protects the activity of the bound enzyme against inhibition by high molecular weight inhibitors.[49] The fact mentioned above, accompanied by the finding that the remaining activity of the enzyme does not result in its release from the complex, indicates that the active site of the enzyme is not involved in the interaction with α_2M. Not only the active site shows the characteristics of steric hindrance. The interaction of many enzymes with their antibodies is almost completely blocked after the binding of the enzyme to α_2M.

The bactericidal activity of cathepsin G, which is independent of this enzymatic activity, is also lost after interaction with α_2M.[50] Interestingly, sometimes the activity of the bound enzyme towards small substrates may increase in the complexed form. Twumasi et al.[51] described an activation of human leucocyte elastase in such instances. Therefore, it has been suggested very early that the enzyme bound to α_2M is almost completely surrounded by the inhibitor, leading to a slight modification in the microenvironment of the active center, at the same time, maintaining its capability to split small substrates. This altered microenvironment may be more favorable for the acylation-deacylation reaction.

4. Proteolytic Cleavage of α_2M

Following the initial noncovalent complex formation, one of the two reversibly bound proteinase molecules initiates the "activation" of the inhibitor by cleaving a "bait" region sequence of α_2M at a specific Arg-Leu bound into 2 subunits. The enzyme converts a quarter subunit (mol. wt. 190,000) to fragments of about 85,000 mol wt. Total fragmentation of all the subunits occurs only in the presence of excess amounts of enzyme. Whatever is the ratio of the enzyme to α_2M, the reaction gets completed within 1 minute. The cleaved subunits are held together by disulphide bonds under nonreducing conditions.[49] This proteolysis in α_2M was proved for cathepsin B (thiol proteinase), cathepsin D (carboxyl-proteinase) and thermolysin, as well as for collagenases (metal proteinase), respectively. Barrett and Starkey[36] demonstrated that the resulting peptides after this limited proteolysis are not the same; furthermore, the site of the attack also differs in cases of various enzymes inhibited by α_2M. This indicates that in 1 subunit of native α_2M, there should be a particular region which is highly susceptible for proteolysis, in general.[35]

a. Conformational Changes in α_2M

Proteolysis results in a conformational change in the α_2M molecule. This occurs as a result of the attacking proteinase becoming physically entrapped in the inhibitor. Concommitant to the entrapment is the appearance of four thiol groups. The native α_2M is generally cylindrical, presenting an ''H'' shape in lateral projection. Movements of the two trapping arms of each functional half-molecule are required for effective trapping. The conformational changes in the inhibitor in the complexed form can be provided by increased electrophoretic mobility, electron microscopy, etc. If two enzyme molecules are inhibited by one molecule of α_2M, 2 subunits are cleaved, but the second enzyme molecule should be in a convenient position for binding and cleavage to occur, i.e., the orientation of the second enzyme is important.

Therefore, the entrappment of proteinases into α_2M is displayed in two steps: the first is a proteolytic attack of the enzyme directed towards α_2M, which requires catalitically active molecules. This step may be inhibited by the presence of competing substances. In the second step, the proteolytically modified α_2M undergoes a conformational change in such manner that the enzyme(s) is enclosed within the inhibitor, thus preventing the escape of the enzyme(s) and hindering the access of substrates, inhibitors, and antibodies to the enzyme. This step is irreversible and does not involve the active site of the enzyme. The appearance of thiol groups that are extremely susceptible to nucleophilic attack is also a sign of a conformational change. The exact positions of the intramolecular thioester bonds, as well as the structure around the thioester bond, have recently been characterized, and their role in the increased conformational stability of the enzyme-inhibitor complex have been elucidated.[52-54] After the appearance of free thiol groups, the enzyme-α_2M complex will be stabilized covalently. The free SH groups react rapidly with the acyl groups of the enzyme, thus forming a covalent complex. This sequence of reactions have been suggested by Wang and co-workers, Howard, and others.[55,56]

Methylamine cleaves thioester bonds in α_2M, followed by a conformational change in the inhibitor that is nearly equivalent to the change observed after the reaction with proteinases.[19] (Recently, it has been demonstrated that it loses the ability to bind proteinases.)[57] In contrast to this, a similar cleavage takes place in the presence of dinitrophenyl cyanate, a reagent that cyanylates the liberated thiol groups, but does not change the electrophoretic mobility of α_2M, and the inhibitor also retains its activity. Björk has studied extensively the minor conformational changes in the inhibitor and concluded that thioester as such is not required for maintaining stability in the gross conformation of α_2M for binding proteinases.[55] Nevertheless, they participate in the maintainance of certain structural features that are necessary for the full proteinase-binding ability. Disruption of these structures results in a less-efficient trapping. Since the nature of this inhibition is totally different from the normal enzyme-inhibitor interactions, conventional kinetic investigations cannot be used.[69]

Wu and his co-workers emphasized the importance of intact lysyl ϵ-amino groups in the proteinases, with special reference to trypsin.[58] They have found that the covalent modification of ϵ-amino groups in bovine trypsin resulted in a reduced binding ability and complex formation. The modified enzyme-α_2M complexes were much more susceptible to dissociation by SDS than complexes formed by native trypsin. They proposed the role of these amino groups in the nucleophilic attack to thiol-esters and the role of these lysines in covalent bond formation.

Fibroblasts have receptors for recognizing α_2M-complexes. The recognition is directed by the conformation of the inhibitor which "traps" proteinase. Interestingly, methylamine treatment of α_2M transforms the inhibitor in such a way that it becomes indistinguishable from the α_2M-protease complex. By modification of the lysines in the α_2M-protease as well as in the α_2M-methylamine complexes, the receptor-mediated endocytosis was blocked, showing the sensitivity of the receptor in conformation of the complexes.[59] Similarly, modification of α_2M by dansylcadaverine and other primary amines changed the recognition by the cellular receptor.[60]

b. α_2M, a Zn-Binding Protein

α_2M is a major serum-zinc-binding protein and this feature has been exploited in the purification of the protein by zinc-chelate affinity chromatography. Pratt and Pizzo have shown by the equilibrium dialysis technique that α_2M has multiple classes of zinc-binding sites; the one with the highest affinity having a site number of 20 and a K_d value of 8×10^{-7} *M*.[62] The trypsin-complexed form of the inhibitor contained comparable amounts of zinc. The proteinase inhibitory activity of α_2M remained unaffected by zinc-binding as well as by the removal of zinc by EDTA. The zinc-binding capacity of α_2M might be involved in the zinc-binding capacity of the serum. The transport of zinc via endocytosis of complexed α_2M has physiological importance.

C. INTERACTION OF α_2M WITH THROMBIN, PLASMIN, AND TRYPSIN

The molar concentration of antithrombin-III and α_2M in normal plasma is roughly equal. The participation and importance of α_2M in the inactivation of thrombin has been discussed extensively.[83] Recently, it has been accepted that α_2M has a minor (about 20 to 23%) role in the total thrombin-inhibiting capacity of plasma under normal conditions, but its role and practical interest increase under pathological circumstances, e.g., nephrotic syndrome and in all situations that are accompanied by low antithrombin-III levels.[63-65]

1. Binding and Inactivation of Thrombin by α_2M

Thrombin and plasmin were reported to bind with α_2M in a 1:1 ratio, but by increasing the enzyme concentration, this ratio could be enhanced only in the case of thrombin. Straight and McKee characterized thrombin binding to α_2M.[66] It was shown that thrombin occupies rapidly the first binding site on the inhibitor, but binding to the second site takes place with some difficulty. Despite its low molecular weight (32,000) it occupies mainly one site. Others have proposed that binding of an enzyme to a site on α_2M results in structural changes in all the 4 subunits, thereby altering the second binding site.[59] They suggested that after a thiol ester bond is broken proteolytic cleavage is less likely to occur, just as is binding. They also thought that thrombin binding to α_2M may involve a functional negative cooperativity, which is caused by thiol ester scission before all binding sites can be occupied and cleaved by thrombin. Wang et al.[67] have also demonstrated that a single thrombin molecule forms two or more covalent bonds to two or more different α_2M chains. They showed that a 260 kD band represents two proteolyzed inhibitor subunits linked to one thrombin molecule. This intersubunit link maintains the integrity of the inhibitor even under reducing conditions. This form of complexation is unique.[67]

The kinetics of the reaction of α_2M with human thrombin can be studied by recording the appearance of thiols as well as PAGE analysis. The kinetics of the reaction of α_2M with human thrombin can be studied by recording the appearance of thiols as well as PAGE analysis. The kinetics of the appearance of thiol groups is biphasic, the early phase showing a second-order behavior. The observed second-order rate constant for thiol group release was found to be faster than the second-order rate constant for the disappearance of the band corresponding to native α_2M.* This may be the reflection of the multiple products formed

* It was 2.39 to 5.88 $\times$ 10^3M/s at pH 8.0.

from thioester. Thrombin may cross-link a variety of subunits internally.[68] α- and β-thrombins are inactivated by α_2M with identical reaction rates.[70]

Heparin does not have any role to play in the thrombin-inhibiting activity of α_2M. Heparin, complexed with thrombin, does not bind to this inhibitor, and if thrombin is entrapped into α_2M, it does not bind heparin.[71] A primary amine, as hydroxylamine, does not prevent the formation of thrombin/α_2M complexes but reduces the covalent binding of the enzyme to the inhibitor depending upon its concentration.[72] The interaction of hirudin with the α_2M-thrombin complex is very much slower than the free thrombin.[73]

2. The Inactivation of Plasmin

α_2M does not have a primary role in the inactivation of plasmin. Along with antithrombin-III, it becomes of importance when α_2-antiplasmin is saturated. α_2-antiplasmin has the capacity to neutralize about 50% of the potential amount of plasmin. Plasmin, trapped within α_2M, also retains its activity towards small, synthetic substrates.[74] Christensen and Sottrup-Jensen studied extensively the rate of interactions of α_2M and plasmin and trypsin because of the controversial kinetic data available in the literature (measuring the thiol-generation, intrinsic protein fluorescene, etc.).[50,66,75] They have found an initial association rate constant for α_2M-plasmin, 5×10^5 M/s, apparently corresponding to the overall rate constants of cleavage of one "bait" region in the native inhibitor. After rearrangements within the complexes, with generation of two possibly thiol groups, a further "bait" region cleavage step was slowed down, the apparent rate constant being 3×10^3/M/s. The same data for trypsin slightly differed. Roche and Pizzo have recently demonstrated that the extent of the subunit cleavage of α_2M is a function of plasmin concentration.[76] It was shown that the 2.5-fold molar excess of plasmin resulted in the cleavage of half of the subunits, whereas a 20-fold excess showed a 90% splitting with no additional plasmin binding. They have also studied the consequence of this finding on the receptor recognition of α_2M-plasmin complex. The ligand binding increased to 140 fmol/mg of cell protein in cases of total subunit cleavage, but K_d remained unaltered. The receptor-binding behavior of the complete subunits was equivalent to that observed in the case of the trypsin-α_2M complex.

3. Inactivation of Trypsin

The interaction of trypsin with α_2M was found to be very fast.[75] The initial association rate constant was 2×10^7 M/s, and the second, slower cleavage of the next "bait" region was also faster than in the case of plasmin, i.e., it was $1.3 \times 10^6/M$/s. Several authors have studied the preventing effect of α_2M-complexation on trypsin against other trypsin inhibitors.[77-79] α_2M was most effective in this issue.[77] The α_2M-trypsin complex may react with the soy bean-trypsin inhibitor forming a ternary complex, resulting in a decrease of esterase activity of trypsin, which has remained intact in the α_2M complex. Interestingly, formation of the ternary complex is as follows: trypsin dissociates from trypsin-soy bean trypsin inhibitor complex then reacts with α_2M and finally, the α_2M-trypsin complex reacts with the soy bean-trypsin inhibitor. Not going into details, the soy bean-trypsin inhibitor can react with α_2M-bound protease, and the resulting ternary complex has many characteristics common to soy bean-trypsin inhibitor-enzyme complexes in the absence of α_2M.[79] Similarly, the α_2M-trypsin complex can bind with the pancreatic basis trypsin inhibitor, too, but the enzyme activity exhibits some differences.[80] Christensen and Sottrup-Jensen also studied this system with two inhibitors and they have shown that the soy bean-trypsin inhibitor apparently discriminates between two distinct binding modes of trypsin to α_2M, covalently and the noncovalently α_2 M-bound trypsin.[81] They also supported the finding that binding of the first trypsin makes the access of the second less easy.

Hayes and Harpel pointed out the possibility that under acidic conditions (at pH 5.0), such as at inflammatory sites, trypsin retaining its activity in α_2M-complexes gives some physiological proof to the experiments mentioned above, which came up with recent findings regarding the molecular mechanisms of the α_2M action.[82]

D. INTERACTION OF α_2M WITH OTHER ENZYMES

Earlier, it was thought that there were no direct evidences for the interaction of α_2M with other coagulation enzymes, but recently, it was demonstrated that this inhibitor has a well-circumscribed role in coagulation.

1. Factor XIIa (Hagemen factor) and α_2M

Comparing the effectiveness of various plasma proteinase inhibitors, Pixley et al.[84] have shown that α_2M is a weak but not negligible inhibitor of Factor XIIa. The relative effectiveness in this regard, at plasma concentrations, was as follows: 61:2:3:1 for the CI inhibitor (CINH): α_2-anti-plasmin:α_2M: and antithrombin-III. CINH functions as the predominant inhibitor of Factor XIIa in plasma. The second-order rate constant of inhibition for α_2M was 5×10^3 *M*/min.

2. Factor Xa and α_2M

Utilizing synthetic, small molecular weight substrates, Ellis et al.[85] have found that α_2M inhibited Factor Xa, and Factor Xa exhibited amidolytic activity towards this substrate. They did not investigate the prothrombin-activating capacity of Factor Xa in a α_2M-complexed form, but they emphasized the possible differences in the effectiveness of various proteinase inhibitors if they exert their activity in the prothrombinase (Factor Xa-Factor Va phospholipid) complex.

3. Urokinase and α_2M

Ogston et al.[87] have indicated that the activation of plasminogen by urokinase is inhibited by α_2M. Vahtera and Hamberg demonstrated that α_2M was capable of binding some amount of urokinase in a nonspecific manner which could be disrupted by isoelectric focusing, but not gel filtration.[86] Along with pancreatic and urinary kallikreins, urokinase and some enzymes with very limited proteolytic action are unable to form true inhibitor complexes with α_2M.

4. Miscellaneous

Mosher described that besides cold-insoluble globulin in plasma, α_2M may also be transamidated by the fibrin-stabilizing factor (Factor XIIIa).[88]

Human leukocyte elastase became more active in a complexed form with α_2M towards various synthetic substrates.[51] This phenomenon was mentioned earlier. Its clinical significance might be there in cases of genetic deficiencies of α_1-antitrypsin, where a greater portion of elastase would be expected to complex with α_2M leading to a further exacerbation of lung destruction.

The macrophage activation factor, partially purified and complexed with α_2M and albumin, was shown to be more active. This phenomenon has not yet been clarified, but it was suggested that α_2M is a protective carrier for only the small molecular weight active substances.

α_2M was found to have an activating effect on immune haemolysis in the presence of calcium.[90] An interaction between the highly basic and cytotoxic eosinophil cationic protein and α_2M has also been described.[91] This binding was shown to be competitive with proteinase cathepsin G. This phenomenon has an importance in hypereosinophilic syndrome in the elimination of this highly cytotoxic protein.

VI. α_2M IN DISEASES

The concentration of α_2M correlates with chronological age. Its serum level is high in the young and decreases gradually to a minimal level in the 40s. Following this, its serum concentration increases with increasing age.[92] The mean concentration is about 210 to 250 ± mg/100 ml. Its level increases significantly in pregnancy and in women taking oral contraceptives.[93] However, oestrogen treatment does not cause an increase in α_2M.

A. DISEASES ACCOMPANIED BY HIGH LEVELS OF α_2M

The sera of patients suffering from the following diseases contain elevated levels of α_2M: ataxia teleangiectasia,[96] atopic dermatitis,[14,96] Down's syndrome,[95-97] nephrotic syndrome,[63,95,99] carcinoma of the prostate,[14,99] diabetes mellitus,[96] agammaglobulinaemia,[95] various pulmonary disorders,[14] and liver damage.[101]

Twining and Brecher measured the proteinase inhibitor content of normal and malignant breast, colon, stomach, etc. tissues and they found a significant elevated α_2M content in malignant breast and colon tissues.[94] α_2M may limit the activity of intercellular proteases or may interact with cell surface proteases or may interact with cell surface proteases to regulate cell proliferation. Zinc deficiency is commonly associated with high levels of α_2M, either in congenitally zinc-deficient dwarfs or, in cases of nephrotic syndrome, where the zinc levels are extremely low. The role of α_2M in trace element transport is also under speculation.[95] It is also questionable whether α_2M is a so-called "acute-phase protein." In animal experiments, a variety of nonsteroidal antiinflammatory drugs reduce the rapidly elevated levels of α_2M after an injection of turpentine.[100] On the other hand, it does not increase in patients with rheumatoid arthritis who are known to have high haptoglobin and C-reactive protein levels.[97] Surgical patients, who usually show an increase in acute-phase protein reactants in the postoperative period, do not show an increase in α_2M concentration during this time period.

B. DISEASE WITH LOW α_2M

The concentration of α_2M decreases rapidly during cardiopulmonary bypass.[101] The lowest levels were shown to be normalized within 240 min after the operation was over. This latter is the result of a release of unrecognized stores and a rapid new synthesis. The following diseases are commonly associated with low levels of α_2M: multiple myeloma,[96] rheumatoid arthritis in women,[97] pre-eclampsia (in the absence of proteinuria only),[102] and fibrinolytic therapy.[103,104]

In cystic fibrosis, the metabolism of α_2M is defected.[105]

1. Inherited Deficiency of α_2M

Bergquist and Nilsson first reported an inherited deficiency of this inhibitor; however, the total absence of this protein might not be compatible with life.[106,107] The defect is apparently inherited as a dominant trait. Persons with low levels of α_2M seem to be in perfect health; another propositus has also been described with Ehlers-Danlos syndrome. All of them are probably heterozygous. As it was hypothesized by these authors, the deficiency might be dangerous in cases undergoing fibrinolytic therapy, due to the exhaustion of the antiplasmin activity of the blood and since α_2M is the secondary defense mechanism against plasmin activity; in these patients, it might be hazardous.

VII. α_2-PROTEINASE INHIBITOR — INTRODUCTION

α_1-Proteinase inhibitor (α_1-PI) or α_1-antitrypsin, the inhibitor present at highest concentration in human plasma, belongs to the serpin protein family.[108] α_1-Antitrypsin received its name from its identification as an α_1-globulin and from the original method used for measuring its activity.[122] Since α_1-antitrypsin is actually capable of interfering with the action of a variety of proteolytic enzymes, Johnson et al.[123] recommended the term α_1-proteinase inhibitor. It has become the preferred label. Interest in α_1-PI was further stimulated by the discovery of its hereditary deficiency.[125] The genetic polymorphism of α_1-PI was recognized first by the work of Laurell and his colleagues.[125,126] However, the complexity of this system was elucidated by the combined efforts of Fagerhol and Laurell.[127] α_1-PI inhibits some enzyme(s) of the blood coagulation system, but its role as an important modulator of the coagulation system remains questionable. No thrombotic tendency has been noted in congenitally deficient patients in whom liver and pulmonary destruction by uncontrolled leukocyte enzymes dominate the clinical picture.[110] α_1-PI has been shown to inhibit thrombin slowly *in vitro,* as it was described by Gans and Tan.[111] However, despite its high concentration, it does not contribute any significant part to the overall antithrombin activity of whole plasma.[112,113] For its role being questionable as antithrombin, α_1-PI will be discussed briefly here and only its relation to the coagulation system will be described in more details.

VIII. BIOCHEMISTRY OF α_1-PI

α_1-PI is a single-chain glycoprotein of 394 amino acid residues with three carbohydrate chains.[128,129] The molecular weight varies from 54,000 to 58,000 and has an overall high negative charge. The cDNA studies carried out by Kurachi et al.[130] show that α_1-PI has a 24-residue hydrophobic pre- or signal peptide. α_1-PI functions as an inhibitor of the serine proteases in general, but the critical targets are the proteases released by stimulated neutrophil leukocytes: cathepsin G and, more particularly, neutrophil leucocyte elastase.[114] Analysis of the amino acid structure of α_1-PI revealed a definite homology with a number of inhibitors of the coagulation and fibrinolytic systems and other proteins, such as chicken ovalbumin. This observation led to the concept of the serpin superfamily.[108,115]

The first of the family to have their amino acid sequences determined were antithrombin III and α_1-PI.[116,117,118] These two plasma protease inhibitors were noted to be homologous with 30% identity. The homology did not include the first N-terminal portion of the molecule, but did extend to the C-terminus.

The serpins are a superfamily of proteins having evolved from a primitive ancestral serine protease inhibitor over a period of more than 500 million years.[119] The plasma serpins are ''suicidal'' proteins in the sense that they form a tight 1:1 complex with their target protease, following which the complex is subsequently removed from the circulation and catabolized.

A. MECHANISM OF ACTION

The mechanism of inhibition is best explained in terms of the tertiary (cristallographic) structure of α_1-PI.[120] This shows it as a globular, highly ordered molecule, with 30% of its structure in helical form and 40% in beta-sheets. There are two vulnerable regions in the molecule susceptible to enzymatic attack: an amino-terminal sequence of 20 residues and a loop, containing the reactive center, situated near the carboxy-terminal end. Cleavage of the amino-terminal sequence is known to occur, and there is a suspicion that the released pentapeptide has a physiological role.

The reactive center of α_1-PI is formed by the amino acid methionin at position 358, which is situated on an exposed loop of the molecule forming a ''bait'' for the target enzymes. This 16 residue, the exposed loop of sequence is under considerable tension, as it holds the molecule in a stressed metastable form. This stressed conformation is thought to strain the reactive center 358-359 Met-Ser bond so that it fits the active site pocket of the serine proteases precisely. The specificity of inhibition of each serpin is substantial, though not completely dependent upon the single amino acid at its reactive center. α_1-PI has a methionine fitting into the active center of elastase. This concept explains the ability to change the specificity of α_1-PI by mutations, e.g., replacement of the 358 methionine by arginine-changes α_1-PI from an inhibitor of elastase to an inhibitor of thrombin.[121]

IX. THE SYNTHESIS AND DISTRIBUTION OF α_1-PI

α_1-PI is synthesized in the liver and secreted into the plasma, where it has a half-life of 6 to 7 d.[131,132] It is an acute-phase reactant, the plasma concentration of which increases in response to inflammation or estrogens. The rise in plasma concentration is due to an increased synthesis of α_1-PI, particularly its triantennary isoforms (see below).[133] The normal concentration in plasma is about 1.3 g/l.[134] However, the concentration (measured immunochemically) and inhibitory activity of α_1-PI may differ as it was demonstrated by Miszczuk-Jamska and Pajdak.[163] About 40% of the protein is present in the plasma and most of the remaining 60% in the extravascular compartment. It has been found in varying concentrations in several body secretions, such as amniotic fluid, bronchial secretion, cerebrovascular fluid, cervical mucus, colostrum, duodenal fluid, gall bladder fluid, meconium, saliva, seminal fluid, synovial fluid, urine, and tears. α_2-PI is also present in platelets, alveolar macrophages, mast cells, neutrophils, and lymphocytes.[124] Various chromatographic methods have been described for the isolation of α_1-PI.[164,165,166]

X. NONGENETIC AND GENETIC VARIANTS OF α_1-PI

Human α_1-PI shows multiple banding patterns on acid starch gel electrophoresis (ASGE) or on isoelectrofocusing (IEF). Variation in the carbohydrate composition of the molecule is the major cause of these multiple bands.[133] The three carbohydrate side chains of α_1-PI are linked to asparagine residues at position 46, 83, and 247. A physiologically controlled variation can occur in the structure of these side chains to give isoforms which are nongenetic variant forms. Three isoforms, I, II, and III, have been described and they correspond to three major bands, M6, M4, and M2, respectively, of the α_1-PI phenotypic pattern recognized by IEF.[133,135] There is an increased production of M4 and M2 isoforms during inflammation and after estrogen administration, which could be due to an increased susceptibility to catabolism by the liver.[133]

Apart from this physiological variation, there is also a genetic variation of α_1-PI. More than 50 electrophoretic variants have been described and the nomenclature of the PI system has been standardized.[136]

The inheritance of α_1-PI is autosomal codominant and its structural locus has been assigned to chromosome 14.[137] The PI locus seems to be closely linked with that of the Gm marker of immunoglobulin (IgG) heavy chain.[138] The concentration of α_1-PI in human plasma is mainly determined by the individual's genotype. In the homozygous form of the Null variant, no α_1-PI can be detected in the plasma of the affected patients. Of the other variants, the PI Z and PI S mutants are of particular interest. They are mainly confined to European populations. Both differ from the normal in only a single amino acid and both result in a plasma deficiency: the S variant giving a production of 60% of the normal that is the M allele, the Z variant exhibiting a much more severe plasma deficiency that is 15% of the normal.[116] Gene-mapping studies have shown that the Z mutation probably arose in a single individual in Northern Europe some 6,000 years ago.[139] Since then, the variant has spread through Europe with a frequency gradient extending from North to South. There is a reciprocal distribution of the S variant from 10% in Southern Europe to 5% in the North.

The mutation in the S and Z variant, S 264 Glu→ Val and Z 342 Glu→ Lys, results in the loss of conserved glutamic acids which form ionic bonds that stabilize the molecule in each case. The consequent loss of stability is most marked with the S variant and probably contributes to its low level because of proteolysis of the nascent protein. Point mutation causing the S variant also introduces a false splice site in the gene and may lead to some loss of messenger RNA owing to incorrect splicing.[116]

In the case of the PI Z variant, 15% of the Z polypeptide is secreted into the plasma. However, 85% of the newly synthesized polypeptide appears to be blocked in the endoplasmic production of the hepatocyte, at a stage just prior to final processing of its carbohydrate side chains and to its entry into the Golgi secretion system. The defect lies in the transport of the Z α_1-PI at the final stages of its passage through the endoplasmic pathway. The amino acid replacement in the Z polypeptide may affect recognition, required for the final transport step or more likely, the mutation may cause a minor perturbation of structure affecting the solubility of the incompletely processed material. The failing in transport results in the aggregation of Z α_1-PI, giving rise to microscopically visible inclusions in the periportal hepatocytes.[140]

Multiple genetic variants and microheterogeneity of α_1-PI was observed in other mammals as well.[159,160]

A. PATHOPHYSIOLOGICAL ASPECTS

Two different processes are involved in the pathophysiology of α_1-PI deficient state. The first is directly related to the plasma deficiency, which causes damage to susceptible tissues, especially the lungs because of inadequate protection against proteases. The second is associated with the lungs and seems to be satisfactorily maintained by plasma α_1-PI concentrations up to 40% the normal value; neither the MZ heterozygote having a plasma concentration of 58% the normal nor the MS with a concentration of 80% have significantly increased risk of lung disease.[108] The association with chronic obstructive lung diseases (emphysema) is primarily confined to the 1:1000 Europeans who inherit two deficient genes, i.e., ZZ (concentration: 15% of normal concentration) and SZ (concentration: 38%), but not SS (concentration: 60%).

The association of α_1-PI deficiency with the development of chronic obstructive airway disease led to the hypothesis that protease-antiprotease imbalance is a general contributor to the various conditions leading to this disease.[141] The realization that α_1-PI is an inhibitor of neutrophil elastase strengthened the case because elastase is an endogenous enzyme capable of degrading elastin and collagen. The injury to lung tissues can result on the one hand from a prolonged exposure to leukocyte proteases, as in chronic inflammation, and on the other, from an insufficiency of α_1-PI. Demonstration that α_1-PI could also oxidatively be inactivated by stimulated neutrophils was of great interest, providing the explanation of elastase secretion by the neutrophil granulocytes, even in the presence of normal concentrations of α_1-PI.[142] The oxidative inactivation of human α_1-PI was demonstrated by Johnson and Travis.[167]

Stimulated neutrophils release oxygen radicals which create a zone of oxidation around them, in effect, forming a microenvironment within which α_1-PI is inactivated. This facilitates the localized breakdown of the connective tissue. In the case of smoking, the inactivation of α_1-PI could be a contributing factor for the development of chronic obstructive lung disease. Tobacco smoke contains oxidizing radicals capable of inactivating α_1-PI. However, this is largely a localized event, confined to the immediate proximity of the neutrophil leukocytes with significant damage, resulting from the summation of focal damages over a period of years. The progress of this destruction will obviously be accelerated by the presence of a genetic deficiency of α_1-PI. Indeed, this fact was demonstrated by Janus et al.[143] and Larsson.[144] They investigated the changes in forced expiratory volume (FEV_1), confined to the study of ZZ homozygotes. The ZZ nonsmoker had an annual FEV decrease of 80 ml as compared to that of 36 ml of the nonsmoker control. The first signs of dyspnea did not appear till after the age of 60 to 65. A number of ZZ individuals had a normal life span (up to 87 years) without major respiratory problems. However, the ZZ smoker showed a catastrophic progression, with an average FEV_1 loss of 300 ml/y and an onset of emphysema after 15 cigarette-packed years, often by the age of 50.

As it was mentioned earlier, the Z variant of α_1-PI is associated with liver disease.[145] About 10% of ZZ infants develop neonatal cholestasis. Most recover, but some (2 to 3% overall) progress to juvenile cirrhosis. There is also slowly progressing liver damage found in the adult. Almost all homozygotes show histological evidence of liver damage and about 20% eventually develop cirrhosis. The most probable mechanism of this liver damage is the intracellular accumulation of the Z variant of α_1-PI.[108]

XI. α_1-PI AND BLOOD COAGULATION

The question of the antithrombin activity of α_1-PI is controversial. Heimburger et al.[146] have reported that purified α_1-PI does not inhibit thrombin, whereas several other investigators have suggested that α_1-PI functions as an antithrombin in plasma.[111,147] On investigating normal and α_1-PI-deficient plasmas, a lower progressive antithrombin activity was observed in patients with a genetic α_1-PI deficiency, and this deficiency has been attributed to the lower α_1-PI level in plasma. Rimon et al.[148] have purified an α_1-PI proteolytic inhibitor from human plasma, which comprised about 2% of the plasma proteins and could inhibit plasmin, trypsin, chymotrypsin, and thrombin. This inhibitor appears to be identical with α_1-PI. Lane et al.[149] have found that about 25% of the human plasma antithrombin activity was due to α_1-PI. According to Shapiro and Anderson, α_1-PI does not contribute to the overall antithrombin activity of whole plasma.[113] Later, Matheson and Travis demonstrated the antithrombin activity of α_1-PI in cases of highly purified proteins.[150] Both the clotting and esterase activities of thrombin are inhibited by α_1-PI. The inhibition is a time- and temperature-dependent reaction which is proportional to the molar ratio of thrombin to the inhibitor. α_1-PI forms a 1:1 complex with thrombin, which is comparable to the complex formed with trypsin and other proteinases. Machovich et al.[70] studied the inactivation of α- and β-thrombin by α_2-Macroglobulin, by α_1-PI and antithrombin III, and by heparin. α_1-PI formed a complex with α- and β-thrombin, similarly to antithrombin III, although the inactivation of the enzyme required a high inhibitor concentration and long incubation time.

On the basis of these observations, the psysiological importance of α_1-PI, as an antithrombin, seems to be questionable. The fact that no thrombotic tendency has been noted in patients with congenital α_1-PI deficiencies contradicts its physiological role as antithrombin. The minor, if any, role of α_1-PI as an antithrombin was observed in our own investigations as well.[152] When we studied antithrombin activity of the plasma of a consanguinous patient with an abnormal antithrombin (AT-III) (i.e., AT-III Budapest) we found that this patient had a very low progressive thrombin inactivating activity and this low activity could almost totally be suspended by mixing purified anti-$\alpha_2$macroglobulin IgG.

This observation suggests that AT-III and $\alpha_2$macroglobulin are involved mainly, if not exclusively, in the physiological inactivation of thrombin. α_1-PT may play some role in the inactivation of activated factor X (F Xa).[153] Further investigations supported the inactivation of F Xa by α_1-PI, but these latter studies suggested that α_1-PI was responsible for 28% of the total F Xa inactivating capacity of the human plasma instead of the 60% calculated previously.[154] α_1-PI inhibits factor XIa and contributes nearly 70% to the overall anti-F XIa activity in plasma. Nishkado et al.[155] observed the elevation of F XIa-α_1-PI complexes in the plasma of a patient with disseminated intravascular coagulation. Despite these findings, the absence of thromboembolic episodes in patients with α_1-PI deficiencies contradicts the physiological importance of these reactions. α_1-PI may play a significant role in the pathogenesis of thrombosis in inflammation.[156] A central event in inflammation is the release of both elastase and oxygen radicals by neutrophil leukocytes. The oxygen radicals have a limited radius of activity, but within the radius, they readily oxidize methionine at the reactive center of α_1-PI, which consequently loses its activity to inhibit elastase. The loss of the elastase inhibitory activity of α_1-PI allows released neutrophil elastase to break down local connective tissue and to inactivate other inhibitors, including AT-III and Cl-inhibitor. This sequence of events, with an S-R inactivation of inhibitors, provides a molecular explanation for the observed modification of the proteolytic cascades, such as the coagulation and complement system, that occur locally in the case of inflammation. Both α_1-PI and Cl inactivator are present on washed normal platelets and this fact may contribute to the complex events of inflammation.[157]

A. A BLEEDING DISORDER ASSOCIATED WITH α_1-PI DEFICIENCY

Lewis et al.[158] described in 1978 a unique bleeding disorder. The coagulation abnormality occurred in a young boy who died at the age of 14 with a huge hematoma in his leg and abdomen. This was the final result of lifelong series of intermittent bleeding episodes. The bleeding episodes all followed after trauma. Laboratory examinations showed a prolongation of bleeding, clotting, partial thromboplastin, prothrombin, and thrombin times. These findings could be related to the presence of a potent inhibitor of thrombin-fibrinogen reaction in the plasma. The inhibitor had the electrophoretic and antigen characteristics of 1 variant form of α_1-PI. Further investigations clarified the essence of this abnormality.[121] A variant α_1-PI was identified in which the methionine at position 358 had been replaced by an arginine. This had turned α_1-PI from normal function of an inhibitor of elastase to that of an inhibitor of thrombin. The reactive center of α_1-PI is methionine 358, which acts as a bait for elastase, just as the normal reactive center for AT-III is arginine 393, which acts as a bait for thrombin. The episodic nature of the bleeding was the consequence of the mutant protein behaving as an acute-phase reactant, the level of which increased several-fold after trauma.

ACKNOWLEDGMENT

The authors are very indebted to Susanna Turi Blaskó, M.D., for her help in the preparation of this manuscript and for her valued criticism.

REFERENCES

1. **Laskowski, M., Jr. and Kato, I.,** Protein inhibitors of proteinases, *Ann. Rev. Biochem.*, 49, 593, 1980.
2. **Schultze, H. E., Göllner, I., and Heide, K.,** Zur Kenntnis der α-Globuline des menschlichen normalserums, *Z. Naturforsch. Teil B:*, 10, 463, 1955.
3. **Müller-Eberhard, H. I., Kunkerl, H. G., and Franklin, E. C.** Two types of γ-globulins differing in carbohydrate contents, *Proc. Soc. Exp. Biol. Med.*, 93, 146, 1956.
4. **Bourillon, R. and Razafimahaleo, E.,** α_2-macroglobulin, in Glycoproteins, Vol. 5, Gottschalk, A., Ed., Elsevier, Amsterdam, 1972, 699.
5. **Cochran, C. D., Revak, S. D., and Wuepper, K. D.,** Activation of Hageman factor in solid and fluid phases. A critical role of kallikrein, *J. Exp. Med.*, 138, 1564, 1975.
6. **Rinderknecht, H., Fleming, R. M., and Geokas, M. C.,** Effect of α_2-macroglobulin on some kinetic parameters of trypsin, *Biochim. Biophys. Acta*, 377, 158, 1977.
7. **Ratnoff, O. D.,** Some relationships among haemostasis, fibrinolytic phenomena, immunity and the inflammatory response, *Adv. Immunol.*, 10, 145, 1969.
8. **Gauthier, F. and Mouray, H.,** Rat α_2-acute phase macroglobulin. Isolation and physicochemical properties, *Biochem. J.*, 159, 661, 1976.
9. **Bieth, J. and Klumpp, T.,** Purification of α_2-macroglobulin with trypsin-like activity from pleural fluids, *Biochim. Biophys. Acta*, 439, 363, 1976.
10. **Hall, P. K. and Roberts, R. C.,** Physical and chemical properties of human plasma α_2-macroglobulin, *Biochem. J.*, 171, 27, 1978.

11. **Pellegrini, A., Zweifel, H. R., and von Fellenberg, R.,** Isolation and characterization of horse α_2-macroglobulin protease inhibitor, *Int. J. Biochem.*, 15, 1003, 1983.
12. **Virca, G. D., Travis, J., Hall, P. K., and Roberts, R. C.,** Purification of human α_2-macroglobulin by chromatography on Cibacron Blue Sepharose, *Anal. Biochem.*, 89, 274, 1978.
13. **McEntire, J. E.,** Purification of alpha-2-macroglobulin by immunoadsorbent chromatography, *J. Immunol. Methods.*, 24, 39, 1978.
14. **Harpel, P. C. and Rosenberg, R. D.,** α_2-macroglobulin and antithrombin-heparin cofactor: modulators of haemostatic and inflammatory reactions, in Progress in Haemotasis and Thrombosis, Vol. 3., Spate, T. H., Ed., Grune and Stratton, New York, 1976, 145.
15. **Sottrup-Jensen, L., Stepanik, T. M., Kristensen, T., Wierzbicki, D. M., Jones, C. M., Lønblad, P. B., Magnusson, S., and Petersen, T. E.,** Primary structure of human α_2-macroglobulin. V. The complete structure, *J. Biol. Chem.*, 259, 8318, 1984.
16. **Welinder, K. G., Mikkelsen, L., and Sottrup-Jensen, L.,** Appendix. Structural prediction on α_2-macroglobulin from the amino acid sequence, *J. Biol. Chem.*, 259, 8328, 1984.
17. **Sottrup-Jensen, L., Gliemann, J., and VanLeuven, F.,** Domain structure of human α_2-macroglobulin, Characterization of a receptor-binding domain obtained by digestion with papain, *FEBS Lett.*, 205, 20, 1986.
18. **Arakawa, H., Muto, Y., Arata, Y., and Ikai, A.,** Proton nuclear magnetic resonance study of human α_2-macroglobulin, *Biochemistry*, 25, 6785, 1986.
19. **Feldman, S. R. and Pizzo, S.,** A three-dimensional model of a unique proteinase inhibitor: α_2-macroglobulin, *Semin., Thromb. Haemost.*, 12, 223, 1986.
20. **Pochon, F., Favaudon, V., and Tourbez-Perrin, M.,** Localization of the two protease-binding sites in human α_2-macroglobulin, *J. Biol. Chem.*, 256, 547, 1981.
21. **Van Leuven, F.,** Human α_2-macroglobulin: structure and function, *Trends Biochem. Sci.*, 7, 185, 1982.
22. **Starkey, P. M., Fletcher, T. C., and Barrett, A. J.,** Evolution of α_2-macroglobulin. The purification and characterization of a protein homologous with human α_2-macroglobulin from plaice (Pleuronectes platessa L.) plasma, *Biochem. J.*, 205, 97, 1982.
23. **Berg, K. and Bearn, A. G.,** An inherited X-linked serum system in man — the Xm system, *J. Exp. Med.*, 123, 379, 1966.
24. **Leikola, J., Fudenberg, H. H., and Kasukawa, R.,** A new genetic polymorphism of human serum: α_2-macroglobulin, *Am. J. Hum., Genet.*, 23, 134, 1972.
25. **Gallango, M. K. and Castilo, O.,** α_2-macroglobulin polymorphism: a new genetic system detected by immunoelectrophoresis, *J. Immunogenetics*, 1, 147, 1974.
26. **Saunders, R., Dyce, B. J., and Wannier, W. E.,** The separation of alpha-2-macroglobulin into five components with differing electrophoretic and enzyme-bonding properties, *J. Clin. Invest.*, 50, 2376, 1971.
27. **Frénoy, J.-P. and Bourrillon, R.,** Studies on the structure of human α_2-macroglobulin. IV. Analysis of the microheterogeneity by isoelectric focusing, *Biochim. Biophys. Acta*, 371, 168, 1974.
28. **Barrett, A. J.,** α_2-macroglobulin, *Methods Enzymol.*, 80, 737, 1981.
29. **Gitlin, D. and Biasucci, A.,** Development of γG, γA, γM, β1C, β1A and $C_1$1 esterase inhibitor, coeruloplasmin, transferrin, haemopexin, haptoglobin, fibrinogen, plasminogen, α_1-antitrypsin, orosomucoid, β-lipoprotein, α_2-macroglobulin and prealbumin in the human conceptus, *J. Clin. Invest.*, 48, 1433, 1969.
30. **Tunstal, A. M. and James, R.,** Preliminary studies on the synthesis of alpha-2-macroglobulin by human lymphocytes *in vitro, Clin. Exp. Immunol.*, 17, 697, 1974.
31. **Mosher, D. F. and Wing, D. A.,** Synthesis and secretion of α_2-macroglobulin by cultured human fibroblasts, *J. Exp. Med.*, 143, 462, 1976.
32. **Gliemann, J. and Davidsen, O.,** Characterization of receptors for α_2-macroglobulin-trypsin complex in rat hepatocytes, *Biochim. Biophys. Acta*, 885, 49, 1986.
33. **Blatrix, C., Amouch, P., Drouct, J., Steinbuch, M., and Friess, A.,** Study on the plasmatic elimination of the alpha$_2$-macroglobulin/proteinase complexes, *Pathol. Biol. Suppl.*, 21, 11, 1973.
34. **Sugihara, J., Nagasawa, S., and Suzuki, T.,** Studies on α_2-macroglobulin in bovine plasma. III. Its action on bovine plasma kallikrein, plasmin and thrombin, *J. Biochem.*, 70, 649, 1971.
35. **Starkey, Ph. M.,** α_2-macroglobulin. A review, in The Physiological Inhibitors of Coagulation and Fibrinolysis, Collen, D., Wiman, B., and Verstraete, M., Eds., Elsevier, Amsterdam, 1979, 221.
36. **Barrett, A. J. and Starkey, P. M.,** The interaction of α_2-macroglobulin with proteinases, *Biochem. J.*, 133, 709, 1973.
37. **Nagasawa, S., Han, B. H., Sugihara, H., and Suzuki, T.,** Studies on α_2-macroglobulin in bovine plasma. II, *J. Biochem.*, 67, 821, 1970.
38. **Jacquot-Armand, Y. and Krebs, G.,** Amidase activity of NE-acetyl-trypsin free or bound on the α_2-macroglobulin, *Biochem. Biophys. Res. Comm.*, 36, 815, 1969.
39. **Steinbuch, M., Blatrix, C., and Josso, F.,** Action antiprotease de l' α_2-macroglobuline. II. Son role d'antithrombine progressive, *Rev. Eur. Etud. Clin. Biol.*, 13, 179, 1968.

40. **Ogston, D., Bennett, B., Herbert, R. J. et al.,** The inhibition of urokinase by alpha-2-macroglobulin, *Clin. Sci.,* 44, 73, 1973.
41. **Baumstark, J. S.,** Studies on the elastase-serum protein interaction. II. On the digestion of human α_2-macroglobulin — an elastase inhibitor by elastase, *Biochim. Biophys. Acta,* 207, 318, 1970.
42. **Brown, S. I., Hook, C. W., and Tragakis, M. P.,** Presence, significance, and inhibition of lysosomal proteoglycanases, *Invest. Opthalmol.,* 11, 149, 1972.
43. **Yu, R. J., Grappel, S. F., and Blank, F.,** Inhibition of keratinases by α_2-macroglobulin, *Experientia,* 28, 886, 1972.
44. **Starkey, P. M. and Barrett, A. J.,** Human Cathpsin Bl. Inhibition by α_2-macroglobulin and other serum proteins, *Biochem. J.,* 131, 823, 1973.
45. **Werb, Z., Burleigh, M. C., Barrett, A. J., and Starkey, P. M.,** The interaction of α_2-macroglobulin with proteinases. Binding and inhibition of mammalian collagenases and other metal proteinases, *Biochem. J.,* 139, 359, 1974.
46. **Boyle, T. R. C. and Pryme, I. F.,** Alpha-2-macroglobulin binding of trypsin, chymotrypsin, papain and cationic aspartate aminotransferase, *Clin. Chim. Acta,* 2, 9, 1968.
47. **Saunder, R., Dyce, B. J., Vannier, W. E., and Haverback, B. J.,** The separation of α_2M into five components with differing electrophoretic and enzyme-binding properties, *J. Clin. Invest.,* 50, 2376, 1971.
48. **Sakamoto, S., Goldhaber, P., and Glimcher, M. J.,** Maintenance of mouse bone collagenase activity in the presence of serum protein by the addition of trypsin, *Proc. Soc. Exp. Biol. Med.,* 139, 1038, 1972.
49. **Starkey, P. M. and Barrett, A. J.,** α_2-macroglobulin: a physiological regulator of proteinase activity, in Proteinases in Mammalian Cells and Tissues, Barrett, A. J., Ed., North-Holland, Amsterdam, 1977, 663.
50. **Venge, P., Olsson, I., and Odeberg, H.,** Cationic proteins of human granulocytes. V. Interaction with plasma proteinase inhibitors, *Scand. J. Clin. Lab. Invest.,* 35, 737, 1975.
51. **Twumasi, D. I., Leiner, I. E., Galdstone, M., and Levytska, V.,** Activation of human leucocyte elastase by human α_2M, *Nature,* 267, 61, 1977.
52. **Sottrup-Jensen, J., Petersen, T. E., and Magnusson, S.,** A thiol-ester in α_2-macroglobulin cleaved during proteinase complex formation, *FEBS Lett.,* 121, 275, 1980.
53. **Sottrup-Jensen, L., Hansen, H. F., Mortensen, S. B., Petersen, T. E., and Magnusson, S.,** Sequence location of the reactive thiol ester in human α_2-macroglobulin, *FEBS Lett.,* 123, 145, 1981.
54. **Björk, I. and Jörnvall, H.,** The structure around the thioester bond in bovine α_2-macroglobulin. Possible implication for the conformational stability of the inhibitor on thioester cleavage, *FEBS Lett.,* 205, 897, 1986.
55. **Wang, D., Wu, K., and Feinman, R. D.,** α_2-macroglobulin-protease reactions: relationship of covalent bond formation, methylamine reactivity, and specific proteolysis, *Biochem. Biophys. Res. Comm.,* 211, 500, 1981.
56. **Howard, J. B.,** Reactive site in human α_2-macroglobulin: circumstantial evidence of a thiolester, *Proc. Natl. Acad. Sci. U.S.A.,* 78, 2235, 1981.
57. **Björk, I.,** Binding of proteinases to human α_2-macroglobulin with its thioster bonds cleaved by methylamine in the presence of a thiol-group cyanylating reagent, *Biochem. J.,* 231, 451, 1985.
58. **Wu, K., Wang, D., and Feinman, R. D.,** Inhibition of proteases by α_2-macroglobulin. The role of lysyl amino groups of trypsin in covalent complex formation, *J. Biol. Chem.,* 256, 10409, 1981.
59. **Marynen, P., Van Leuven, F., Cassiman, J. J., and Van den Berghe, H.,** Proteolysis at a lysine residue abolishes the receptor-recognition site of α_2-macroglobulin complexes, *FEBS Lett.,* 137, 241, 1982.
60. **Van Leuven, F., Cassiman, J. J., and Van den Berghe, H.,** Functional modification of α_2-macroglobulin by primary amines. I. Characterization of α_2M after derivatization by methylamine and by Factor XIII, *J. Biol. Chem.,* 256, 9016, 1981.
61. **Blatrix, C., Amouch, P., Druet, J., and Steinbuch, M.,** Study on the plasmatic elimination of alpha-2-macroglobulin/proteinase complexes, *Pathol. Biol.,* 21, 11, 1973.
62. **Pratt, C. W. and Pizzo, S. V.,** The effect of zinc and other divalent cations on the structure and function of human α_2-macroglobulin, *Biochim. Biophys. Acta,* 791, 123, 1984.
63. **Lebreton de Vonne, T. and Mouray, H.,** Human α_2-macroglobulin and its antitryptic and antithrombin activities in serum and plasma, *Clin. Chim. Acta,* 99, 83, 1978.
64. **Fischer, A. M., Tapon-Bretaudiere, J., Bros, A., and Josso, F.,** Respective roles of antithrombin-III and alpha-2-macroglobulin in thrombin inactivation, *Thromb. Haemost.,* 45, 51, 1981.
65. **Abildgaard, U.,** Role of α_2-macroglobulin as an inhibitor of coagulation, in The Physiological Inhibitor of Coagulation and Fibrinolysis, Collen, D., Wiman, B., and Verstrate, M., Eds., Elsevier/North-Holland, Amsterdam, 1979, 239.
66. **Straight, D. L. and McKee, P. A.,** Characterization of thrombin binding to α_2-macroglobulin, *J. Biol. Chem.,* 259, 1272, 1984.
67. **Wang, D., Yua, A. I., and Feiman, R. D.,** Covalent thrombin-α_2-macroglobulin complexes. Evidence for bivalent cross-linking of inhibitor by a single enzyme molecule, *Biochemistry,* 23, 2807, 1984.

68. **Feinman, R. D., Yuan, A. I., Winder, A. R., and Wang, D.,** Kinetics of the reaction of thrombin and α_2-macroglobulin, *Biochem. J.*, 231, 417, 1985.
69. **Duke Virca, G. and Travis, J.,** Kinetics of association of human proteinases with human α_2-macroglobulin, *J. Biol. Chem.*, 259, 8870, 1984.
70. **Machovich, R., Borsodi, A., Blaskó, Gy., and Orakzai, S.,** Inactivation of α-, and β-thrombin by antithrombin-III, α_2-macroglobulin and α_1-proteinase inhibitor, *Biochem. J.*, 167, 393, 1977.
71. **Pochon, F., Lambin, P., and Steinbuch, M.,** Heparin and the progressive anti-thrombin activity of α_2-macroglobulin, *Thrombin. Res.*, 26, 307, 1982.
72. **Lambin, P., Pochon, F., Fine, J. M., and Steinbuch, M.,** The α_2-macroglobulin/thrombin interaction in the presence of hydroxylamine, *Thromb. Res.*, 32, 123, 1983.
73. **Pochon, F. and Steinbuch, M.,** Interaction of α_2-macroglobulin-bound thrombin with hirudin, *FEBS Lett.*, 177, 109, 1984.
74. **Gyzander, E. and Teger-Nilsson, A. C.,** Activity of the α_2-macroglobulin-plasmin complex on the plasmin specific substrate H-D-Val-Leu-Lys-p-nitroanilide, *Thromb. Res.*, 19, 165, 1980.
75. **Christensen, U. and Sottrup-Jensen, L.,** Mechanism of α_2-macroglobulin-proteinase interaction. Studies with trypsin and plasmin, *Biochemistry,* 23, 6619, 1984.
76. **Roche, P. A. and Pizzo, S. V.,** Characterization of α_2-macroglobulin-plasmin complexes: complete subunit cleavage alters receptor recognition *in vivo* and *in vitro, Biochemistry,* 26, 486, 1987.
77. **Takada, A., Fukuda, S., and Takada, Y.,** Inhibition of bovine trypsin with human plasma inhibitors, *Thromb. Res.*, 14, 413, 1979.
78. **Krebs, G. and Jacquot-Armand, Y.,** Interactions between trypsin, α_2-macroglobulin and soybean trypsin inhibitor, *Biochem. Biophys. Res. Comm.*, 55, 929, 1973.
79. **Wang, D., Wu, K., and Feinman, R. D.,** The reaction of α_2-macroglobulin-bound trypsin with soybean trypsin inhibitor, *J. Biol. Chem.*, 256, 10934, 1981.
80. **Tourbez, M., Dimicolli, J. L., Pochon, F., and Bieth, J.,** The two α_2-macroglobulin bound trypsin molecules have different affinities for the basic pancreatic trypsin inhibitor, *Biochim. Biophys. Acta,* 789, 74, 1984.
81. **Christensen, U. and Sottrup-Jensen, L.,** Enzymatic properties of α_2-macroglobulin-proteinase complexes. Apparent discrimination between covalently and noncovalently bound trypsin by reaction with soybean trypsin inhibitor, *Biochim. Biophys. Acta,* 747, 263, 1983.
82. **Hayes, M. B. and Harpel, P. C.,** Effect of acid on α_2-macroglobulin-trypsin complex, in The Physiological Inhibitors of Coagulation and Fibrinolysis, Collen, D., Wiman, D., and Verstraete, M., Eds., Elsevier/North-Holland, Amsterdam, 1979, 273.
83. **Downing, M. R., Bloom, J. W., and Mann, K. G.,** Comparison of the inhibition of thrombin by three plasma protease inhibitors, *Biochemistry,* 17, 2649, 1978.
84. **Pixley, R. A., Schapira, M., and Colman, R. W.,** The regulation of human Factor XIIa by plasma proteinase inhibitors, *J. Biol. Chem.*, 260, 1723, 1985.
85. **Ellis, V., Scully, M., MacGregor, J., and Kakkar, V. V.,** Inhibition of human factor Xa by various plasma protease inhibitors, *Biochim. Biophys. Acta,* 701, 24, 1982.
86. **Vahtera, E. and Hamberg, U.,** Interaction of urokinase with α_2-macroglobulin investigated by isoelectric focusing, *Biochem. J.*, 171, 767, 1978.
87. **Ogston, D., Bennett, B., Herbert, R. J., and Douglas, A. S.,** The inhibition of urokinase by α_2-macroglobulin, *Clin. Sci.*, 44, 73, 1973.
88. **Mosher, D. F.,** Action of fibrin-stabilizing factor on cold-insoluble globulin and α_2-macroglobulin in clotting plasma, *J. Biol. Chem.*, 251, 1639, 1976.
89. **McDaniel, M. C., Laudico, R., and Papermaster, B. W.,** Association of macrophage-activation factor from a human cultured lymphoid cell line with albumin and α_2-macroglobulin, *Clin. Immunol. Immunopathol.*, 5, 91, 1976.
90. **Dumitrescu, A., Ganea, D., Olinescu, A., Ghitescu, L., and Szégli, G.,** Effect of human α_2-macroglobulin on immune haemolysis. Importance of α_2-macroglobulin-bound clacium, *Rev. Roum. Biochim.*, 14, 167, 1977.
91. **Peterson, G. B. and Venge, P.,** Interaction and complex formation between the eosinophil cationic protein and α_2-macroglobulin, *Biochem. J.*, 245, 781, 1987.
92. **Ganrot, P. O. and Scherstén, B.,** Serum α_2-macroglobulin concentration and its variation with age and sex, *Clin. Chim. Acta,* 15, 113, 1967.
93. **Horne, C. H. W., Howie, P. W., and Wier, R. J.,** Effect of combined oestrogen-progestogen oral contraceptives on serum levels of α_2-macroglobulin, transferrin, albumin and IgG, *Lancet,* 1, 49, 1970.
94. **Twining, S. S. and Brecher, A. S.,** Identification of α_1-acid glycoprotein, α_2-macroglobulin and antithrombin III as components of normal and malignant human tissues, *Clin. Chim. Acta,* 75, 143, 1977.
95. **McBean, L. D., Smith, J. C., Berne, B. H., and Halsted, J. A.,** Serum zinc and alpha$_2$ macroglobulin concentration in myocardial infarction, decubitus ulcer, multiple myeloma, prostatic carcinoma, Down's syndrome and nephrotic syndrome, *Clin. Chim. Acta,* 50, 43, 1974.

96. **James, K., Johnson, G., and Fudenberg, H. H.,** The quantitative estimation of α_2-macroglobulin in normal, pathological and cord sera, *Clin. Chim. Acta,* 14, 207, 1966.
97. **Housley, J.,** Alpha$_2$-macroglobulin levels in disease in man, *J. Clin. Pathol.,* 21, 27, 1968.
98. **Kluthe, R., Hagemann, U., and Kleine, N.,** The turnover of α_2-macroglobulins in the nephrotic syndrome, *Vox Sang.,* 12, 308, 1967.
99. **Hitzig, W. H.,** Normalwerte in der postnatalen Period, in Die Plasmaproteine in der klinishen Medizin, Vol. 3, Springer Verlag, Berlin, 1963, 110.
100. **Baldo, B. A.,** Additional inhibitors of rat serum acute phase α_2-macroglobulin levels. Effect of 6-merkaptopurine and some lipoxygenase and cyclo-oxygenase inhibitors, *Agents Actions,* 12, 3, 1982.
101. **Pickering, J. J., Brody, J. I., Fink, G. B., Finnegan, J. O., and Ablaza, S.,** The behavior of antithrombin III, alpha$_2$-macroglobulin and alpha$_1$-antitrypsin during cardiopulmonary bypass, *Am. J. Clin. Pathol.,* 80, 459, 1983.
102. **Horne, C. H. W., Howie, P. W., and Goudie, R. B.,** Serum alpha$_2$-macroglobulin, transferrin, albumin and IgG levels in pre-eclampsia, *J. Clin. Pathol.,* 23, 514, 1970.
103. **Damus, P. S. and Wallace, G. A.,** Immunologic measurement of antithrombin-III-heparin cofactor and α_2-macroglobulin in disseminated intravascular coagulation and hepatic failure coagulopathy, *Thromb. Res.,* 6, 27, 1975.
104. **Spöttl, F. and Holzknecht, F.,** The influence of inhibitors of plasmin and plasminogen activation of the streptokinase-induced fibrinolytic state, *Thromb. Diath. Haemorrh.,* 24, 100, 1970.
105. **Wilson, G. B. and Fudenberg, H. H.,** Role of polyamines in regulation of proteinase and proteinase inhibitor function: Emphasis on a defect in α_2-macroglobulin and polyamine metabolism in cystic fibrosis, in Advances in Polyamine Research, Vol. 2, Campbell, R. A., Ed., Raven Press, New York, 1978, 281.
106. **Stenberg, S.,** Inherited alpha$_2$ macroglobulin deficiency, *Thromb. Res.,* 22, 491, 1981.
107. **Bergquist, D. and Nilsson, I. M.,** Hereditary alpha$_2$-macroglobulin deficiency, *Scand. J. Haematol.,* 23, 433, 1979.
108. **Carrel, R. W.,** α_1-antitrypsin: molecular pathology, leukocytes and tissue damage, *J. Clin. Invest.,* 78, 1427, 1986.
109. **Morse, J. O.,** Alpha$_1$-antitrypsin deficiency (First of two parts), *N. Engl. J. Med.,* 299, 1045, 1978.
110. **Morse, J. O.,** Alpha$_1$-antitrypsin deficiency (Second of two parts), *N. Engl. J. Med.,* 299, 1099, 1978.
111. **Gans, H. and Tan, B. H.,** α_1-Antitrypsin, an inhibitor of thrombin and plasmin, *Clin. Chim. Acta,* 17, 111, 1967.
112. **Learned, L. A., Bloom, J. W., and Hunter, M. J.,** The antithrombin activity of α-1-protease inhibitor: the antitrypsin activity of antithrombin III, *Thromb. Res.,* 8, 99, 1976.
113. **Shapiro, S. S. and Anderson, D. B.,** Thrombin inhibition in normal plasma, in Chemistry and Biology of Thrombin, Lundblad, R. L., Fenton, J. W., and Mann, K. G., Eds., Ann Arbor Science Publishing, Ann Arbor, MI, 1977, 361.
114. **Travis, J. and Salvasen, G. S.,** Human plasma proteinase inhibitors, *Ann. Rev. Biochem.,* 52, 655, 1985.
115. **Hunt, L. T. and Dayhoff, M. O.,** A surprising new protein superfamily containing ovalbumin, antithrombin-III and alpha$_1$-proteinase inhibitor, *Biochem. Biophys. Res. Comm.,* 95, 864, 1980.
116. **Carrell, R. W., Boswell, D. R., Brennan, S. O., and Owen, M. C.,** Active site of α_1-antitrypsin: homologus site in antithrombin-III, *Biochem. Biophys. Res. Comm.,* 93, 399, 1980.
117. **Petersen, T. E., Dudek-Wojchiehowska, G., Sottrup-Jensen, L., and Magnusson, S.,** Primary structure of antithrombin III (heparin cofactor) partial homology between alpha-1-antitrypsin and antithrombin III, in The Physiological Inhibitors of Coagulation and Fibrinolysis, Collen, D., Wiman, B., and Verstraete, M., Eds., Elsevier/North Holland Press, Amsterdam, 1979, 43.
118. **Carrell, R. W., Owen, M., Brennan, S., and Vaughan, L.,** Carboxy terminal fragment of human alpha-1-antitrypsin from hydroxylamine cleavage: homology with antithrombin-III, *Biochem. Biophys. Res. Comm.,* 91, 1032, 1979.
119. **Carrell, R. W. and Boswell, D. R.,** Serpins: the superfamily of plasma serine protease inhibitors, in Proteinase Inhibitors, Barrett, A. and Salvasen, G., Eds., Elsevier, Amsterdam, 1986, 47.
120. **Loebermann, H., Tokuoka, R., Deisenhofer, J., and Huber, R.,** Human alpha$_1$-proteinase inhibitor. Crystal structure analysis of two crystal modifications, molecular model and preliminary analysis of the implications for function, *J. Mol. Biol.,* 177, 531, 1984.
121. **Owen, M. C., Brennan, S. O., Lewis, J. H., and Carrell, R. W.,** Mutation of antitrypsin to antithrombin. α_1-antitrypsin Pittsburgh (358 Met-Arg), a fatal bleeding disorder, *N. Engl. J. Med.,* 309, 694, 1983.
122. **Schultze, H. E., Heide, K., and Haupt, K.,** α_1-antitrypsin and human serum, *Klin. Wochenschr.,* 40, 427, 1962.
123. **Johnson, D. A., Pannell, R. N., and Travis, J.,** The molecular stoichiometry of trypsin inhibition by human α_1-proteinase inhibitor, *Biochem. Biophys. Res. Comm.,* 57, 584, 1954.
124. **Kamboh, M. I.,** Biochemical and genetic aspects of human serum α_1-proteinase inhibitor protein, *Dis. Markers,* 3, 135, 1985.

125. **Laurell, C. B. and Eriksson, S.,** The electrophoretic α_1-globulin pattern of serum in α_1-antitrypsin deficiency, *Scand. J. Clin. Lab. Invest.*, 15, 132, 1963.
126. **Axelsson, O. and Laurell, C. B.,** Hereditary variants of serum α_1-antitrypsin, *Am. J. Hum. Genet.*, 17, 466, 1965.
127. **Fagerhol, M. K. and Laurell, C. B.,** The Polymorphism of pre-albumin and α_1-antitrypsin in human sera, *Clin. Chim. Acta,* 16, 199, 1967.
128. **Mega, T., Lujan, E., and Yoshida, A.,** Studies on the oligosaccharide chains of human α_1-protease inhibitor. I. Isolation of glycopeptides, *J. Biol. Chem.*, 255, 4053, 1980.
129. **Carrell, R. W., Jeppson, J. O., Vaughan, L., Brennan, S. O., Owen, M. C., and Boswell, D. R.,** Human α_1-antitrypsin: carboyhydrate attachment and sequence homology, *FEBS Lett.*, 135, 301, 1981.
130. **Kurachi, K., Chandra, J., Degen, S. J. F., White, T. T., Marchioro, T. L., Wood, S. L. C., and Davis, E.,** Cloning and sequence of cDNA coding for α_1-antitrypsin, *Proc. Natl. Acad. Sci. U.S.A.*, 78, 6826, 1981.
131. **Laurell, C. B., Nosslin, B., and Jeppson, J. O.,** Catabolic rate of α_1-antitrypsin of Pi type M and Z in man, *Clin. Sci. Mol. Med.*, 52, 457, 1977.
132. **Jones, E. A., Vergalla, J., Steer, C. J., Bradley-Moore, P. R., and Vierling, J. M.,** Metabolism of intact and asialylated α_1-proteinase inhibitor, *Biochem. Biophys. Res. Comm.*, 57, 584, 1974.
133. **Vaughan, L., Lorier, M. A., and Carrell, R. W.,** α_1-antitrypsin microheterogeneity. Isolation and physiological significance of isoforms, *Biochem. Biophys. Acta,* 701, 339, 1982.
134. **Jeppson, J. O., Laurell, C. B., and Fagerhol, M. K.,** Properties of isolated α_1-antitrypsin of Pi types M, S and Z, *Eu. J. Biochem.*, 83, 143, 1978.
135. **Vaughan, L. and Carrell, R. W.,** α_1-antitrypsin isoforms: structural basis of microheterogeneity, *Biochem. Inst.*, 2, 461, 1981.
136. **Cox, D. W., Johnson, A. M., and Fagerhol, M. K.,** Report on nomenclature meeting for α_1-antitrypsin, *Hum. Genet.*, 52, 429, 1980.
137. **Darlington, D. W., Astrin, K. H., Muirhead, S. P., Desnick, R. J., and Smith, M.,** Assignment of human α_1-antitrypsin to chromosome 14 by somatic cell hybrid analysis, *Proc. Natl. Acad. Sci. U.S.A.*, 79, 870, 1982.
138. **Gedde-Dahl, T., Frants, R. R., Olaisen, B., Eriksson, A. W., Loghem, W. V., and Lamm, L.,** The Gm-Pi linkage heterogeneity in view of PiM subtypes, *Ann. Hum. Genet.*, 45, 143, 1981.
139. **Cox, D. W., Woo, S. L. C., and Mansfield, T.,** DNA restriction fragments associated with α_1-antitrypsin indicate a single origin for deficiency allele PI Z, *Nature London,* 316, 79, 1985.
140. **Bhan, A. K., Grand, A. J., and Colten, H. R.,** Liver in α_1-antitrypsin deficiency: morphologic observations and in vitro synthesis of α_1-antitrypsin, *Pediatr. Res.*, 10, 35, 1976.
141. **Lieberman, J.,** Elastase, collagenase, emphysema and alpha$_1$-antitrypsin deficiency, *Chest,* 70, 62, 1976.
142. **George, P. M., Vissers, M. C. M., Travis, J., Winterbourn, C. C., and Carrell, R. W.,** A genetically engineered mutant of α_1-antitrypsin protects connective tissue from neutrophil damage and may be useful in lung disease, *Lancet,* 2, 1426, 1984.
143. **Janus, E. D., Phillips, N. T., and Carrell, R. W.,** Smoking, lung function and α_1-antitrypsin deficiency, *Lancet,* 1, 152, 1985.
144. **Larsson, C.,** Natural History and Life Expectancy in Severe Alpha$_1$-Antitrypsin Deficiency, Pi Z, *Acta Med. Scand.*, 204, 345, 1978.
145. **Sharp, H. L.,** α_1-antitrypsin deficiency in Medical Genetics, McKusick, V. A. and Caliborna, R., Eds., HP Publishing Co., New York, 1974, 131.
146. **Heimburger, N., Haupt, H., and Schwick, H. G.,** Protease inhibitors of human plasma, in *Proc. Int. Res. Conf.* Proteinase Inhibitors, Fritz, H. and Tschersche, H., Eds., Walter de Gruyter, Munich, 1970, 1.
147. **Borsodi, A. D., Bradshaw, R. A., Rughani, I. K., and Bruce, R. M.,** Structural and functional relationship of human antithrombin III and alpha$_1$-antitrypsin, *Adv. Exp. Med. Biol.*, 52, 249, 1974.
148. **Rimon, A., Shamash, Y. and Shapiro, B.,** The plasmin inhibitor of human plasma: IV. Its action on plasmin, chymotrypsin and thrombin, *J. Biol. Chem.*, 241, 5102, 1966.
149. **Lane, J. L., Bird, P., and Rizza, C. R.,** A new assay for the measurement of total progressive antithrombin, *Br. J. Haematol.*, 30, 103, 1975.
150. **Matheson, N. R. and Travis, J.,** Inactivation of human thrombin in the presence of human α_1-proteinase inhibitor, *Biochem. J.*, 159, 495, 1976.
151. **Hörl, M., Sperling, M., Majer, J., and Hörl, W. H.,** Plasma proteinases, proteinase inhibitors and other selective plasma proteins following aortofemoral bypass operation, *Eur. Surg. Res.*, 18, 69, 1986.
152. **Sas, G., Blaskó, G., Bánhegyi, D., Jákó, J., and Pálos, L. A.,** Abnormal antithrombin III (antithrombin III "Budapest") as a cause of a familial thrombophilia, *Thromb. Diath. Haemorrh.*, 32, 105, 1974.
153. **Scully, M. F., Ellis, V., and Kakkar, V. V.,** Studies of anti-Xa activity, *Thromb. Res.*, 29, 387, 1983.
154. **Ellis, V., Scully, M. F., and Kakkar, V. V.,** Inhibition of prothrombinase complex by plasma proteinase inhibitors, *Biochemistry,* 23, 5882, 1984.

155. **Nishikado, H., Komiyana, Y., Masuda, M., Egawa, H., and Murata, M.,** Factor α_1-antitrypsin complex-elevation in the patients with DIC, *Thromb. Res.,* 41, 489, 1986.
156. **Carrell, R. W. and Owen, M. C.,** Plakalbumin, α_1-antitrypsin, antithrombin and the mechanism of inflammatory thrombosis, *Nature,* 317, 730, 1985.
157. **Endresen, G. K. M.,** Immunological studies of plasma protease inhibitors associated with human blood platelets, *Thromb. Res.,* 19, 157, 1980.
158. **Lewis, J. H., Iammarino, R. N., Spero, J. A., and Hasiba, U.,** Antithrombin-Pittsburgh: an α_1-antitrypsin variant causing hemorrhagic disease, *Blood,* 51, 129, 1978.
159. **Ikehara, Y., Miyasato, M., Ogata, S., and Oda, K.,** Multiple forms of rat-serum α_1-protease inhibitor, *Eur. J. Biochem.,* 115, 253, 1981.
160. **Nathoo, S. A. and Finlay, T.,** Immunological and chemical properties of mouse α_1-protease inhibitors, *Arch. Biochem. Biophys.,* 246, 162, 1986.
161. **Pellegrini, A. and von Fellenberg, R.,** Fractionation and partial characterization of α-1-protease inhibitors of horse, *Biochem. Biophys. Acta,* 616, 351, 1980.
162. **Koj, A., Hatton, M. W. C., Wong, K. L., and Regoeczi, E.,** Isolation and partial characterization of rabbit plasma α_1-antitrypsin, *Biochem. J.,* 169, 589, 1978.
163. **Miszczuk-Jamska, B. and Pajdak, W.,** Comparison of the inhibitory activity and concentration of alpha$_1$-antiprotease in normal human serum, *Experientia,* 35, 116, 1979.
164. **Glaser, C. B., Karic, L., and Fallat, R.,** Isolation and characterization of alpha-1-antitrypsin from the Cohn fraction IV-I of human plasma, *Prep. Biochem.,* 5, 353, 1975.
165. **D'Souza, S. and Ananthakrishnan, R.,** Affinity chromatography in the separation of human alpha$_1$-antitrypsin (α_1-AT) and antithrombin-III (AT-III), *Austr. J. Exp. Biol. Med. Sci.,* 57, 245, 1979.
166. **Kurechi, T., Kress, L. F., and Laskowski, M.,** Purification of human plasma α_2 macroglobulin and α_1-proteinase inhibitor using zinc chelate chromatography, *Anal. Biochem.,* 99, 415, 1979.
167. **Johnson, D. and Travis, J.,** The oxidative inactivation of human α-1-proteinase inhibitor, *J. Biol. Chem.,* 254, 4022, 1979.

INDEX

A

G

H

I

J

K

L

M

N

O

P

Q

R

S

T

U

V

W

Z